THE GEOLOGY OF THE MODERN CANCER EPIDEMIC: THROUGH THE LENS OF CHINESE MEDICINE

THE GEOLOGY OF THE MODERN CANCER EPIDEMIC: THROUGH THE LENS OF CHINESE MEDICINE

TAI LAHANS

Cornerstone Cancer Clinic, Washington, USA

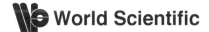

World Scientific

NEW JERSEY · LONDON · SINGAPORE · BEIJING · SHANGHAI · HONG KONG · TAIPEI · CHENNAI

Published by

World Scientific Publishing Co. Pte. Ltd.

5 Toh Tuck Link, Singapore 596224

USA office: 27 Warren Street, Suite 401-402, Hackensack, NJ 07601

UK office: 57 Shelton Street, Covent Garden, London WC2H 9HE

Library of Congress Cataloging-in-Publication Data
Lahans, Tai, author.
  The geology of the modern cancer epidemic : through the lens of Chinese medicine / by
Lahans Tai.
    p. ; cm.
  Includes bibliographical references and index.
  ISBN 978-9814436304 (hardcover : alk. paper)
  ISBN 978-9814436311 (softcover : alk. paper)
I. Title.
  [DNLM: 1. Neoplasms--therapy. 2. Environment. 3. Environmental Pollution--adverse effects.
4. Medicine, Chinese Traditional. 5. Neoplasms--etiology. QZ 266]
  RA645.C3
  614.5'999--dc23

                                   2013024670

British Library Cataloguing-in-Publication Data
A catalogue record for this book is available from the British Library.

Cover:

The Neijing Tu ("Diagram of the Inner Scripture") from the original stele at the Bai Yun Guan, or White Cloud Temple, in Beijing.

Cover layout and design by Adam Vick.www.adamvick.com

Typeset by Stallion Press
Email: enquiries@stallionpress.com

Printed in Singapore

Dedication

This book is dedicated to my maternal grandparents:

Emily McAllister, a Highlander Scot who immigrated to Canada as a very young woman; and my grandfather, Arenaquohatse — a First Nations Saulteaux from Quebec, Canada.

Their spirits live on in me, as do the spirits of all my ancestors back to our beginnings in Africa.

I am forever grateful.

Endorsement

"The Taoist school of Chinese medicine has long advocated the concept of a body ecology, where being in harmony with the environment cultivates harmony in the body. If readers of Tai Lahans' book heed her message to become advocates for political, social, and personal change, they will address the urgent issues of today and help both themselves and their patients achieve the most effective way to address cancer — that is, through prevention. While being consistent with the messages of the Chinese medical tradition, they will also join the ranks of famous doctor–activists, such as Sun Yat Sen. Stewardship of the land and being a part of our Earth are both connected to universal sacred relationships and to human health."

Michael McCulloch, L.Ac., M.P.H., Ph.D.
Pine Street Foundation
San Anselmo, CA, U.S.A.

"In this book Tai Lahans combines the wisdom of perennial systems of medicine with modern knowledge and presents the greater message the cancer epidemic stands for. She takes a bird's-eye view perspective to illustrate how the 'cancers' inflicted on our planet by the modern disconnected world directly relate to the disease of cancer. By employing a micro-macrocosm approach, she explains why the 'fight-the-cancer' approach is no real solution and how humans and human health are part of the intricate and fascinating web of life. In addition, Tai Lahans offers her profound experience of Chinese medicine treatment approaches for cancer patients and pre-cancerous conditions. However, more than anything, this book deepens the understanding of the world as a whole, the Great Chain of Being and the Sacred."

Simon Becker, L.Ac.
Academy of Chinese Healing Arts
Switzerland

"Dr. Tai Lahans, a living treasure, presents a refreshingly unique perspective in this book. By interweaving Chinese medicine philosophy, modern scientific theories and data, and economic/political/social principles she has created a comprehensive book on cancer prevention. Dr. Lahans emphasizes that precaution is the only way to meet the medical imperative 'do no harm.' Kudos to Dr. Lahans for her vision."

Misha Cohen, L.Ac., O.M.D.
Research Specialist in Integrative Medicine, U.C.S.F.
Institute for Health and Aging
Associate Member, U.C.S.F. Comprehensive Cancer Center
Director, M.R.C.E. Foundation
Clinic Director, Chicken Soup Chinese Medicine,
San Francisco, CA, U.S.A.

Contents

Dedication   v

Endorsement   vii

Foreword   xiii

Introduction   1

Chapter One: Water: The *San Jiao*   21

After the introduction, this chapter opens into
the lowest common denominator of life and
of pollution — water. It defines the status of
waters across the earth and how they are constantly being attacked in terms of quantity,
quality, and their ability to support life. The
latter part of the chapter is a discussion on
how water is the energetic and material
equivalent of the San Jiao of Chinese medicine — one step up from the Source.

Chapter Two: Air — Lung Cancer   75

Following the discussion of water comes that
of air and millions of ways that air is currently
becoming contaminated. Then the chapter
goes into the discussion of the lungs from a
Chinese medicine perspective and how the
lungs are connected to our immunity, to our
emotions, and to the San Jiao.

Chapter Three: Earth — Colorectal Cancer   131

The Earth is the ground for life. We are sustained by water, air and earth. The equivalent

of earth within the human body is the entire gastrointestinal tract. Whatever happens to the Earth outside of us happens also to the earth within us. Loss of species, heritage crops, habitat, sustainability, and health are all one.

Chapter Four: *Yin* and *Qi* — **Breast Cancer**   **199**

Women hold up the world. When the Earth is denigrated it is but an expression of how women are denigrated. Women live multitudes of lives within their one lifetime — wife, lover, caregiver, mother, career person, provider. The breast has become Mother Earth, Goddess, Seductress, life giver. How can the female breast be all of these things and remain healthy?

Chapter Five   *Yin* and *Yang* — **Prostate Cancer**   **301**

The flip side of the coin. If women are oppressed, so are men. Boys don't cry. Men must succeed. Only men go to war. Rage is male; depression is female. Only women raise children. Where is compassion? What happens to our male children? The Heart has been beaten out of men.

Chapter Six   *Fire* — **Chronic Viral Infection and Cancer**   **357**

Many cancers are caused by chronic viral infection. HCV and HBV are now the main causes of liver cancer. These viruses are considered epidemic worldwide. The public health system barely exists in the US. Some states do not have a public health cancer registry. In 1974 the NCI at the NIH was mandated by the Congress to put 10% of its research dollars into prevention. Since then the NCI has never utilized more than 4% of its research dollars on prevention and it defines prevention only as early screening. Lung cancer kills more people than all other cancers combined but there is no early screen for lung cancer. We need to re-establish a broadened public health structure in the United States and globally.

Chapter Seven: **Epigenetics, the *Source*, and the Precautionary Principle** **401**

When the Native Americans speak of the Seventh Generation, they are speaking of prevention, conservation, and protection of all who are to come — human and animal and plant species. Epigenetics is showing that as far back now as five generations there are impacts on the yet to be born offspring of all of life. These impacts include environmental, emotional, climate, starvation, and so on. The San Jiao and the Source are deeper concepts of Chinese medicine that speak to and expose this perennial philosophy. The Precautionary Principle is a modern way of speaking to this perennially true way of viewing life.

Chapter Eight **The Geology of Hope** **439**

Science and religion have been at odds for a long time. They have been placed at odds with one another, and used by modern corporate economics to mire us all in a profit-driven world where contamination is possible because of free speech laws applied to corporations. The reductionist science of the Enlightenment has taken single pieces of the universe and of life out of relationship to the ecosystem and sacred universe in which they live. The knowing side of life must come together with the meaning side of life. It is a immensely necessary first step in saving ourselves.

Chapter Nine   **Connections**   **489**

What is health? How we can remake our world.

Addendum: Books and websites that are worth reading and monitoring   **517**

Index   **521**

Foreword

The Science of Life
By Dr. Vandana Shiva

Life, and the knowledge of living systems and living processes, have become the epicenter of conflicts over resources and paradigm wars.

On the one hand is the myopic, mechanistic paradigm that sees nature as dead, living systems as machines, and other ways of knowing as primitive and outmoded. The imposition of the mechanistic, reductionist world on life and life forms is being called "the life sciences industry." On the other hand are the many streams from ancient sciences like Ayurveda (which translates into "The Science of Life"), Chinese systems of medicine, and new sciences of life which see living systems as complex, self-organized, and dynamic. These emerging life sciences include Gaia theory, agroecology, gene ecology, and epigenetics.

Across the world, the ancient, time-tested, perennial knowledge systems are being resurrected and are being reinforced by new breakthroughs in science. A paradigm shift is taking place — from one based on *terra nullius* ("empty earth") to one based on *Terra Madre* ("Mother Earth"). It is a shift from separation to interconnection, from eco-apartheid to unity and harmony with the earth. Seeking this path of harmony has become an imperative for the well-being of the earth and the well-being of humans.

The U.N. Secretary-General, in his report on "Harmony with Nature," has elaborated on the imperative of "the route back to the future," which involves "reconnecting with nature."

Separatism is at the root of disharmony with nature, and violence against nature and people. Tagore, India's national poet and winner of the Nobel Prize in Literature, saw in separation the roots of both bondage and poverty. As he wrote, "I could understand how great the concrete truth was in any plane of life, the truth that in separation is bondage, in union is liberation…. Poverty lay in separation and wealth in union." (Sabyasachi Bhattarcharya, 2008, *The Mahatma and the Poet,* National Book Trust, India, p. 108.)

Today, we need to overcome the wider and deeper apartheid, an eco-apartheid based on the illusion of separateness — the separation of humans from nature in our minds and lives. This eco-apartheid is an illusion because we are *part* of nature and earth, not *apart* from it.

The war against the earth begins in the mind. Its contemporary seeds were sown when the living earth was transformed into dead matter to facilitate the Industrial Revolution. Reductionism replaced holism, monocultures replaced diversity and complexity, "raw material" and "dead matter" replaced a constantly renewing and vibrant earth, and *terra nullius* replaced *Terra Madre*.

According to Bacon, called the father of modern science, "the nature of things betrays itself more readily under the vexations of art than in its natural freedom." The discipline of scientific knowledge and the mechanical inventions it leads to do not "merely exert a gentle guidance over nature's course; they have the power to conquer and subdue her, to shake her to her foundations."

In *Tempores Partus Masculus* (*The Masculine Birth of Time*), translated by Farrington in 1951, Bacon promised to create a blessed race of heroes and supermen who would dominate both nature and society.

The Royal Society, inspired by Bacon's philosophy, was clearly seen by its organizers as a masculine project. In 1664, Henry Oldenberg, Secretary of the Royal Society, announced that the intention of the society was to "raise a masculine philosophy… whereby the Mind of the Man may be ennobled with the knowledge of solid truths." And, for Glanvill, the masculine aim of science was to know "the ways of captivating Nature, and making her subserve our purposes, thereby achieving the Empire of Man Over Nature."

Robert Boyle, the famous scientist who was also the Governor of the New England Company, saw the rise of mechanical philosophy as an instrument of power not just over nature but also over the original inhabitants of America. He explicitly declared his intention of ridding the New England Indians of their ridiculous notions about the workings of nature. He attacked their perception of nature, "as a kind of goddess," and argued that "the veneration, wherewith men are imbued for what they call nature, has been a discouraging impediment to the empire of man over the inferior creatures of God."

The death of nature in the mind allows a war to be unleashed against the earth. After all, if the earth is merely dead matter, then nothing is being killed. As Carolyn Merchant points out, this transformation of nature from a living, nurturing mother to inert, dead, and manipulable matter was eminently suited to the exploitation imperative of growing capitalism. The nurturing earth image acted as a cultural constraint on exploitation of nature. "One does not readily slay a mother, dig her entrails or mutilate her body." But the mastery and domination images created by the Baconian program and the scientific revolution removed all restraints and functioned as cultural sanctions for the denudation of nature.

Modern science was a consciously gendered, patriarchal activity. As nature came to be seen more like a woman to be raped, gender too was recreated. Science as a male venture, based on the subjugation of the female sex, provided support for the polarization of gender. Patriarchy as the new scientific and technological power was a political need of emerging industrial capitalism.

The exclusion of nonreductionist, nonmechanist systems of knowledge has narrowed the knowledge base of our actions; it has shrunk our intellectual capacities to adapt. Humanity is poorer in excluding the wealth of knowledge of indigenous communities and women on how to live lightly on a fragile continent.

Barry Commoner gave us the first law of ecology: "Everything is connected to everything else." (*The Closing Circle, Nature, Man and Technology*, Alfred Knopf, pp. 33–39.) Yet the mechanical worldview has created the illusion of separation and fragmentation. It has tried to divide an indivisible unity of nature. It has tried to separate us from the earth.

We are made up of the same five elements (the pancha mahabhuta — earth, water, fire, air, and space) that constitute the earth. The water that circulates in the biosphere circulates in our bodies. The oxygen which the plants produce becomes our breath. The web of life is woven through interconnectedness. The food that is produced by the soil and the sun's energy becomes our cells, our blood, our bones. Biologically and ecologically we are one with the earth. It is the disease of separatism and eco-apartheid that denies it and then creates the diseases of loneliness, depression, alienation. As Arthur Robbins has observed in his book *Paradise Lost, Paradise Regained*, "To live without a context, to live outside of rather than within the community, is to live in a state of ekstasis, to be out of place, to be without a place. *Ekstasis* is to be separated from the stability of forces seeking balance, equilibrium, harmony or 'stasis.' In medieval times the Greek *ekstasis* became *alienato mentis*, which is the basis for the English word 'alienation.' '*Lien*' is the French for tie. The insane person is known as an *aliene*, 'he who is without ties'. "Thus insanity and separation have a common origin."

The U.S., the richest country of the world, has the highest rate of depression. Depression rates have increased tenfold over the last 50 years. (E. Diener and MEP Seligman, 2004, Beyond money: toward an economy of well-being, Psychol. Sci. the Publ. Interest **5**: 1–31.)

Interconnectedness is the nature of reality. While separation was intrinsic to the old science based on Cartesian, Baconian, and Newtonian assumptions, nonseparability is built into the new science of quantum theory and the new biology. I did my Ph.D. on the Foundations of Quantum Theory, especially the aspect of nonlocality or nonseparability which acknowledges the interconnectedness of the universe.

The Einstein–Podolsky–Rosen paradox (A. Einstein, B. Podolsky, and N. Rosen, 1935, Can quantum mechanical description of physical reality be considered complete? *Phys. Rev.* **47**: 999) has shown that when a quantum system is subdivided, and the two subsystems are separated in space and time, their state is nonseparable. Physicists like Bohr, Pauli, and Bohm stressed the nonseparable wholeness of the universe of physical phenomena.

Nonseparability and wholeness is also intrinsic to Bohr's view that one can meaningfully ascribe properties such as a position or momentum to a quantum system only in the context of some well-defined experimental arrangement suitable for measuring the corresponding property (N. Bohr, 1934, *Atomic Theory and the Description of Nature*).

Pauli interpreted Bohr's correspondence theory to be inspired by correspondention, the perception of a world in harmony and resonance.

Even in biology, nonseparability is being recognized through fields like epigenetics and gene ecology.

The term "gene ecology" was born in Tormso. Gene ecology is a new interdisciplinary field that is unique in its combination of genetics and biochemistry with bioethics, the philosophy of science, and social studies of science and technology. It builds on innovative work in the areas of genomics, proteomics, food science, ecology, and evolution. It goes beyond the reductionist approaches of the individual scientific disciplines (www.genok.com//gene-ecology).

Epigenetics is another emerging field shows that there is no separation between genes, the organism, and the environment. The reductionist view is that the DNA carries all our heritable information and is insulated from the environment. Epigenetics adds new dimensions to the behavior of genes. It proposes a control system of "switches" that turn genes on or off — and suggests that things people experience, like nutrition and stress, can control these switches and cause heritable effects in humans. (Epigenetics: DNA isn't everything; www.sciencedaily.com/releases/2009/04/090412081315.htm).

The illusion of separation from nature is at the heart of mechanistic thought, which treats nature as dead. This gives license to exploit and violate nature. As I wrote in *Staying Alive*, if nature is dead, and the earth is empty — terra nullius — then all violence against nature is defined as "human progress." Technologies based on the mechanistic paradigm, such as the "green revolution" and "genetic engineering," tear apart the interconnectedness of the earth at the ecosystem, the cellular, the genetic level, and have no method for assessing the damage. Economics based on the mechanistic paradigm, with its mismeasures of "growth," GDP, GNP, separates it from ecology and sustenance, even though both have their roots in "*oikos*," or home.

The mechanistic and reductionist worldview involves violence against science and knowledge itself. Quantum theory has taught us that the world is not a machine, and that there is no separability. The new biology of complexity, self-organization, and epigenetics points to the interrelatedness of life. The violence of the mind begins with fragmenting that which is whole, separating that which is connected, thus violating nature and the web of life. Mechanistic science also violates women and non-Western societies and indigenous communities by denying them a status as knowing subjects. Today this violence has taken the form of biopiracy. We have fought and won three cases of biopiracy — of neem, basmati, and wheat. Violent ways of knowing dominate by violently destroying nonviolent alternatives.

Paradigm wars also include the emerging conflicts between economic growth and human and planetary well-being. Across the world, people are questioning the "growth" model. Limitless growth on a limited planet is an ecological impossibility. The more the "economy" grows, the faster our ecosystems, species, and communities are destroyed. The more the "economy" grows, the fewer the creative opportunities for people, especially young people. That is why people around the world are questioning "growth" and instruments that falsely measure destruction as growth.

The radical shift that movements around the world are making is a shift from an earth-degrading, human-degrading economic system based on greed, profits, and financial growth to earth-centered, human-centered systems which reduce the ecological footprint while increasing well-being. Not only will this shift that is already underway bring harmony with nature, it will sow the seeds of social justice and equity, both in terms of sharing the earth's resources and recognition of work that goes into caring for the planet and people.

It will recognize women's work in sustenance. It will also recognize the knowledge creation and production of Third World and indigenous communities. It will create space for future generations.

Activities that provide sustenance and well-being for all are currently called unproductive. In a green economy whose aim is to maximize well-being, not profits, serving the earth and community becomes the most important work we are called on to do. Activities that rejuvenate the earth and human communities become the core of a truly green economy.

Making peace with the earth must begin in our minds and our consciousness, by changing our paradigms and worldviews from those based on war with nature to those which recognize that we are a strand in the web of life. It involves a shift from fragmentation and reductionism to interconnectedness and holistic thinking. It involves a shift from violence, rape, and torture as modes of knowing to non-violence and dialogue with the earth and all her beings. It involves inclusion of biodiversity of knowledge systems — of women, of indigenous communities, of our grandmothers.

This is what the International Commission on the Future of Food and Agriculture, which I chair, has said in the Manifesto on Knowledge Systems.

We need other ways of thinking and knowing to overcome the separation from nature. As Tagore reminded us, "The language of Nature is the eternal language of creation. It penetrates reality to reach the deepest layers of our consciousness, it draws upon a language that has survived thousands of years with the human…it is the musical instrument of nature; it replicates the rhythm inherent in life itself. If we listen carefully we will be able to trace within them the murmurs of eternity where the spirit of liberation, peace and beauty lurk, it reminds us of the sea that is *santam, shivam, advaitam*…it reminds us of our bond with the world…if we can accept this music of the wild within us, we can perceive the great music of oneness.…" (Rabindranath Tagore, "Introduction," to Bonobani, *Rabindra Rachanavali*, Vol. 8, p. 87).

Eco-apartheid refers to the ecological separation of humans from nature in the mechanical, reductionist worldview which is resulting in the multiplicity of the eco-crisis that is threatening human survival — climate catastrophes, species extinction, water depletion and pollution, desertification of our soils, and acidification and pollution of our oceans. It also refers to the apartheid created between corporations and citizens, and between rich and poor on the basis of the appropriation of the earth's resources by a few and denial to the rest of their rights to access the earth's gifts for sustenance of all life, including human life.

I am very happy to write this foreword to Tai Lahans' book, in which she combines ancient and emerging sciences of life to offer multidimensional solutions to multidimensional problems like the cancer epidemic. As she writes, "The modern science of genetics and epigenetics is laying a foundational language for concepts within many perennial forms of medicine that have to do with the paradigm of a source for all of life. Ayurvedic and Chinese medicine, in particular, have very sophisticated explanations of how life comes about and is changed by the act of living itself. But, because these perennial systems never had to analyze the effects of environmental and sociocultural contamination, they do not have the modern tools for understanding the specifics of that contamination. Combining bioscience with perennial sciences to understand our pathway in this morass is essential. On one side we have the biochemical and genetic/epigenetic understanding of how these things work. On the other side we have the prelinear understanding of how nature works and how to protect and rehabilitate life. Each perspective is equally valuable. They are the Yang and the Yin of understanding."

Introduction

When a human being views a painting of an individual, the brain knows that what it is viewing is a two-dimensional representation of a three-dimensional object. It knows that what is being viewed is a collection of paints accumulated in various ways to give depth and perspective to the painting. But when the viewer moves around the canvas of the painting, it appears that the eyes of the portrait are following him or her. This phenomenon is a metaphor for modern science. Modern science tries to explain that which we can see but typically the view is two-dimensional and linear. All of the complexity of perspective and interrelationships through time, the ecology and the geology of the subject, is missing. Through the work of separating, science today pulls things apart in order to explain the truth of them but fails to put them back together within the larger context in which these things came to evolve and continue to become what they are in that moment.

This book is an effort to bring into focus the many perspectives necessary, in my view, for understanding the steep rise in the incidence of cancers in the developed world in our time. Without knowing the reasons for this rise it becomes impossible to act upon that knowledge and prevent those cancers that are now occurring more than ever before. The discussion goes beyond the biochemical and molecular mechanisms of cancer causation. It looks at the way we live, the decisions we make, the emotions that drive us, the history of our relationships to one another, ourselves, and the environment. And so this is a book about anthropology, history, sociology, psychiatry, politics, economics, medicine, nature, and the commons.

The Importance of Cancer Prevention

In the United States as of 2010, one in every two men and one in every three women are diagnosed with cancer in their lifetime. Since

1

1974, the incidence of testicular cancer has risen by 115%, and that of non-Hodgkin's lymphoma by 67%. Breast cancer occurred in 1 out of 22 women in 1940, and in 2000 it occurred in 1 out of 8 women. Childhood leukemia has the greatest rate of increase of any cancer. Cancer is now the only killing disease in the developed world whose incidence is rising. When adjusted for an increased population and longevity, the rates for cancers in the developed world are far above what is traditionally expected. It appears that during the 20th century something of profound significance occurred to greatly increase the risk of cancer not just in an aging population but in everyone, including children.

The primary rationale in conventional Western medicine is that cancers are predominantly caused by a variety of factors and sometimes multiple factors that include genetic predisposition, aging, chronic viral infections and environmental factors. This last category includes immunodeficiency, environmental carcinogens, and lifestyle. Immunodeficiency is often linked to aging and oxidative stress on the DNA of cells but also occurs as a result of chronic underlying disease. Type II diabetes, a condition now occurring in children, is an example of a chronic disease that may be a predisposing factor for some cancers; a link between insulin secretion and cell proliferation has been found in breast and colorectal cancers, the only two cancers studied in this regard to date.

Cancer has long been considered a disease of aging. In the US there is a burgeoning population of aging adults, making this factor alone look more responsible than any other for the rise in the incidence of cancers. But cancers in the young are also occurring more frequently. Childhood leukemias, as stated, have the highest rate of increase of any cancer, except for lung cancer. Testicular cancer, a cancer of younger men, was never even mentioned in the 1960s because it was so rare. And it is now one of the cancers whose incidence is considered medically epidemic. Non-Hodgkin's lymphomas are also now considered medically epidemic and occur in children as well as adults. Breast cancers are occurring in younger and younger women, including teenagers and women in their 20s. Cancer is no longer just a disease of aging.

The realm of environmental carcinogens and multiple chemical exposures is a growing and complex area of carcinogenic exposure. The rate of increase in the production and dissemination of new chemicals used in manufacturing, solvents, plasticizers, cosmetics, fire retardants, fertilizers, medicines, herbicides, and pesticides has exploded since the mid–20th century. Today there are over 100,000 new chemicals on the earth never before seen by living beings. Approximately 33,000 of them are in daily use and, of those, only about 1500 have been studied for human health effects. The intricate biochemical defenses that living beings have developed to cope with their environment are now being constantly violated by foreign materials introduced into the environment. Many of these products drift from their original place of application via the movement of air and/ or water. They accumulate, often far from the locale of their original application and sometimes up to one million times the original amounts. Many have a very long half-life; for example, DDT was banned from use in the US in 1972 and is still found in the environment and in the breast tissue of women who have been diagnosed with breast cancer. Many of these chemicals are fat-soluble and lipophilic, meaning that fat tissue in living animals, including humans, becomes a repository for these chemical molecules. The higher the animal is placed on the food chain, the greater the possible exposure. Since the food chain in the ocean and other waters is longer than the food chain on land, fish at the top of the food chain, for example tuna, tend to be more highly contaminated than land-based animals.

More than ever before, lifestyle factors also play a major role in cancer risk. Diet has been linked to breast cancer, colorectal cancer, prostate cancer, and lung cancer — the top four cancers in the US in terms of incidence. High-fat, low-fiber diets with little vegetable nutrients and fiber cause obesity, a primary concern for these cancers. A high-vegetable diet has been found in several studies to be protective against lung cancer, even in smokers. In terms of colorectal cancer, a diet high in fat leads to higher levels of bile acids, which then promote anaerobic bacteria which secrete a carcinogenic enzyme that contributes to colorectal cancer. Hyperinsulinemia, a form of type II diabetes also called insulin-resistant diabetes, has been linked to colorectal and breast cancer. This condition is primarily caused by a diet high in sugar and refined carbohydrates. Animal fats and uric acid from red meat have been found to promote prostate cancer. Diet is a contributing factor to cancers. It is something that people partake in three times daily every day of their lives. A good and clean diet is immensely important to health.

When conventional medicine looks at prevention of cancers, it looks primarily at early detection. The belief is that the latency period of most cancers is so long, often ten years until symptoms occur which would result in a diagnosis, that it becomes impossible to identify the original injury or exposure that caused the genetic mutation leading to that cancer. Because of this orientation Western scientific research does not invest a great deal of time in research on individual cancers' causes; it looks primarily at the result of the cause. The identification of carcinogens and lifestyle hazards has been left to private institutions and nonprofits. And the idea that an individual can reduce their risk of cancer and possibly prevent a cancer diagnosis is rarely discussed in conventional medical practice.

In Chinese medicine the foundations of good health drive the practice and are always the starting place for the patient–doctor relationship. The fundamentals of good health are considered to be those elements of daily living that are easily observable by an individual — regular stools and good sleep. Regular stools indicate a good diet and that the digestive tract, a primary source of acquired *Qi*, is working well. Proper sleep indicates that the body has the capacity to rehabilitate itself. Many people have come to believe that sleep is an unnecessary waste of time but nothing could be further from the truth. During sleep the human body cycles in and out of REM sleep. During REM sleep a deeper cycle occurs in the delta phase that allows the liver, a major detoxifying organ, to repair and detoxify itself. It is also the only time when growth hormone is secreted. Without growth hormone our bodies do not repair function. This loss of repair contributes to aging, oxidative stress, hormone imbalances, and immune deficiency. In Chinese medicine terms, the

Wei Qi (protective energy) circulates 12 times externally and 12 times internally during a daily cycle. In the night cycle the *Wei Qi* is internal and circulates to protect and clear the *liver Qi*. This is the only time when the liver has time to recuperate and detoxify both physically (conventional science) and psychically (the *Hun* aspect of Chinese medical science). These fundamentals of health — good digestion and good sleep — are taught in Chinese medicine practice but are rarely even discussed in conventional medical practice.

Working too much, sleeping too little or poorly, eating a poor diet, and emotional discontent intertwine with one another to form knots of deficiency and constraint. They are expressions of a belief pattern in the West that is a primary generator of the cancer environment. And they are the result of an emotional underlay that understands the meaning of life in a particular way. No other system of medicine has such a profound and accurate iteration of how this underlay of beliefs and unresolved emotions can cause injury in the physical body as does Chinese medicine. This iteration will be a basis for discussion of many of the cancer types covered in this book.

Every one of the primary causes of cancer except for genetic pre-disposition is preventable; the chapter on epigenetics may address the possibility that even genetics is changing and can be changed both from the Western science point of view and from the perspec-tive of Chinese medicine. Diet and lifestyle are within our control on the personal levels. The chemical exposures that injure us via food, water, and air are all within our control on the practical and political levels. Exposure to chronic viral infection is also within our control, and education and world public health works can be primary tools in this prevention. Aging is not within our control and it is true that we begin aging as soon as we are born. However, many of the illnesses of aging reflect a loss of vitality that results from failing to live actively. We become more and more sedentary as we age, and then we lose our fitness as we live our lives passively. Fitness is not only musculoskeletal in nature. It is whole-body wellness and includes our spirit. The loss of vitality is more of a cultural and per-sonal phenomenon than it is a given biological phenomenon. This lack of movement, of fitness, of vitality translates into *Qi* and *blood stasis* in Chinese medicine — the main underlying etiological factors that create the cancer environment. The chronic diseases of aging are often the result of poor lifestyle habits that compound blood stasis syndrome and inflammation. We program our bodies for a cancer diagnosis by the way in which we live.

The Internal/External Mechanisms of Disease

Every disease has an internal and an external mechanism in nature. In previous times most diseases were a result of public health issues and the lack of a cultural and social means of addressing these issues — the external mechanisms. This led to infections, and the internal mechanisms were usually ascribed to scientific and medical explanations. These infections then sometimes became plagues. Plagues were the result of pathogens that still exist in nature but no longer cause a great threat, particularly in the developed world because of public infrastructures that limit them, especially public hygiene in the form of clean water, good nutrition, adequate housing, maternal health care and, to a lesser extent, vaccinations and antibiotics. In modern times, cancers are sometimes caused by biological pathogens, especially chronic viruses. But more frequently they are caused by carcinogenic exposures, the effects of which are made worse by certain lifestyles. In other words, there are carcinogenic hits from outside the body that are made worse by internal promoting factors, almost all of which are related to lifestyle — diet, exercise, stress, poor sleep, unhappiness. The external mechanisms come through the environment, and the internal mechanisms come through belief and the resulting lifestyle. Belief as an internal mechanism and the environment as an external mechanism are currently becoming more and more entwined.

The frenetic and out-of-control nature of cancer and the loss of normal controls on damaged cells make cancer a modern day canary in the coalmine. Cancer, as an overall rubric of more than 100 different diseases, is emblematic of how we live in modern life and of the world we have constructed. Cancer is a public health issue, but in a different way from past epidemics. The external factors mingle with the internal factors, but all boil down to how we live: the burgeoning of the human population living in unusually crowded conditions without connectedness to one another or to the natural world and driven by the need to survive comes close to describing the condition of modern life. It also describes the ecology and natural history of most cancers. The external mechanisms are our current lifestyle and all of those things we engage in that are destructive. The internal mechanisms are all of the measurable impacts regarding growth factors, genetic injuries, immune deficiency, chronic inflammation, and so on — the results of that destructive behavior. Modern medicine treats the internal mechanisms but pays little attention to the external mechanisms. Conventional medical providers see themselves as disease treatment purveyors but not as guardians of people's lives; they have only half of the story as the basis for their interventions. Unlike infectious diseases, a distinction is made regarding the obvious public health issues of cancers. No public health measures are taken when it comes to cancers. There are many economic, political, and social reasons why this is true. There are no scientific reasons why cancers should not be considered within the public health domain except that public health equals prevention, and cancers, according to modern biomedicine, are not preventable.

Historical Underpinnings

The philosophy of life, the internal meaning mechanism, that brought about this condition began in the late prehistory of humankind, and, in the West, reached its zenith during the Age of Enlightenment. It was during the Age of Enlightenment in Europe that a philosophical conclusion was reached, beginning the final separation of the receptive from the initiatory, male from female, nature from science, the rational mind from meaning given by the heart — and the spirit residing in the heart. This philosophy is a metaphor for and the driving motivator of a way of life that exemplifies the characteristics of cancer according to Chinese medicine — uncontrolled growth, imbalances that cause loss of proper function, ulceration and decay, emptiness of *Qi* in the viscera, smoke in the channels, separation of Yin and Yang.

When Sir Francis Bacon made the statement that "modern science has the capacity to not only control Mother Nature but to bring her to her knees," the mechanical school represented by him created the final dichotomies between culture and nature, soul and matter, and male and female. As part of a long history moving toward complete separation, this school of thought devised a conceptual strategy that ended in domination of the receptive, and thus over nature, as though humankind was not part of and an element within nature. It was not seen at that time that this domination would be over ourselves, as a part of nature; nor were the consequences even remotely visible. This philosophy of life continues to drive much of our modern dilemma. The 20th century produced many institutions and their offspring that have brought us to the brink of life. We are living in life-threatening times in a multitude of ways, all of which are connected.

The European contest between the mechanical and hermetic traditions was won by a strictly masculine project of the upper class, mainly of England. This culture war occurred within the context of the beginnings of the Industrial Revolution. Those who owned resources utilized industrialism as a means to build empires upon the backs of those who did not. This class system has persisted to this day, even within democratic societies. And reductionism in science became the major agent of political and economic change to engender and deepen the separation dichotomizing gender and class relations and humankind's relationship with nature.

For more than three centuries now, reductionism has ruled the only validated scientific method and system, distorting the history of the West. The ideology of reductionism hides behind projected objectivism, neutrality, and progress. This ideology has been sold to the rest of the world as a superior tradition. And the parochial roots of science in patriarchy and in a particular class and culture have been concealed behind a claim to universality. Within these roots is the subjugation of women, of nature, of natural resources, of non-Western and nonwhite peoples who live as a part of nature, and perhaps even the human body. With this subjugation have come ecological destruction and the colonization of peoples of the earth who have been framed as subhuman and "part of the natural world," thus being rendered savage, small, and powerless, as though the framers themselves were not part of the same natural world.

The violence of reductionism has been expressing itself for centuries. Some will say that reductionism is not in itself violent but rather that the consciousness of those people who utilize its objective truths causes violence. However, another way of looking at this problem is to approach consciousness as an evolution in itself, and to determine whether the consciousness that developed reductionism as a philosophical technique was itself incomplete. This incompleteness, linear rather than circular, engendered an incomplete and violent form of thinking and way of understanding. Should reductionism truly be let off the hook? Some see reductionism as the culmination of a long history of separation of the mind and the soul. Therefore, explanations derived from this form of thinking, based solely on observable facts that only the eye can see, are necessarily incomplete. And their incompleteness is what causes the violence of DDT, biomedicine that treats the disease but not the patient or the cause, wars fought in lieu of diplomacy and understanding, industrial agriculture that grows food but wreaks havoc on the natural environment and causes species annihilation. Some might even say that this way of knowing and living creates the disease of cancer and, therefore, only it has the capacity to treat it.

Whatever the conclusions are on this subject, the fact remains that there is necessarily a kind of violence inherent in separating the external measurable truths of life from the internal immeasurable truths of life. One of the deepest and most destructive ways in which this separation worked to destroy early cultures where this separation had not yet occurred was to declare as evil, outdated, folklore, savage, or nonprogressive anything that threatened this way of thinking. Natural healers, land-based peoples and cultures, natural farming techniques, holistic religious beliefs and wisdom traditions were all made small, wrong, and antiprogress. Modern Western patriarchy's special epistemological tradition of the "scientific revolution" reduced the capacity of humans to know nature by excluding both other knowers and other ways of knowing, and it reduced the capacity of nature to creatively regenerate and renew itself by manipulating it as inert and fragmented matter. This is violence.

This discussion is not about the war of the sexes, although the patriarchal systems of governance and knowing were and have been manifestations of this separation. Women have participated in this separation as well. More deeply, this discussion is about the loss of connection to the receptive that occurred for everyone. The inner meaning aspect of the physical world has been lost, and the connection to broader immaterial spheres of enlivenment of the physical world is increasingly tenuous. Modern science tends to foster this tenuousness, because its ability to know truth is limited to the observable world. Reductionism has driven this phenomenon, and reductionism is a manifestation of an evolution of human consciousness that is as yet incomplete. We are all incomplete — men and women. This incompleteness is not a gender issue. It is a spiritual issue. And the science that we are looking for must become complete by incorporating the spirit into knowing. This will result in institutions and philosophies that are whole, much as the perennial philosophies are whole. The perennial philosophies, an example of which is Chinese medicine, evolved from societies where humankind still lived in connection to nature. As such, they have much to offer the deep injuries that are responsible for the modern cancer epidemic.

The mechanistic metaphors of reductionism have reconstituted nature and society. Organic metaphors are based on interconnectedness and reciprocity. The reality of the natural world of which we are all part is not mechanistic but is rather that of a living organism. We are cells within that organism. No one part of the organism can be dominated without violence to every other part. The integrity of the whole organism cannot be violated without injury. Just as the theory and resulting modalities of Chinese medicine as expressed in the five phases are holistic in nature, it is the loss of this cyclical reality of life by Western science that is responsible for the loss of species, environmental degradation and human health decline in the developed world. It is the nature of mechanistic reductionism, and many of the philosophical ways of understanding that have grown out of reductionism, that the fundamental unity of all life is undermined, leading to only half-truths. When a living network is taken out of the relationship to itself, It becomes impossible to know the complete truth about that network.

The philosophy of reductionism and its offspring in modern science fails to perceive the interconnectedness of nature, or the connection, for example, of women's and children's lives, and work and knowledge, with the creation of wealth — wealth of all kinds. This paradigm is less of a cognitive evaluation of its efficacy and more of a political rationality. It is a philosophy of domination rather than of partnership. With the mediation of the state involved, citizens become objects of change rather than the determinants of change, and consequently lose both the capability and the right to assess progress. One need only look at the curricula driving our public school education to know that what children learn is based on what corporate needs are prevalent in terms of the projected workforce. To a large extent in the US, music and the arts have been eliminated from school curricula; creativity has been eliminated. The ability to project corporate needs and, therefore, a well-trained workforce is what keeps nations in power, and this drives history. Modern China is an example of how the politics of a few have run the political reality of many to benefit only some. The people at the bottom are truly slaves. The Shanghai skyline we see now was nonexistent 20 years ago, and the people who built it will never live anywhere near it or partake in the financial realities that this skyline stands for. As China has opted for a combination of oligarchical communism in its politics and state-sponsored capitalism in its economics, the same hierarchy of humanity persists, with some buying a greater right to life than others. The Chinese and many other nations have bought into the linear truths of a reductionist philosophy that separates meaning and agency from action.

We are currently in need of a process by which we, humanity, can assess what has worked and is working and what is not. Are people in the West living longer merely because we are pickled into old age with preservatives coming through the food stream? Do we agree that *all* of our lives are improved by the ways in which we now live? Does the current generally poorer status of peoples of color in the world have anything to do with activities and beliefs coming from Europe and North America? Does the rising incidence of cancer in the developed world over the last 100 years have anything to do with actions generated by a philosophy of domination and exploitation that has also driven the separation of humanity from nature? What will become of the rest of the world as this philosophy of domination and exploitation spreads?

If we were to look at only one common denominator — water — it might provide a bridge of understanding about our predicament. Water has been used by every spiritual tradition on earth as a metaphor for the sacred and for the soul. Water is the essence of life. Water is the Mother. From the ancient literatures, including the Bible, the Koran, the Torah, and the Upanishads, the belief was imparted that "the waters must be taken" in order to heal the physical and subtle body. These waters were both physical and metaphorical for the sacred. Certain wells and springs were reserved for making medicines and for healing all ills. Water is the mother of life as we know it on earth. And the inner water of wisdom that comes from quiet and listening is the mother of a truthful life.

The "war against cancer" is emblematic of this conflict between acting out of wisdom and acting out of ignorance, greed, and progress. Cancer does not, as Nixon stated in 1972, require a war; it requires a revolution in our way of living. Acting out of the wisdom traditions implies actions driven by a realization that connectedness and integration are essential to all life, and that maintaining the purity of the essence of that life is absolute. Acting out of greed in modern times implies actions driven by the philosophy coming out of the Age of Enlightenment that drove the Industrial Revolution and the notion of science as we understand it today. The split between the external expression of reason — through modern science, capitalist economics driven by growth and not sustainability, agribusiness, trickle-down politics — and the interior expression of wisdom and all that it offers to the morality, values, agency, and knowing of humanity is what allows the destruction now rampant in our world. We make that destruction. And cancer is a material example of the violence of that destruction. Since we are part of the world, this violence is against ourselves. It is a form of insanity.

The view of water as a precious essence of life containing sacred qualities and the ability to heal has now been relegated to the waste heap of ancient beliefs. Water is now only the elemental substance known by science as H_2O and nothing else. All sacred qualities of water have been stripped away. It is not that they have ceased to exist; it is that science has no way to view them and, therefore, refuses to acknowledge them. The philosophical conflicts surrounding water arise from the same conflicts between science based on reductionism and its underpinning of ownership — ownership of everything including knowledge, ownership of the seeds of life, and ownership even of the perennial cultures of peoples who have for millennia lived as part of the earth, not on the land but as part of and within the land as part of the local ecology sharing in all of its blessings along with all of the other members of that ecological family of life.

The Great Chain of Being

Huston Smith, who many consider the world's leading authority on comparative religion, has pointed out in his book *Forgotten Truth* that virtually all of the world's great wisdom traditions subscribe to the belief in the Great Chain of Being. According to this universal world-view, reality is a rich tapestry of interwoven levels reaching from matter to body to mind to soul and spirit, and back. Each level envelops or enfolds its under dimensions, a series of nests within nests within nests of Being. Every thing and event in the world is interwoven with every other, and all are ultimately enveloped and enfolded by Spirit, God, Goddess, Tao, Brahman, Absolute Self, or whatever we choose to call it.

With the rise of modernity in the West, the Great Chain of Being almost entirely disappeared, gone the way of extinction. Starting with the Enlightenment, the modern West became the first major civilization to deny entirely the existence of the Great Chain of Being. One of the contributions of the science of the Age of Enlightenment is the double-blind randomized placebo-controlled study that takes one item out of the relationship to all other items in order not to skew the truth about that item through the bias of relationship. This way of seeking truth is a crystallization of the break in the Great Chain. The philosophy of the science that engendered the double-blind randomized placebo-controlled study is, in many ways, responsible for our current problematic state precisely because it destroyed the ecology of knowledge by splitting knowledge into a million pieces and by fracturing the relationship of knowledge and wisdom.

Contrast again the words of Francis Bacon from 17th century England with those of Chief Sealth of the Duwamish tribe of the northwestern state of Washington in the 1800s. Bacon said: "The discipline of scientific knowledge and the mechanical inventions it leads to, does not merely exert a gentle guidance over nature's course; it has the power to conquer and subdue her, to shake her to her foundations." Notice the change from a nongendered identification in the quotation to the female gender. Chief Sealth said in part: "This we know — the earth does not belong to the people, the people belong to the earth. All things are connected like the blood that unites one family. Whatever befalls the earth befalls the sons and daughters of the earth. Humanity did not weave the web of life; humanity is merely a strand in it. Whatever is done to the web is done to humanity." These two quotes are emblematic of the conflict inherent in our current condition, philosophically and pragmatically. Bacon's philosophy drives all of the major decisions regarding economics, scientific research, medicine and how we understand diseases, politics, ecology, and the environment. This is the ground zero out of which we are now trying to dig ourselves.

In the place of the Great Chain of Being has come what Ken Wilber calls "flatland." Flatland is the place where the universe is composed basically of matter, including material bodies and material brains, all of which are studied best by science as we now know it, or scientific materialism. The Great Chain of Being could not stand up to the truth as offered by modern science. And this is where we find ourselves today. It is an immensely confusing place to be. The State can no longer be viewed as the custodian of the dream of justice, nor can the dream be left to the rule of the market and the domination of commercial interests on a global scale with the single principle of profit maximization, also part of the philosophy coming out of the Age of Enlightenment. Where is the deeper meaning? Where is the inner truth that gives vitality to life and preserves it?

Our environment is becoming an ultimate expression of flatland. This environment is not expressed only outside of us. It is not just the natural environment, the water, the forests, the salmon, orca, and spotted owl. It is the economic environment, the political environment, and the philosophical and spiritual environment. It is the meaning, or lack of it, by which we live. If we continue as we have, we will be committing suicide. If we do not, we will be recommitting ourselves to the adoration of the receptive in life and the powerful transformation that can bring. If we do not honor, adore, respect, and live in connected *Yin* and *Yang*, in a web of receptivity to active response and meaning, action moving from meaning based on the wisdom of the heart, then this world cannot endure. Reductionism is a revolutionary form of science based on a consciousness that must continue to evolve and find a way to interweave the exterior realities of measurable existence with the interior realities of wisdom and intuition and meditation states whose effects are observable but not the process through which they were arrived at.

Water again becomes emblematic of this struggle. Following in Chapter 1 are myriad ways in which water and the world it creates is a reference for our predicament. These examples lead to questions about the link between the health of our bodies and spirits and the health of our waters and surroundings. In a world understood as a Great Chain of Being, there can be no separation.

Responsibility

The world has changed so dramatically just in our lifetime. Even the constancy of nature has begun to shift. And as it does, I realize how afraid I am in my deeper self about our common future. Not just the human future but the future of our world — Earth. All of the premonitions that drove my earlier life seem to have come true. And I understand now that the pathway I walked as a younger person was a pathway through and into this understanding — of how we, and our world, are one and have made one another.

There is a Hopi story of creation that ends with the sentence "We are the people we have been waiting for." This story and the ending sentence are emblematic of a belief that each time and place between the infinities has a story of its own, and the people born into that time and place have the answers for all of the difficulties encountered there. I realize now that the deep underlying sadness that has permeated my life has been the product of a symbiotic reality of loss in this world — the loss of nature and of our place in it. As a part of nature, my own short life has absorbed through osmosis the intense pain of the loss of species, the change in weather, the diminishment of pure living water, the embedding of pollutants in every material of life, and the terrible loss of any relationship to the world that has given us so much.

Into this mixture of modern reality comes the plague. Plagues have been a part of human history ever since there were enough of us to call a common affliction a plague. They have almost always been the result of a combination of exposure to climatic factors, the proliferation of a pathogen, and public health issues like hygiene and a clean water supply. Because of these issues they have often been confined to the poorest of humans, who had no recourse for escape. But in modern life and in the developed world, where generally a public health infrastructure exists to protect us from plaguelike diseases, a modern epidemic is taking hold and it is attacking the poor and the wealthy alike. The public health issues that drive the cancer epidemic are of a new order and ultimately come out of how we live separate from the natural world that supports us. The pathogens are coming not from nature but from humanity and the mind of humanity.

As we learn more about everything, it becomes clearer that the landscape we are studying is a shifting reality with shifting truths. And the pictures derived from the snapshots we have to date change our view of what intelligence is and how it is manifested. It may be that intelligence even as we define it now, in terms of brain capacity, is ubiquitous in all forms of life — brain or not. Perhaps it is consciousness that is evolving and brain capacity is a manifestation on one strand of evolution that is only part of what drives consciousness. In our attempts to design and redesign various scales of intelligence, perhaps it is consciousness that we are really trying to define and quantify. The evolution of consciousness may be common to all species — elephant, *T. rex*, human, primate, deodar cedars, mosquitoes.

Modern science, as a linear form, looks primarily at that which is observable and measurable. When we read the words of the plant spirits from the writings of the Findhorn community in northern Scotland, they tell us that plants came to this world first in order to prepare it for higher forms so that those forms could feel at ease in the natural and material world. Looking at the writings left by Mirra Alfassa, the spiritual partner of Sri Aurobindo, we learn that many flowers have very specific healing powers — physical, emotional, and psychic. Even the Bible tells us that all of the needed medicines for diseases are contained in water and the plants of earth. Beyond modern science there are many points of view about how life occurs and the functions of each form.

The concept that diseases have a spirit tied to the nature of the time in which it occurred is not a new one. In the past, many epidemic diseases were understood as expressions or manifestations of how that particular culture or society interpreted the meaning of life and, therefore, lived their lives. For example, many of the plagues of Europe in the Dark and Middle Ages were caused by public health issues that no one understood were problems — lack of clean water (especially in cities), lack of waste removal, poor food quality due to no refrigeration and other issues, and overcrowding, all of which were driven by more and more people being forced to leave the land and enter the cities; this exodus continues even today, with negative effects. The microscope had not yet been invented and no one knew in 800 CE about microscopic waterborne and airborne pathogens. No one knew that fleas living on rats were the vector for bubonic plague. What is remarkable to me is that in Tibet during this same time, an accurate map was drawn of the developing human fetus from one cell to birth. Without a microscope, how did this map come about? The spirit of the plagues in Europe was very much a combination of ignorance and lifestyle factors driven by a particular way of life. In Tibet the realizations that resulted from a meditative life enabled at least certain people to know the evolution of the germination of a human egg and that the human egg even existed as part of the life cycle.

We live in a complex and small world where the isolation of cultures and societies is past history. What people believe and how they live now affects everyone else. We are moving as a species from a tribal orientation to a global orientation. And the spirit of the diseases we see now is no longer just local or simple.

This book is an attempt to understand and share the spirit of the modern cancer epidemic. We can be aware, through the observation and measurement techniques of modern science, of many of the modern day exposures and lifestyle habits that drive the numbers. But this text is an attempt to also delve into and describe the underlying psychic mechanisms of our lives that drive the decisions we make that ultimately contribute to our demise and that of many others. Is there anything about the very nature of how we live and think now that is responsible for the modern epidemic of cancer in the developed world? What is the spirit of the cancer epidemic and how did we get here? How can we understand the terrain of the modern world that we have created and are part of in relation to this manmade epidemic?

Chinese medicine, a logical and ecological form of medicine that still contains elements of the Great Chain of Being, has survived into the 21st century, and has a lot to offer this discussion. It is one of the few perennial forms of medicine based on a philosophy of interconnectedness that continues to evolve and simultaneously is stimulated by the reality of modern biomedicine. Balance of Yin and Yang, connection of the interior and the exterior of life, and the resultant harmony between the two are components of the theoretical foundations of Chinese medicine. And the concept of *Qi* as an interface between energy and form, the enlivening force for creation, contributes greatly to the understanding of these issues in our modern world.

If we are at a crossroads of life and death, the ancient consciousness that evolved the system of Chinese medicine out of an ecology of connectedness and interrelationship, and, very importantly, out of meditation and inner listening technologies, may have a great deal to offer our dilemma. We are, no doubt, the people we have been waiting for. And we are the composite of all of our ancestors. They lived in order to bring us here. Chinese medicine is itself a product of those peoples who lived across an expanse of time bridging the perennial cultures and modern cultures. It comes partially from a hierarchical and sexist system but still retains, at least philosophically, the seeds of equanimity and balance and the goal of a unified whole that requires the nourishment of and respect for all of its parts.

The hope for our future lies in the deeper process of discovering our own disconnection from self, soul, spirit, and nature. These aspects of truth are the only pathways into which and through which we might rediscover ourselves and heal the great torn world we have made. We cannot live separate from the natural world, and the natural world cannot live separately from us, because we are one and the same. We are one. Our hope lies in once again knowing this, not in our minds, but in our hearts and souls. It requires that we regain an inner silence, at a time when action seems the only possible solution, in order to hear the perennial truth of life — our world and our selves are one. Without first realizing this, we cannot know what our next step is. Without knowing this again, we cannot hope to find a cure for cancer — the scourge of our time.

CHAPTER 1

Water — The *San Jiao*

> Ecstatic love is an ocean, and the Milky Way is a flake
> of foam floating on it.
>
> — Rumi

Water is the basis of life and the lowest common denominator. Everything flows downward to water. And all actions taking place within the global atmosphere and on the Earth eventually find their way to water. Water makes it impossible to get away with any misuse or abuse that takes place in our world. Eventually payment comes due, usually via the lack of clean and pure water with which to sustain life. Water is the basis for the circle of life — the hub.

Only about 3% of the world's water is fresh. And it is becoming more and more precious. We are initiating wars for water. Water is no longer emblematic of life — a much-overused metaphor. Water, air, and Earth *are* life. And we are at the edge of the world looking for a bridge to span the inevitable chaos that will accompany the loss of pure water because of drought, global climate change, misuse, lack of recharge in our aquifers due to overuse, contamination by industrial wastes that have used our waterways as a dump, and agricultural techniques that waste and abuse water as though it would last forever.

As the lowest common denominator, water has become a delivery system for most contaminants that are known to be carcinogenic and those whose health effects are unknown.[1-4] Even contaminants released into the air eventually end up in water. Since the human body is largely made up of water, and since we are at the top of most food chains in the modern world, and since many contaminants are bioaccumulative, we are at high risk for injury from contaminants coming through water. This is the primary reason that this discussion of cancer prevention begins with water and the attitudes toward it that drive decisions that end up fouling and drying up waters across the world — decisions that ultimately cause diseases that end in death.

Not all of such discussions are about carcinogens. They are about all of the conditions that result from a limited view about water. Cancer is often a multifactorial disease, no matter what type. The multiple factors that can be taken into account about water, water use and contamination are manifestations of an underlying condition of the human mind and heart that overlooks and is in denial about these issues. This is the real and first injury. The waste of water and the modern cancer epidemic are but symptoms.

Water and Africa

The continent of Africa is the largest continent below the equator. As such, it is at greater risk for the effects of climate change. For many reasons, including climate change, the desertification of Saharan Africa is spreading into sub-Saharan Africa.[5] The large landmass of the continent is primarily below the equator and absorbs heat from the sun more than any other continent. The Nile watershed carries approximately 30% of all the runoff from sub-Saharan Africa, more than any other watershed in Africa. The concentration of the water-sheds of Africa into only two or three major river systems makes for a higher risk of water shortages, flooding, salination of the soil, desertification, and famine. Africa is far more delicately balanced to begin with.[6]

Central Africa is home to one of the world's largest rainforests, and serves as one of its most important carbon sinks.[7] Carbon sinks capture carbon dioxide from the atmosphere, thus reducing global greenhouse gas levels since carbon dioxide is the main greenhouse gas.[2] Climate change is already diminishing Central African rainforests. These rainforests are under the same pressures as the Amazon rainforest.[8] Besides climate change, deforestation for lumber (much of which is sent to Japan and the United States for construction purposes) and deforestation for local agricultural needs and fuel will have depleted three-quarters of the forest cover in Central Africa by 2025. This leads to downstream flooding, reduced water quality, sedimentation in rivers and lakes, dust storms, air pollution, health problems, and an increased effect on climate change. It is a vicious circle.[9]

Water has gone scarce in India and sub-Saharan Africa partly because the World Bank, run primarily by the US and other developed, well-funded, and mostly European countries, has prescribed the mining of groundwater in areas that are very arid; these groundwater sources have an extremely low recharge.[10] This is why the ancient system of agriculture in these areas is a profound design of balance between crops that require less water, recharging the groundwater, and the use of hand-dug wells rather than deep tube wells. Areas in northern India that have fed thousands of people for millennia are now in drought and famine because modern techniques of irrigation and modern genetically engineered food crops have wasted the water and failed in the long term to feed the people.[11]

The great dams of Africa have also been funded by the World Bank as a means of providing drinking water and energy in places where water and energy are scarce.[12] Only well-funded corporations or landowners have been able to afford this water and energy for the drilling of deep tube wells for irrigation water. Poor farmers, for whom this intervention was supposedly meant, cannot afford to drill the wells, buy the water, or irrigate their farms. Almost 100% of the income of the poor is spent on nutrition. These people cannot afford to buy water provided by a dam or from a deep well. As a result, in India and Africa people are starving and unable to grow enough food as they once did, only 50 years ago.

These issues are issues of the commons.[13] Every living thing on Earth has a right to live. Air, water, and sustenance are all part of the commons — that part of life that contains the essentials that sustain life. When these essentials are owned and then sold, not everyone has equal access. The individual human body also has a right to the commons; and defining what the commons are now is a major task not only in the developing world but also in the developed world.[14] Clean air, clean water, clean soil, and clean food are all essential to everyone, living anywhere. Cancer is a disease often caused by contamination of these essentials and, as such, is a public health crisis that requires a definition of what the commons in the developed and the nondeveloped world will look like. What should the commons be based on in the prevention of chronic diseases and the many forms of cancer? These questions on the commons are political, social, moral, and spiritual. They include the exterior truth as we know it now, combined with the interior truth, the wisdom of a holistic view that combines exterior and interior — spirit and science, meaning and identified need.

Over the last several centuries the exterior truth has changed based on knowledge and information that is itself continually changing. Wisdom truths do not change. They are based on inner knowing that is perennial in nature. They tend to be moral, intuitive, and essentially complete. Consciousness is not the same as wisdom but is part of wisdom. Consciousness as it drives the scientific view is limited by the evolution of humanity at any given time. Wisdom is perennial in that it remains whole and has as its foundation grounding in the connectedness of inner and outer life and of humanity and nature.[15]

The history of Africa regarding colonialism and the slave trade has contributed immensely to the "meaning side" of its current condition. There is no way to quantify the damage done to the commons, the consciousness, and the spirit and local wisdom traditions of Africa by the colonial rape of the land and its peoples over the centuries by people looking to own the African commons. In fact, it has consistently been mostly European peoples who have colonized areas of the world where the concept of the commons in each case made it inconceivable that another people would arrive and cause such destruction and actually steal land and resources they themselves had always considered sacred and as part of their commons open to everyone and for which everyone was responsible.[16–18]

Paul Rohrbach, as head of German immigration in South-West Africa,[19] in his bestseller, (1912), German thought in the World,[8] stated:

"No false philanthropy or racial theory can convince sensible people that the preservation of a tribe of South Africa's kaffirs...is more important to the future of mankind than the spread of the great European nations and the white race in general. Not until the native learns to produce anything of value in the services of the higher race, i.e. in the service of its and his own progress, does he gain any moral right to exist."[20]

This intensely racist and arrogant quote tries to justify the European Christian white man's usurpation of the right to life of African peoples and the lands on which they and their ancestors had lived since the advent of humankind. The racism and colonialism that all of Africa has had to endure for so long, not unlike the native first peoples of North and South America and many people of color, exacts a deep wound that takes many generations to heal and recover from.[21–24] These wounds are in the people and in the land, and continue today. These wounds were perpetrated by people who were so split from the truth in their hearts that they actually thought that they were right in dominating and destroying cultures of people unlike themselves. Of course, the primary purpose was to own the land and extract the resources from it by using the labor of the people who knew and lived as a part of that land.

The Africa we find now is not the same Africa of even 200 years ago. The climate change driving the desertification of northern and now sub-Saharan Africa is not due to activities taking place in Africa based on African peoples' philosophies of life but is due to activities taking place primarily in North America and Europe and based on philosophies of North American and European peoples. The climate change occurring in Africa is due to greenhouse gases formed in the developed world, where policies usually formulated by non-Africans for Africa result in deforestation, the products of which are then used primarily in the developed world and not in the part of the world from which they came. A modern colonization continues to occur.[25,26]

Water Around the World

Climate is the generator of water. When climate changes, it exacerbates all other changes that also contribute to a lack of clean and available water. Through a complex hydrology cycle, weather, climate, and the land relate to one another in a ballet of movement and energy.[27] One could say that the global hydrology cycles and all that they create are the *San Jiao* ("triple burner") of the Earth. Water physiology, temperature regulation, immune function, interconnected bodily communications, absorption, and the very spirit of the Earth are expressed in the Chinese medicine theory of the *San Jiao* as manifested by the global hydrology cycles.[28] The Taoist map of the macrocosm and the human microcosm expresses very beautifully this ancient theory of ecology and the ubiquitous nature of the *San Jiao* of Chinese medicine as it weaves together every organ and tissue of the human body and every ecological system of the Earth and the microcosm. When we look at injuries to our water systems on the Earth, we are viewing injuries to the *San Jiao* of the globe, at once related to water, to temperature, to cooling, to *Yin*, and to the Earth's ability to heal itself.

Coastal areas are essential to the Earth's *San Jiao* and provide the foundation for clean water, for fisheries and inland fresh waters. As of 2000 C.E., in many countries around the world — Europe, South America, Africa, Australia, and North America — there had been an 80% loss of estuaries and coastal wetlands.[29] These are areas where salt water meets and becomes fresh water. The mangroves in most countries, including the United States, have been reduced by more than 30% in just the last 20 years. The 2004 estimate regarding coral reefs was that 20% of the world's coral reefs were damaged and unlikely to recover, and that a total of 70% were destroyed, critical, or threatened. Coral reefs contain the greatest abundance of sea life of any water ecosystem.

All of the above are due to manmade causes — primarily climate change, pollution, and degradation by improper use. The desire to live near the ocean has destroyed many wetlands that have traditionally acted as buffers for tidal surges that result from hurricanes and other types of storms. The Hurricane Katrina damage was made far worse by the fact that so much of the coastal wetland area has been lost to fill and construction of homes in areas where the wetlands have traditionally preserved life by absorbing and filtering sea water surges.[30] Nowhere is this loss of wetlands more severe than in Florida, where coastal wetlands are lost along with the Everglades connected to them acre by acre, day after day, year after year.[31] These areas are part of the Great Chain of Being, the Earth *San Jiao*, and protect life and clean water. People have lived in these areas for thousands of years because of the abundance of life in these systems. They have lived there without destroying these systems because they lived as perennial cultures in the land as part of it and its systems, and not on or off the land as do modern humans. They saw themselves as part of the cycle of life and not as manipulators of that cycle.[32]

The sea grass beds are also accelerating in degradation, and major losses have been incurred in the Mediterranean, Florida, the Caribbean, and Australia. Do not buy sea grass rugs or furniture even if they are advertised as sustainably harvested. Sea grass beds, kelp beds, saltwater marshes, and coastal wetlands all provide ecosystems for fish and other aquatic species to live. Coastal peoples have for millennia used these smaller systems for food and other products. This is as true in the Pacific Northwest as it is in South Asia. It is true everywhere where land meets water.

Fish

If you have noticed over the last 20 years that more and more exotic fish species are available for your dinner plate, it is because the local fisheries that used to provide cod, halibut, and other local species in northern fisheries are fished out. You may have noticed also that your swordfish steaks are getting smaller and smaller. This is because the larger fish, the only ones that can breed, are almost gone. Depleting the smaller fish ensures that someday soon we will no longer be eating swordfish.[33,34] Taking fish from other parts of the world will ensure that those fish will also be gone. And the local fishermen and peoples who used to fish for and eat them will also be out of fish as we eat their stocks.

The decline in worldwide catches of fish is due largely to the loss of large, slow-growing predators at high trophic levels. These are gradually being replaced, in global landings, by smaller, short-lived fish, at lower trophic levels. Until a few decades ago, depth and distance from coasts protected much of the deep ocean fauna from the effect of fishing. However, fleets now fish further offshore and in deeper water with greater precision and efficiency, thanks to modern technology, compromising areas that acted as refuges for the spawning of many species of commercial interest to both industrial and artisanal fleets. The Atlantic was the first ocean to be fully exploited in this way and eventually overfished. The Pacific is now in the process — a process that is almost completed. The people who suffer from this more immediately are the small fishermen, as their life bread is taken from them by larger industrialized fleets.[35] But soon all of us will suffer. The high–omega-3 content of fish will not be available to us or will have to be weighed against pollution of these same fish, making it a complex decision to even eat fish.[36,37]

In the Pacific Northwest, the local marine ecosystem fisheries and especially salmon fisheries are depleted because of loss of habitat in the smaller streams due to logging practices, because of overfishing, and because of pollution. There are now 14 species of salmon that are considered endangered. Two years ago the Puget Sound orca whales (the largest of the dolphins) were finally found to be a species separate from the Inland Passage orcas because they speak a different language than their northern cousins and this meant that they could be evaluated as a separate group. The Puget Sound orcas — the J, K, and L pods — are now considered an endangered species. The primary reasons for their demise are starvation and malnutrition due to depleted salmon runs and contamination by primarily PCBs. The Puget Sound orca pods are now considered the most contaminated whales in the world.[38] Washington state has the highest rate of breast cancer in the United States. Although it may be more complex than this, my question is: If this is what is happening to the whales, which are also mammals, what is happening to us since we are part of the same ecosystem?

From 1950 to 1990, the world's oceanic fish catch climbed from 19 million tons to 89 million tons. But, since 1990, there has been no growth in the catch. The world can no longer rely on the oceans for an expanding food supply.[39] In 1997, the United Nations Food and Agriculture Organization reported that 11 of the world's 15 major fishing grounds had gone into serious decline as a result of overfishing. They also found that 34% of all fish species were vulnerable to, or in immediate danger of, extinction.[40] These insults to the Great Chain of Being are ubiquitous. There is no place to go anymore where the problems of habitat loss, overuse, and pollution are not visible and impacting local ways of life. These impacts dramatically affect the local peoples first, and then trickle up to the most affluent, who can yet afford to buy from distant fisheries when their own are depleted. Industrialization, a component of reductionism, and separation of one thing from the many and the whole — whether it is on land or in the sea — is a major culprit in the demise of the Earth and those living as an integral part of the Earth.

All of these insults are emblematic of a way of thinking that separates us from our world even when we are actually living as part of it. The same insults that result in the demise of the environment also result in the demise of our health and in the symptom of this way of thinking that we call cancer.

The World's Largest Hydraulic Civilization

From Denver to Tijuana and the Oregon border to Tucson is the world's largest hydraulic civilization. Pumps and shunts take water from the Colorado River and the rivers of California to increase soil moisture to grow monocrops. Unfortunately, irrigation accelerates the salting of soil. It took 2500 years for the Tigris–Euphrates societies to ruin their soils with salt. In the western United States, agriculture irrigates with salty water, adds salty fertilizers, cultivates salty soils and thereby forces the water table into the root zone through irrigation. Irrigation has degraded arid land soils in 50 years or less.[41] This is also what is happening in Africa and India as they use more and more the modern Western style of industrial agricultural techniques. These techniques require hybrid seeds that must be purchased each year, more water use, petrochemical inputs because of destruction of the soil fertility, and loans from the World Bank on an annual basis in order to grow crops that do not feed one's family, contain less nutrition, and are contaminated with herbicides and pesticides that are carcinogenic. The idea that the food produced in this way is cheap is a complete lie.

Here in America 50–60 million acres have been degraded by salination.[42] This salination is caused by inappropriately growing crops
in a climate unsuited for that crop, thus requiring irrigation in large
amounts and the use of pesticides, all of which cause mineral salts to
build up in the soil. Tens of thousands of acres need to be overirri-
gated to leach salts to drain below the root zone. In San Luis districts
in California, some of these drains are seven feet below the surface.[43]
The leached water must then be carried to a river or internal basin.
How to dispose of the brine has not been resolved in California or
Arizona. Well pollution and wildlife poisoning are common.

In the eastern US and the Mississippi Delta region, very wet areas
of our country, drains have had to be placed for agricultural crops
grown in areas with too much water. These drains are used to manage
soil water. Applied fertilizers and other additives like herbicides seep
into the drainage networks. Tail waters released into a river from the
drainage networks harm downstream people and life. The Mississippi
Delta is one of the most contaminated areas in the world as a result
of runoff from the drainage networks placed to handle too much
water. Hurricane Katrina added to this toxic soup, creating a dead
zone that may never recover.[44]

In the Minnesota River Basin, 40% of farm soils are also overwet
for desired crops. The drainage from these soils fast-tracks fertilizers
and pesticides into the river. To a large extent it is from these waters
draining into the Mississippi River that pollution finally settles out in
the Mississippi Delta.[45] Like the Nile Delta, the Mississippi Delta
used to be one of the most fertile places on the Earth. Because of
industrial agricultural processes based on the science of reductionism, which fails to see the whole ecosystems in which it operates, the
Delta is now one of the most-polluted places in the United States.[46]
The pollution from agriculture up north hyperstimulates the growth
of plant and microbial life. The fast-growing plants consume the
Delta's oxygen and asphyxiate local fish and shellfish. This upstream
drainage creates a downstream dead zone about the size of
Connecticut at the Mississippi's mouth.[47] What happens in one place
has repercussions in another, distant place. The pollution along the
Mississippi and in the Delta is mainly responsible for the rising rates

of cancer over the last 100 years all along the Mississippi and in the Delta. The ubiquitous *San Jiao* of the Earth is continually injured in this way and this results in distant impacts that create disease in the ecosystem and disease in those who live there. Mississippi and Louisiana have some of the highest rates of cancer of any state in the country.

Modern agricultural techniques are supposed to bring progress and feed the world. In fact, they are polluting the soil and water, stripping away the topsoil, and providing food that may not be fit to eat.

Water and Erosion

Soil erosion remains a persistent problem in the US.[48] Topsoil helps to retain moisture and its loss makes the soil more sensitive to drought. Plowing is a major wound that leads to topsoil loss. Less organic matter and nutrients drives up production costs as yields go down. If topsoil is lost, the subsoil becomes the surface. Subsoil has less organic material, too much clay, and reduced phosphorus, and limits root extension as the depth of bedrock decreases. Eroded soil is called sediment. American farmland still loses topsoil 17 times faster than it builds it, because of modern agricultural techniques. As the topsoil erodes away it carries with it every input that agriculture has used on it.[49]

Soil erosion varies perversely with the price of soy, corn, wheat, and cotton. Higher prices for these commodities result in more erosion, not less. Farmers still receive greater government payments for growing high-erosion monocrops. The use of biodiesel and ethanol as fuels may actually exacerbate this problem and may not end up being the rescue from imported petroleum we had hoped for.[50] Monsanto and ADM are lobbying for these alternative fuels, because they will sell more seeds for these crops. Most of the seeds are genetically engineered, adding to the confusion about whether or not this is a good way to solve our long-term fuel problems. These large companies, along with the USDA and government subsidies, are most responsible for driving out small farmers. They exemplify the relationship of government and corporations in taking over the commons and degrading life for many by destroying land quality, water quality, and the ability to make a life in the land while simultaneously contributing to climate change through the addiction to petroleum and carbon-based fuels. These companies and the policies of the government are also responsible for draining the non-renewable aquifers in the Midwest by growing high-priced monocrops in ways that demand irrigation and use of the Ogallala Aquifer, the largest in the US.

Farmers are punished financially for good soil-retaining practices like crop rotation and the shortening of the time that bare soils are exposed to the weather. Some farmers now replace the plow with herbiciding weeds. In no-till systems, the cover "weeds" that naturally come back to re-establish a healthy soil cycle are poisoned and this is claimed to be no erosion. The herbicides used end up in the drainage water and then in our rivers, multiplying many times over from the original site of application.[51] Atrazine is a major herbicide used for this purpose. The Environmental Working Group found that of 29 Midwestern cities, 28 had public tap water that was contaminated with atrazine.[52,53] Atrazine ia a presumed risk factor for breast cancer. It is no longer legal for use in Europe and Israel.[54,55] These chemicals come out of the history of the early 20th century, where chemicals were used in warfare and then extended for use in industry. The long-term problems of using chemicals that kill in varying ways were not and continue not to be looked at in terms of the inner truths regarding their use. The meaning, the wisdom side, the moral side, and the whole systems side of their use were separated from the science of their actions and an incomplete truth was come to about the efficacy of their use. Is this a problem of consciousness letting modern science off the hook? Many of these chemicals used in agriculture are carcinogens. And all of them disrupt the *San Jiao* of the Earth in some way. As part of that same cycle, the human microcosm is also disrupted.

The Mississippi Delta is the most obvious case in point but there are literally hundreds of other hot points all along the Missouri and Mississippi Rivers. In industrialized agriculture, the Earth is used as an anchor on which to grow plants that draw their sustenance from chemicals and water added to the Earth. The Earth no longer has any other purpose than to act as an anchor to hold plants, and the quality of the soil itself no longer matters. This loss of soil quality drives in many ways the loss of biodiversity in the world. Plant species requiring certain kinds of soil and climate are grown just about anywhere under these new conditions. The loss in species that results from these insults, in turn, degrades the quality of our lives as human beings, leading to human health crises. The honeybee is a primary example of how the extinction of a pollinator may change the history of life on the Earth.[56] And the quality of modern fruits and vegetables grown under an industrial agricultural system is lacking in vitamins and minerals and many other nutrients.[57-62] They are developed and grown for size and shape, looks, and shelf longevity, but not for nutritional quality. It is not known what effects genetically modified foods will have over time on human and soil health, let alone the entire ecosystem in which they are grown. Round-Up Ready corn or soybeans may look good as a science experiment but it is unknown what the long-term effects of this engineering of plant crops will have. In the developed world, where we can afford to raise our food in these ways, the resulting health crisis takes the form of chronic diseases and cancers. Another example concerns farmers who as a group have a fivefold increase in non-Hodgkin's lymphoma (NHL).[63] This data applies only to farmers who live on their own land, and not to farm workers who migrate from farm to farm. The rate for NHL in migrant workers working on these same farms is unknown, because those people are not part of any health-monitoring system. But, in fact, they are part of subsidization of modern farming and are part of the invisible cost of agribusiness. A known cause of NHL is 2,4-D, a pesticide commonly used in agriculture. People living and working in farm communities have multiple hits during their lifetimes from agricultural inputs, only some of which are known to have human health effects. The lack of public health research into these communities and the true costs of agribusiness amount to a societal and moral decline.

In many ways, water becomes the deliverer of chemicals that cause disease and take life. The Great Chain of Being exists whether we acknowledge it or not, and we are part of it. The consciousness that drives the philosophy and science that enables these actions is disconnected from meaning evolved in the heart — from wisdom. The heart and the mind are no longer connected.

Water Quality — Petrochemicals, Fertilizers, and Pesticides

Since the end of World War II, we have been addicted to synthetic fertilizers. These chemicals were never seen on the Earth before the mid–20th century. The current baby boomers are the first generation of humans to grow up exposed to all of these chemicals.

Synthetic fertilizers:

- Encourage the loss of organic matter that builds and saves soils;
- Damage soil resistance to soilborne diseases;
- Can increase soil acidity;
- Leach quickly, contributing to downstream pollution;
- Are not efficient, with only 50% contributing to crop growth.[64]

By 1997, 72% of our waterways were affected by agricultural pollution, mostly from synthetic fertilizers.[65] And farmers directly inject or fumigate pesticides into the soil. In the 1980s, the EPA began severely restricting soil-injected pesticides because many were carcinogens, and were resistance increasing and wildlife-damaging. Soil solarization has taken the place of injected pesticides. Plastic sheets try to co-opt IPM (integrated pest management) by replacing natural biological control organisms with engineered processes. Why is it that the simplest ways of growing and managing croplands are frequently thrown out for more costly inputs? The answers almost always have to do with financial gain; educational resources that support research on high-intensity and expensive solutions are in contrast to little or no resources for research on or training in simple and sustainable farming techniques. Only very recently (and in small settings) has this begun to change. What is driving it is the public demand for clean and nutritious food.

Pesticides, herbicides, and foliar techniques diminish soil diversity and the complexity of the soil communities. The Great Chain of Being includes circles within circles of dynamic processes, and agricultural chemical inputs destroy these circles of life.[66] Amazingly, some microbes actually ingest pesticides, and transform contaminants by breaking off CO_2 groups. The new molecule is usually more soluble in water. One hopes, that this occurs rapidly, because some breakdown molecules are more toxic than the original. On the other hand, some microbes are being studied by plant biologists to learn how to detoxify lands containing chemicals and return them to organic status.[67] Just as water becomes a carrier molecule for many chemicals, one would hope that some similar means would be found to depurate chemicals in the human body, particularly from fat cells — the most common site of pollution repose. The all-encompassing truth is that what happens in the macrocosm is happening also within the microcosm, including the human body. If we look at the health of our farms, we are simultaneously looking at the health of our own bodies and spirits.

DDT is a ubiquitous example of a pesticide that was outlawed for use in 1972 but still persists in the environment. Its breakdown product is DDE. Both are implicated in breast cancer and both have been found in higher amounts in the breast tissue of women diagnosed with breast cancer. Both are fat-soluble, bioaccumulative, xenoestrogenic, and carcinogenic. DDT is still produced in the United States for export to countries with weak environmental laws, where it remains legal for use. We then import it back in the form of the produce grown with DDT as a pesticide input in the rapidly expanding monocrop agriculture of those countries.[68]

Almost 800 million pounds of pesticides per year end up in run-off.[69] In 1998, the National Water Quality Assessment (NWQA) found pesticide contamination in all of its river and stream samples from all over the US. One half of these samples were taken from groundwater wells. Each sample contained multiple pesticides. Eighty-three pesticides were found. And 66% of the stream samples contained five or more pesticides.[70] The pollutants were originally sprayed or spread on cropland and then washed into nearby streams or were absorbed by underground aquifers. Dangerously high concentrations exist in the drinking water of many people who live in rural agricultural areas or downstream from them.

Soil microbes produce 85% of the atmosphere's greenhouse gases. Soil conservation could reduce the production of US greenhouse gases by up to 42%.[71] These concerns may drive a new emphasis on reducing plowing and soil outgassing. The agricultural techniques of the 20th century have drastically contributed to many forms of pollution and climate change.[72] Most of them, in one way or another, contribute to water reduction due to climate change and draining of our groundwater systems, and to water quality reduction due to pollution from runoff. All of these factors contribute to human health. The loss of species is a harbinger of our own decline in health. And cancer is the canary in the coalmine in the developed world.

Water Depletion

Forty percent of the world's food comes from irrigated land. The only desert civilization that has survived uninterrupted into modern times is Egypt. Egypt irrigates the Nile River Valley based on the river's natural flood cycle. Thus there is no depletion of the water resources. The Nile floods also replenish the soil by washing fertile silt from the Ethiopian highlands down into the valley's croplands. The Aswan Dam has changed all of this. It was built primarily for the purpose of generating electricity to drive certain petroleum and mining operations.[73] These activities have little to do with the land-based people of this region. These people will be forced off their land as the water shortages, loss of fertility, and costs of irrigation water from the dam projects drive them away. Climate change has already begun contributing to water shortages in North Africa, including Egypt. Much of the unrest in the Middle East caused by foreign oil interests is of less concern to the local people than their rights to water. The technology is already available to answer many of the questions regarding water and energy for rural peoples. The will, however, is lacking. Mind, heart, and will are interconnected truths that when in concert could make the Earth a paradise.

Unnatural irrigation-based farming requires a steady source of water but does not replenish this *Source*. Depletion of aquifers far exceeds the natural rate of renewal, and underground water reserves are shrinking.[74] California's Central Valley overdrafts groundwater at a rate of 1.6 billion cubic meters per year, which equals 15% of California's groundwater use. In other words, each and every year 1.6 billion cubic meters of water are used from the aquifer, which is never replaced. The Central Valley produces one half of the fruits and vegetables grown in the US, including almost all of the organic produce sold by Trader Joe's and Whole Foods. Being grown organically is only one part of all of the issues about which we should be thinking when we buy organic produce. The issues with farming and water, irrigation and water, groundwater depletion, water pollution, water and energy production, climate change, slavery of people of color, and human health are all connected. Food and water are part of the Great Chain of Being. Science, in its incompleteness, cannot solve every problem without making sure that it is connected with the larger truths of life.

To maintain the Great Chain of Being, what is required is that we think about water and how the food we are eating was grown, about where it was grown, about the costs of transporting food across state and national borders, environmental and climate costs, and whether it was grown in an area that can support the agricultural use put on the land to grow that produce without harm to the local community and any other community of people and life. Support locally grown produce and foods, and support the Chain of Being. This way you can ask all of the questions needed to make clear choices that save our world and your own and others' health. Begin to question where something came from, how it was made or grown, and who is profiting from it. Food is our first insurance against disease in so many ways.

Groundwater depletion is a problem in India, China, North Africa, South America, and North America. It is due primarily to improper agricultural practices and irrigation. Overuse of nonrenewable aquifers leads to[75]:

- Wells running dry;
- Increased costs of pumping the water above ground;

- Small farmers being squeezed out because of increased costs;
- An increase in wealthy large monocultural operations with technology to pump;
- "Water flows uphill toward money";
- A change from staple crops to high-priced luxury crops to recoup expenses;
- A change in demographics in arid areas like California, Arizona, and Idaho, where water has been traditionally scarce;
- Urbanization versus farmland in competition for water;
- Competition that will end in farming losses and loss of or modifications to the Endangered Species Act.

Water covers two-thirds of the Earth. And yet only 3% of this water is fresh. It is rare and precious. The perennial cultures were right — water is sacred.

Water Safety

Chlorine is the primary means of killing bugs in our public drinking water. It is the cheapest way of providing a clean water supply but it is also a known carcinogen. There are no long-term studies on how the daily drinking of water treated with chlorine affects the human body. It is added to water treatment in quantities that are deemed safe in parts per million. The factor of time and also of timing of exposures is a factor generally not being considered. Before the mid-20th century, most people drank water from ground wells. It was not until the 1930s and 1940s that our municipal water utilities introduced chlorination to the public water supplies of small and larger cities.[76]

Chlorine ions evaporate off treated water and enter the atmosphere, contributing to the weakening of the ozone layer.

Drug-resistant strains of bacteria are promoted by the constant use of chlorine in water treatment,[77] antibiotic use in poultry and livestock production,[78] and antibiotic overuse in medicine.[79] The intricate web of human activity promoting the evolution of bacteria is partially driven by the use of chlorine and other antiseptic products.

Oxygenation is a far better means by which to ensure safe drinking water. It is more expensive in upfront costs but far less expensive in long-term costs including health for humans and our public waterways.[80,81] Do not use chlorine bleach for cleaning. It degrades our public water. Buy a good water filter that will filter chlorine, cryptosporidium, giardia, heavy metals including lead, PCBs, PBDEs, pesticides, and herbicides, and use it for all your drinking water needs. Put small filters on your shower and faucets to filter chlorine and lead. Your skin is your largest organ. It breathes, and the pores of your skin are open during washing with hot or warm water. Chemical contaminants like chlorine can enter through the pores of your skin.

The drinking water you buy in bottled form, as you probably already know, is an unregulated area. There is absolutely no way to know the veracity of the claims being made about it. We all believe that water quality is an important part of health and with good reason. But unless you go to a deep-water spring and get the water yourself, you will not know what you are getting.

Cryptosporidiosis and legionella are most dangerous to our elders and others with compromised immunity. The increased growth in numbers of the elderly population in the global community increases the demand for pure water. Beyond these issues, standard water quality safety tests are for coliforms and miss newer threats. These include pesticides, herbicides, pharmaceutical drugs flushed in toilet water after leaving the human body, and chlorine-resistant bugs. Most of these pathogens and contaminants are not treated at water treatment facilities and are flushed untreated into our local watersheds and sometimes into our public water supplies to be recycled.[82]

Water and Plastics

Water coming to us in plastic bottles raises another issue of contamination and pollution. Many plastics off-breathe endocrine disruptors and other chemicals, which are then infused into the water and contaminate it.[83] Done on a daily basis and over a period of time this exposure can lead to health problems or directly contribute to health problems. Nalgene bottles are a member of this type of plastic bottle that off-breathes. Although Nalgene now makes a better bottle, these Nalgene bottles also come out of an industry that designs plastic contraptions for holding animals used in medical research. Supporting this company by purchasing and using Nalgene bottles does not contribute to the health of animals or humans. It is interesting to note how many chemicals initially designed to be used in warfare then became the basis for commercial uses. Pesticides and herbicides are in this class of chemicals. And the same state of mind that gave birth to the forerunners of modern day pesticides also has given birth to the modern chemical research industry that utilizes animal bodies for experimentation.

Xenoestrogenic chemicals are endocrine disruptors that impact our own hormonal balances. The doses necessary for some of these chemicals to have an effect are often minute. They are sometimes more toxic in small amounts than in larger amounts. These chemicals are found not only in plastics but also in many other petrochemical-based products. The pollution of our waters by ever-smaller pieces of plastic breaking down enters the food chain first of the waters and then the food chain on land. All of life is paying the price. And the number of hits through negative exposures to unclean water keeps accumulating. When they are added to all of the other hits mentioned in this book, the overall effect is overwhelming.[84]

Another reason not to use plastics for storage of water or food is the issue of recycling. To date, only 4.7% of plastics are recycled.[85] The problem is that they are ubiquitous but so varied in composition that it is impossible to design an automated process by which they can be separated. Right now, most of the recyclable plastics of the US go to China. There they are hand-separated and then melted down in open vats, where the workers are exposed to various chemicals released by the heated plastics. In China, that plastic which is not recycled is left lying in the fields.[86] We have once again impacted another culture with our wasteful habits. In the Great Chain of Being this will come back to haunt us.

Even reusing our plastic water bottles is not a good idea, Owing to contamination of the plastic container by whatever is stored in it, and reactions that can cause human harm, including the generation of bacterial strains that are resistant to treatment.[87] Do not use plastic. As manufacturers use more and more plastics to contain their products, often switching from glass, write them mass letters to convince them to stop this wasteful and harmful behavior.

The Law of Ceaseless Cycles

In nature, all life is tuned to the minutest and precisely graduated differences in the particular thermal motion within every single body, which continually changes in rhythm through pulsation. This unique law is the law of ceaseless cycles, which says that every organism is linked to a certain time span and a particular tempo of life. The slightest disturbance of this harmony can lead to the most disastrous consequences for the major life forms.[88] In order to preserve this state of equilibrium, it is vital that the characteristic inner temperature of each of millions of micro-organisms contained within macro-organisms be maintained. All life can be understood in this way, from the gut microflora to the body as organism to a water body to ecosystems to the Earth, and outward and upward into the universe. This law is a modern day expression of the Great Chain of Being. It is also an expression of the inner essence of many meditational paths.[89]

In 1993, a study done under the direction of John Whitelegg, Ph.D., at Lancaster University in England found that the temperature in ambient air and the number of green spaces in major European cities correlated with the number of dust particles and bacteria counts.[90] For example, London was found to have 14% green space and, using tuberculosis bacteria as a reference, 1.9% tuberculosis bacteria were found in each cubic meter of air. In Berlin, where there was 10% green space in the city, 3.1% tuberculosis bacteria were found in each cubic meter of air. In Paris, with 4.5% green space in the city, the street air contained 4.1% tuberculosis bacteria. In the city of Paris, the street air contained 36,000 pathogenic bacteria per cubic meter, whereas the forest and surrounding fields near Paris contained 490 airborne bacteria per cubic meter. From this Whitelegg concluded that cities with less green space, and therefore higher temperatures, tended to have a higher percentage of bacteria. Is it true that the greater content of bacteria in cities contributes to chronic immune system stressors which then contribute to some modern illnesses? Although conclusions cannot be directly drawn from this data, it would seem that many intuitive concerns regarding health effects relative to high-density living in cities could be substantiated if one were to look into it.[91,92]

Similar but unrelated studies here in the US have shown that inland urban air temperatures in the southeastern states have risen over time and are partially responsible for drafting or pulling hurricane winds and water surges deeper into the interior coastal states than recorded previously.[93] As a remedy, several large coastal and interior cities in the southeast are now planting trees, removing asphalt parking lots and replacing them with permeable cover and trees, and placing burms on roofs of high-rise buildings to grow plants in order to increase green space to reduce temperatures to lessen the drafting and damage from hurricanes.[94] This is not being done for human health reasons but the effects could in the end be the same.

When we look at aerial maps of my own city, Seattle, we see that over the past 40 years the aerial photos show less and less green as trees are removed in order to build structures. The biomass of the city itself is a microclimate that contributes to warming, and probably fresh water loss as less water is absorbed by soil, all of which contribute to the growth of pathogens.[95] Seattle has the highest rates of breast cancer and MS in the US. Although it is no doubt more complex than this, is the biomass of the city contributing to these rates?

Warming may contribute to the evolution of circumstances in which higher bacterial and viral levels are stressors on our immune function.[96] Inflammation is a chronic condition that can be measured thermographically and is related to the cancerization of cells.[97] Looking at the macrocosm is as valuable a tool as looking at the microcosm when it comes to understanding diseases. Natural medicine forms derived from perennial cultures have traditionally looked at the macrocosm as part of health. This is a valuable contribution to the modern epidemic of cancer and other chronic diseases, and one that Chinese medicine has consistently made over the past 3000 years.

A New Consciousness

Just like cancer, water — and the modern crisis of water — is emblematic of the predicament in which we now find ourselves. The primary questions in these issues are: Who is profiting? Why do we support them? Are we willing to re-evaluate and lessen our own comfort and desires to support all life everywhere? Have we educated ourselves about food and other products in order to make a life-affirming decision about their purchase? Have we asked the deeper questions about why we allow these things to happen or, even more profoundly, why do we know nothing about them?

As northern Western civilizations have moved forward in time we have lost the Great Chain of Being and what some call the divine feminine, which can be found in every perennial culture. The Goddess, Quan Yin, the Virgin, the Holy Mother, Kali, the Moon, and the Earth itself, are all examples of the power of the receptive in life. All of these examples have made life from the near nonmaterial and have been revered for this capacity. All are examples of the receptive nature of life and of listening for truth rather than using the mind alone and thinking for truth.

This loss of the receptive nature within ourselves, female and male, this degradation of the value of the deep listening traditions, has led us to the brink. The brink is the balance between two enormous forces — truth and meaning. And they are apparently at war. The active truth realm is played out by science and technology, which tells us what is — not what could or should be. It seems to be devoid of meaning and values, and, in fact, is intended to be without meaning and values in order to find "absolute truth" untainted by belief or meaning or relationship. The enormous global scientific infrastructure is, in itself, a valueless skeleton.

Religion has traditionally tried to fill the vacuum by attempting to provide meaning, often by sawing off the branch on which it sits. Leaving out the conundrum of religious traditions and all of the wars that continue to be fought over whose belief is more right, the inner truth of the "meditation and deep listening paths" is receptive in nature and still relies to a large extent on faith — not the faith of belief but the faith required to remain open to whatever may come in. A person lives and meditates holding the faith that achieving a quiet and open state of receptivity will enable that which is greater and more complete to enter and enlighten, or in the silence become visible from within. This faith is based on the idea, hope, concept, intuition that we are part of some greater whole and connection, a connection that can come only through quiet receptiveness, not words, not observation and measurement. And this connection will guide us individually and collectively toward fulfillment. This is the receptive, the inner truth.[98–100]

We find consolation in nature, because it is a pure expression of the faith found in just being. The meaning or deeper interior experience put on it, no matter what our religion or path, springs from the well within us that is part of the receptive. This is why we feel renewed when we are in nature. We listen and be. Being is not something that we should or can be doing only when we are on vacation and finally enter the natural and almost timeless cycle of life. The nature that we must now go to, that we no longer live in, is no longer the web of life that it once was even 50 years ago. This diminishes us and harms our spirit and our ability to know truth. Damage to the spirit of life leads to physical injury. We are currently in the vicious circle of this injury. The physicality of the injury comes out of a deeper and invisible injury.

The reconciliation of science and faith, or spirit, is the dilemma of our modern world. Teilhard de Chardin wrote: "Humanity is being taken to the point where it will have to decide between suicide and adoration." The message being sent to us is: Transform or die. In other words, find a way for the knowledge-based truths brought to us from science to embed themselves in the web of life only in ways that do not destroy it. If science cannot do this, then the truths it is fostering are not whole truths. Find the meaning and wholeness in the partial truths given us by science by finding the spirit in the science. If the spirit and meaning are not part of the scientific truth, know that the science is only a half-truth. Give connection to the external physical world that is being described by science and the internal receptive world within us that tells us the meaning and purpose of life and truth. And know that science cannot go into the receptive and meaning world and measure it. Know that the very act of measuring and taking an entity out of relationship lessens the truth of it. Know that the fact that science cannot measure something in no way makes that something smaller than the mind or the rational; in fact, it is probably the reverse. Make the truth whole again by allowing a relationship with the receptive and the mind of the heart.

Science has answered many questions and has often provided a material consolation in the form of modern medicine and other advances for many people. At the same time, the medicine and science we rely upon today is also creating superstrains of bacteria, is sometimes responsible for the very diseases it treats, is sometimes unwilling to hand over the human body and spirit to a higher power even when it is obvious that no more can be done in the physical realm, and is also often unavailable at any reasonable price to the people who most need it. The pure expression of the sacred receptive exemplified in a calling to medicine and science is commonly lost in the complexity of racism, colonialism, ignorance, greed and intellectual elitism that gradually excludes other ways of knowing.

We may be at the end of so-called civilization. The facts of our global crisis, political and economic, psychological and environmental, spiritual and tangible, show us that only a leap into a new consciousness can engender a vision, a moral passion, joy and energy required to effect the self-sacrifice and change necessary on a scale that is essential. It is from a deep inner transformation and the resolution that springs out of it that outer change occurs. We cannot change what we do not recognize. This requires compassion for our self. Once we have recognized a situation or condition, we must find the meaning that we have placed on it. These conditions start within us and then translate into actions that drive the world in which we live. Cancer is only one canary in the coalmine of conditions that are driven by what we believe and how we live. However, addressing only this one aspect of our predicament will change who we are and how we live, rippling through the Great Chain of Being and re-establishing the connections that have been ripped away in our difficult path to evolve.

Chinese Medicine

Chinese medicine sprang from a perennial culture several thousand years ago but has continued to evolve even into the 21st century. It is a complex evolution fraught with many pitfalls, especially since the rise of European linear science. Chinese medicine is based on a relational science that is best diagrammed by circles and three-dimensional spheres. It contains a fourth dimension — that of time, and how time transforms a disease changing the original presentation and, therefore, diagnosis. Western medicine is exemplified by the double-blind randomized placebo controlled study and is best diagrammed by a straight line from A to Z. It does not have dimensions. Nevertheless, Chinese medicine has incorporated some of the underpinnings of the linearity of Western science. There is much controversy about this amongst practitioners. And some feel that the incorporation of aspects of Western science and medicine occurs because we are not trained well enough in classical Chinese medicine, primarily because of the gaps driven by language and culture. The Western mind does not work like the Chinese mind. Language drives a good deal of this. Akin to the loss of the Great Chain and its philosophy, the path of modern Chinese medicine is a confusing place in which to be walking. Western or conventional medicine may not be confusing but it is so because it lacks the dimensionality of perennial forms like Chinese medicine. We live in a complex world where there are no simple answers.

The modern knowledge about cancers is being driven largely by conventional medicine and Western science. Partially this is appropriate, because it is, at least, the philosophy of Western science and the resulting knowledge and usages derived from that philosophy that is greatly responsible for the modern epidemic of cancer and the tremendous rise in the incidence of cancers in the developed world.[101] Western science and medicine sometimes has the language with which to evaluate the impacts of chemical and other exposures, because it invented those chemicals. However, the science of Chinese medicine also has a language of understanding about how the world and the human body work that is in many ways more complete. Whereas conventional medicine sees the minute pieces of a functional unit, Chinese medicine starts from the macrocosm and the functional relationships of all its units to derive a closer view of what has gone wrong. And Chinese medicine has the capacity to observe and predict the injuries to these relationships over time. One view is from above sweeping in like a GPS locator until the microcosm is seen in that moment — the goal. The other view is from the inside looking out and recognizing all of the interconnections the microcosm has to the whole now and in the future — the goal.

This inside view and relational approach is what makes Chinese medicine, even today, a perennial form of science that has value. It is another way of knowing and is a holistic way of knowing. This is important, because we are stuck in our linear way of thinking. And people across the world intuitively know that studying the inner knowing of Chinese medicine, one of the last extant and organized systems of a perennial form of medicine, is an important part of healing our current world and the diseases it expresses because it acts as a bridge between the holistic world of the past and the modern fragmented world. Chinese medicine is not a religion. But it expresses an ecological view of the world and the human body in the world in a profoundly logical and relationally meaningful way, a view that Western science often works to exclude.

If it is true that many diseases begin primarily in the ethereal body[102] as expressions of the mind and its decisions, then Chinese medicine is the perfect form to be engaged with the healing of this particular wound we call the modern epidemic of cancers. The energetic medicine of some modalities of Chinese medicine — acupuncture, meditation, combined internal and external exercise like *qigong* and *taijiquan* — works with the ethereal body and the invisible flows of energy underlying the ethereal body.[103] Injuries to the ethereal body occur often as a result of unresolved emotional and psychic-level wounds. Although Chinese medicine looks at the individual, some of these wounds are cultural[104]; we have only to look at World War II Germany to understand how a cultural wound can lead to damage to a whole culture and the world (see Chapter 5).[105] I would submit that we are living with what is becoming a global wound cultured in the test tube of the West and its philosophy of the linear one-dimensional mind disconnected from the truth of the heart. For if we know that the chemically contaminated world in which we live was created by us, then why would we continue to do that which kills us? This wound is one that Chinese medicine can partially address.

As we look for primary ways to prevent cancer, the system of Chinese medicine contains several tools that can address not only the emotional injuries caused by loss of connectedness but also the physical injuries caused by lifestyle habits and exposures derived from living an unnatural life and a life that is primarily exterior and lacking in an inner process. The injuries that result from living in this way affect every phase of *Qi* and blood circulation.[106] And it is injury to the circulation of these primary components of health in Chinese medicine that is mainly responsible for the cancerization process. Stagnation, hypercoagulable blood, and inflammation all lead to cancers.[107,108] Nutrition, acupuncture, herbal medicine, internal/external exercises in combination with depuration techniques, nature cures, aerobic exercise, and meditation or quiet listening are the healing tools for the primary and secondary prevention of cancer. All of these tools enable us to regain a relationship with our true selves — a true self that helps us know in our bones what the right way to live is. And living well is the cure for cancer, because it is preventative.

For the past 60 years the Chinese in China and Southeast Asia, the South Koreans, and the Japanese have been studying and clinically applying the system of Chinese medicine in cancer treatment.[109–111] A vast number of pharmaceutical and clinical research studies have been done and are being applied to the overall understanding of how cancer works and how to treat it in combination with conventional medicine.[112] As a result, a kind of hybrid science of the knowledge of cancers according to conventional and Chinese medicine has evolved. This knowledge is being applied in secondary prevention to stave off recurrence in patients treated after a cancer diagnosis and in primary prevention to stave off an initial diagnosis from ever occurring.

It is not yet known how Chinese herbs may act to depurate[113] carcinogens from storage sites in the body. This is an arena of medicine that is of great interest and importance. In primary prevention it is obviously the elimination of exposures to carcinogens that should be first. However, in terms of promoting factors that increase and intensify the impacts of a carcinogenic hit, Chinese medicine offers several thousand years of accrued clinical information, because rehabilitation and maintenance of health has always been the goal of Chinese medicine. Understanding the pathology of cancers according to the system of Chinese medicine is important, because we can then look for and address these general health conditions before they contribute to progression to a cancer diagnosis. Recognizing them in patients who are at high risk is especially important.

Etiological Factors in Cancer Pathogenesis

1. *The Emotions*

When *Qi* and *blood* are imbalanced, stasis results. *Qi* is magnetized by the *blood* and vice versa. *Qi* and *blood* work together to enable movement of the life force within the body and movement of all of those integral elements of *blood* that foster life. *Qi stasis* can lead to *blood stasis*, which can then progress to *blood dryness*, *blood stasis*, and *congealed blood*. *Congealed blood* is one cornerstone of the cancerization process.[114,115] Western medicine analogs for *blood stasis* and *congealed blood* are high fibrinogen levels, hypercoagulability, excessive clotting, and all of the end results of these conditions. These include hypertension and many diseases of the heart. Even in conventional medicine the viscosity of *blood* is a contributing condition in cancers.[116] Many patients are found to have higher fibrinogen levels, and higher platelet aggregation — what the Chinese call *blood stasis* syndrome. This occurs for many reasons, including:

• The aging process and loss of vitality from a sedentary lifestyle pattern;

- Chronic illnesses that lead to *blood stasis* and are left untreated after resolution of the illness;
- Unresolved emotional factors that drive decisions regarding diet and activity levels.

All of the above are saying the same thing. For reasons that are personal to each individual, the mind–body connection is injured by unresolved emotional content, and the resulting unconscious decisions made about lifestyle gradually and over time begin to translate into health conditions that can be promoting factors or precursors to serious illness either for ourselves or for our children. This occurs because, just as we no longer live as part of nature, we no longer live in our bodies except from the head up. What gets our attention is usually some sort of dysfunction, and the resulting symptoms are usually an indication that a long-term process has been in place. Following are some examples of how unresolved emotions can injure the *Qi* and blood according to Chinese medicine theory and contribute to cancer. These emotional and physiological connections can be utilized in reading any of the following chapters on specific cancers.

Lung function[117] can be damaged by continuous grieving and sorrow and, to some extent, any powerful emotion that is repressed. If this grieving and sadness is not expressed and resolved, one common way of compensating is shallow breathing. Deep and full breathing can lead to a discharge of emotional pain, crying, and the feeling of physical and psychic pain. To avoid this, the breath is controlled and suppressed, resulting in shallow breathing. Although this sounds very much like psychotherapeutic analysis, it is also a part of the science of Chinese medicine. This suppression of breathing leads to a lower level of blood oxygenation and contributes to the oppression and the stasis of *Qi* in the chest and then in the body overall.

Breathing involves the action of the diaphragm and this action, in concert with the energetic function of the *lungs*, moves *Qi* and normal fluids up and down in the chest and upper abdomen. The diaphragm is a *dynamic heat exchanger* in relation to the upper and *middle Jiao*. When it is functioning in a lesser capacity, the movement of *Qi* is less, the fluid dynamism in the chest is less, and the exchange or ventilation of heat across the middle and *upper Jiao* is diminished. The *lungs* are the canopy of the human body and act, metaphorically, like the world's rainforests. They cleanse the air, regulate temperature, hold and clean *water*, mist the *upper Jiao*, and form *Qi* and oxygen. Injuries due to emotional constraints create an environment that reduces immune function, contributes to internal heat, lowers fitness levels, changes how fluids are moved, disturbs sleep, and compounds other emotional issues. We could say that global warming has many of the same effects.

If the hydraulic pumping mechanism of the diaphragm is diminished, normal fluids and blood tend to accumulate in the chest. This accumulation leads to stasis, first of *Qi* and then of *blood* and potentially *phlegm*, which is really a form of body fluid that has coagulated. The *lung's* ability to irrigate the *upper Jiao* is intimately connected with breathing and with the *heat* exchange mechanism. Injury at this level leads to internal *heat* and also to static *phlegm*. *Blood stasis, pathogenic heat*, and *static phlegm* are the foundations for most cancer diagnoses, and this is one reason why smoking has been connected with many cancers and not only *lung cancer*. These manifestations of dysfunction also act as magnets for *toxic heat* and *latent pathogenic factors*, shortly to be described and explained.

The *liver*[118] also has a relationship to blood and *Qi stasis*.[119] Everyone has a dream for the precious life they have been given. You can remember the astonishment and joy you felt as a young child being in and discovering the world. However, whatever our beliefs regarding the meaning of life, life itself can have a way of stifling or frustrating our dreams, our being. When we cannot find a way of maintaining our path and cannot cope with these stifling events, the frustration and pent-up emotions can cause injury, especially when we are given no unconditional support to find our way as children. *Lung* and *liver constraints* can walk hand in hand. Smoking can be a way of coping. Smoking restrains the *lungs* and, via the five-phase *ko* cycle, also restrains an overactive and pent-up *liver*. *Liver Qi stasis* occurs for many reasons but all of them can result in *blood stasis*. In the case of breast cancers, the stasis of *Qi* affecting the *liver* can affect the *heart, stomach–spleen axis*, and *lungs*. All of these viscera are important in cancer pathogenesis because of their relationship with blood, with fluids, and with the *Wei Qi* and *Ying* and, therefore, immunity. Many conventional medical studies have shown that the stress of unresolved emotions and loss of relationships can lower immunity. Lowered immunity may not cause cancer but it does contribute to an environment in which cancers can occur more readily because lowered immunity is frequently caused by factors of deficiency and stasis that enable *latent pathogenic factors* to sink more deeply into the body and gain a hold that can smolder for years. A Western science equivalent of this injury is the fact that stress causes increased levels of cortisol (a stress hormone), and women with higher cortisol levels are at higher risk for breast cancer and for metastatic breast cancer. This smoldering is what causes *inverted fire poisons* and other forms of local inflammation that transform into malignancy. Unhappiness and lack of fulfillment are epidemic in the Western developed world. Unhappiness and lack of fulfillment are the true underlying "Western diseases".

The *spleen*[120] is one translation of the Chinese character "*pi.*" An alternate translation is the *pancreas*. The *spleen* function as described by Chinese medicine includes elements of digestion and absorption, including the stomach, pancreas, gallbladder, small intestine, and entire mucosal lining of the gastrointestinal tract. These functional units of the *spleen* are injured by constant worry and resulting obsessive/compulsive disorders. Many of us are poorly parented as children; we lack proper boundaries and unconditional love as children. Some of us are even abused emotionally or physically. The *spleen* orb of Chinese medicine has to do with the ability to parent ourselves as manifested with food, through relationship, through all forms of nurturance, and to find boundaries for all that life has to offer, to nourish ourselves healthily. The *spleen* is the center of the body and, in many ways, the center of the Earth. Issues in this realm can lead to manifestations as adults that prevent us from knowing how to parent ourselves. We choose improper relationships that are unhealthy; we do not know how to nourish our bodies; we do not know how to love ourselves without feeling that we are selfish, or we become narcissistic. These injuries can lead to disrupted eating habits like anorexia, bulimia, overeating, craving sweets, and high-fat diets, all of which are inappropriate ways to try and rebalance *spleen* function. At the supermarket the center isles are full of the expression of this imbalance. Why we shop in the center isles is emblematic of a latent and, to us, invisible cultural disease. In Chinese medicine, this is called *spleen* deficiency of some form and expresses a lack of proper boundaries around choices. When *spleen* function is weakened it leads to:

- *Blood deficiencies* that can affect the other organs and lead to stasis;
- *Damp* accumulations due to impaired metabolic function — like diabetes;
- Stasis arising out of deficiency and accumulations like tumors.

All of these are vicious circles feeding on themselves and one another as they make deeper and deeper tracks in the body. These tracks of injury then become mechanisms for cancer and magnets for carcinogenic influences. Emblematic of this injury is the epidemic of type II diabetes and resulting cardiovascular diseases which are linked to the modern cancer epidemic.

2. *Dampness and Phlegm Accumulations*[121]

There are many reasons why normal body fluids collect and become stagnant. Internally, organ deficiencies due to other illnesses or improper living habits, *Qi and blood disharmonies*, and failure of the transformative processes can all lead to *dampness and phlegm*. *Damp accumulations* can result in *phlegm* and *stasis* and then, under the right circumstances, masses and tumors that are magnets for *toxins*.[122] Dietary irregularity is considered one of the greater promoting factors of *dampness and phlegm*, and also of cancers. And dampness is considered a ground for *latent pathogenic factors*.[123] Just as in *blood stasis*, *phlegm stasis* is resolved by moving the *Qi*, and movement through exercise is a primary tool in remaining healthy. Exercise moves *blood*, transforms fluids, tonifies the *Qi*, discharges pent-up emotions, opens the pores causing sweating, which then discharges *heat* and *toxins*. Exercise and proper diet help to prevent *damp phlegm* conditions from evolving into serious illnesses. From a Chinese medicine perspective, *damp/phlegm* conditions are the underlying cause of many "Western diseases."

3. *Toxic Heat Pathogens, Latent Pathogenic Factors, and Fire Poisons*

This category of external exposures includes infectious agents like chronic viral infections or chemical exposures especially those chemicals that are fat-soluble and lipophilic and remain stored in fat tissue of humans and other animals and bioaccumulate over time. Heavy metals like arsenic, asbestos, nicotine derivatives and additives from smoking, food additives like certain red dyes and saccharin and nitrates, radiation from X-rays and other imaging techniques, and so on are all examples of *toxic pathogens*.

Many of these act like *fire poisons* that ultimately injure the *Yin* and fluids and lead to stasis at the *Qi*, fluid and *blood level*. When stasis is present for a long period of time, it can in itself lead to a *fire poison*. *Fire poisons* continually transform and can affect the DNA and cause mutation. This can happen as part of a long-term process, as in many solid tumors, or it can happen immediately, as in childhood leukemia. Although earlier classical texts, starting with the *Shang Han Lun* (247 CE) and evolving finally into the *Wen Bing Xue* (17th century), speak of *latent pathogens* as external influences, it seems logical to think of chemical exposures and perhaps even chronic viral infections as *latent pathogens* because of the way in which they act over time. In terms of chemicals, few were present for analysis before the 1940s. Since the 1940s over 100,000 new chemicals have been added to the world. Of these, about 35,000 are in everyday use. And of those, only 1500 have been studied in the US for human health effects. We are in effect part of a global uncontrolled study for these chemicals. Endocrine disruptors can cause developmental injuries *in utero* that evolve finally into cancers that manifest in the early 20s of offspring. Chronic viral infections like

HSV, HBV, HCV, EBV, and HPV can remain quiet until moments of immune stress or until a threshold is reached that brings them symptomatically to the surface. Because of these characteristics it seems accurate to call some chronic viral agents and many chemicals *latent pathogenic factors*. No one knows how the accumulation of these many hits in the human body can affect one.

Latent pathogens incur damage especially in the presence of *spleen dampness, Qi stasis,* and *Yin deficiency*. All of these are the bases for promoting factors. It is part of the spirit path of Chinese medicine in the modern world to view these impacts through the window of Chinese medicine in order to reach an understanding of how to resolve them.

4. *Organ Deficiencies*[124]

All of those injuries 1–3 undermine the gastrointestinal tube and the viscera. This continual assault and the onset of chronic disease as the result of aging take their toll. Improper dietary habits can lead to type II diabetes and this has been found to be a risk factor for many cancers. The *spleen–kidney–heart axis* is a major intersection in overall health and a major intersection for damage in adult onset diabetes. Injury to this axis affects blood circulation, fluid metabolism, and the *Source Qi*. Solid tumors tend to develop in those aged over 40 years and in those suffering from various permutations of *Qi* and *blood deficiency* with resulting *Qi* and *blood stasis* and *damp/phlegm*. Strong and healthy *Qi* within each organ and its functional orb is what causes the movement and transformation that we call health.

Many vicious circles turning on themselves and incorporating greater and deeper circles of pathology can cause serious, chronic, and life-threatening illness. When several factors come together with chronic exhaustion, the body's ability to circulate blood effectively and transform *Qi* can become injured.

It is when combinations of the above factors are present in one individual that the terrain — the damaged ecological environment — is present for a cancer to take place. Cancer is a transformation from a healthy cell to one in which regulatory functions no longer occur. It is the environment promoted by *dampness* and *phlegm* and *blood stasis* that provides the soil for a *toxin* to transform the body's efforts at normal function into a malignancy. From the perspective of Chinese medicine, it is not the DNA mutation that is the cause of cancer. It is the long-term and constant assault of combinations of the above four activities in an individual's life combined with a carcinogenic hit or hits that is the cause of cancer. The DNA mutation is the injury from these actions. The result is cancer.

The *San Jiao* and the *Source*

The *San Jiao* is an anatomical and functional paradigm of Chinese medicine that contains the pathways for injury in all of the above causative factors for cancer.[125] Although it is considered a *Yang* "organ" and of the *fire* element, it is ultimately primarily *Yin* and *Yang* by nature, and partially of the *water* phase in that it flows and contains many fluids that are lymphatic and hormonal and are ubiquitous throughout the body. It also theoretically contains activities that are *Yang* in nature that have to do with immunity, digestion and digestive fluids, *water* metabolism in all three burners, the *Ying* (immunogloulins) and the *Wei Qi*.[126] Therefore, it is valuable to study the *San Jiao* as a theoretical entity in this chapter. The Earth also is made up of a *San Jiao*, or triple burner. When referring to the Earth, it speaks to oceans, swamps, rivers, estuaries, rain, forests, soil, weather, temperature, nutrients, water, and transformative activities that keep the cycle of life going. Analogs for injuries to the *San Jiao* include ocean acidification, global climate change and warming, loss of the ozone layer, loss of species, loss of our human cousins (especially those who live in the Third World), global poverty, constant war, and loss of connection. The *San Jiao* in reference to the Earth is an expression of the Great Chain of Being. The *San Jiao* is the link that binds all of these systems on the Earth.

According to the *Su Wen* (Chapter 8), the *San Jiao* is considered one of the six *Yang* organs. The function of the *San Jiao* is referred to by the Chinese word "*tong*" which means enabling things to go through." It is also expressed by the word "*chu*" which is translated as excreting or letting out. "Tong" implies form. "*chu*" refers to function and is in relation to the *Wei Qi* in the *upper Jiao*, the *Ying Qi* in the *middle Jiao*, and the body fluids in the *lower Jiao*. In terms of the human body it refers to many of the modern analogs to be covered as part of this section: fascia, lymph, secretory organs of the endocrine system, neuropeptides, immunopeptides, and the rhythms that move these entities. When referring to the Earth, it speaks to oceans, swamps, estuaries, rain and arboreal forests, rivers and lakes, soils across the world, upper and lower atmosphere weather patterns and their relationship to mountains and deserts and the topography in general. It refers to the Earth's ability to transport nutrients from one place to another, and to its ability to repair itself. It refers to all of the Earth's ecosystems and their function.

According to the *Ling Shu* (Chapter 18), "The ability of the *Wei* and *Ying* (protective entities conventional science calls pertaining to immunity) to spread depends on the letting out function of the *San Jiao*. The *upper Jiao* lets out *Wei Qi* directing it to the *lung*; the *middle Jiao* lets out *Ying Qi*, directing it to all of the organs (especially digestive); and the *lower Jiao* lets out body fluids, directing them down to the *urinary bladder*." In many ways, the Taoist map of the universe is the map of the *San Jiao*, or triple burner.

The *Nan Jing*[127] (Chapter 66) states that the *San Jiao* has a name but no form. It also states that the *Source Qi* resides in the *moving Qi between the kidneys* and is spread to the five *Yin* and six *Yang* organs via the *San Jiao*. The *moving Qi between the kidneys* is the "gate of breathing," according to the *Nan Jing*. This means that the act of inhaling draws energy and movement into the abdomen especially the lower abdomen, where there is a space between the two *kidneys* — hence the *moving Qi between the kidneys* and the *San Jiao* may be the pathway for this movement of energy. It is a receptive conduit. In many of the yoga, meditation, and martial arts disciplines it is breathing into this gate or place that provides the grounding and energy for transformation because breath is at once Earthly and heavenly. The *San Jiao* is the ubiquitous formless ground that provides a medium for the movement of this transformation.

The *master of the heart* (*Ling Shu*, 71: 494),[128] the *heart wrapping* channel, the *pericardium channel*, functions energetically as a communication pathway for the *shen* (or spirit) between the *heart* and the *moving Qi between the kidneys*. It refers to grounding of the sacred within the foundation of the body at the place between the kidneys. The "*small heart*" referred to in the *Su Wen*[129] is *mingmen, fire within water* — the gate of light. The light is the sacred. It is from here that the *San Jiao* comes out — out of the place of sacredness within the human body. Although there is controversy about the *pericardium* and *San Jiao* internal/external relationship in the "*five phases*" theory, it is perhaps here in this relationship that the connection occurs. It is perhaps a place where spirit and substance meet, and it is a template for the mind/body or the sacred and physical world connection.

The energetic center of the body is the *Source*.[130] The *Source* is the *moving Qi between the kidneys*. The *Source* is the gate of breathing. "The organs, stems and branches, the phases are all ripples out from this energetic center." Shallow breathing, for whatever reason, weakens the *Source*. Physical imbalances affect the *Source*. Emotions affect bodily energetics, which in turn affect the *Source*. Dietary problems are manifested because of the close energetic link between the *Source* and the energies derived from food. And so there is a link between the *Source*, the *San Jiao*, and all of the causative factors for cancer.

The continuum that links the *Source* to all of the other energetic orbs in the body is the *San Jiao* along with the master of the *heart* — the *pericardium*. The magnetism of heaven *Qi* into an individual and the resulting creation of *shen* that protects the body is part of the physical act of breathing. On the macrocosmic Earthly level, breathing is the analog of climate. And on the microcosmic human level, breathing exercises are a part of many internal/external exercise regimens from perennial cultures that cultivate *Qi* and *shen* in an effort to bring larger forces into reality within the human being. No other scientific iteration speaks so elegantly of how the one becomes many; of how heaven enters the human body and makes us spiritual beings. And of how this connection is essential to health.[131]

Modern Analogs

In the *Ling Shu* and *Nan Jing*, the *gao* and *huang* were linked to *Source* theory and the *San Jiao*. The *gao* and *huang* refer to fatty, greasy tissues like ubiquitous fascia and connecting membranes. There are many modern references to the fascia, the ligaments, the lymph system (including the mesenterium and the cysterna chyli), the thymus gland, and other "netlike greasy membranes." Thus far, *San Jiao* connections have been made to the *Wei Qi* and *Ying Qi* — both elements of protection and immunity; to the *shen;* to the *jing* — (or inherited DNA); to the *Source Qi* — the primary basis of enlivenment in the human body; and the *moving Qi between the kidneys* — the gate of breath; to *mingmen* — the gate of brightness or light; and to several possible analogs in conventional science and anatomy. In a nutshell, this is the Chinese medicine essential theory of the Great Chain of Being. It explains, in a language that we are unfamiliar with, how the universe or heaven or the sacred makes life and enters into it on the physical plane.

The *San Jiao* and Osteopathy

In osteopathy the role of the fascia and connective integument is given a profound function.[132] The fascia is a slightly mobile continuous laminated sheath that extends through the entire length of the body. It wraps every organ and all of the somatic structures. "By some means, probably via the nervous system, this fascia system is normally kept in constant motion in correspondence with the cranio-sacral rhythmic motion."[133] There are several models as to how this motion and rhythm maintains itself, but most of them have to do with fluid hydrostatics.

Enervation of the fibrous collagen complex of the fascia is both sensory and motor. There is a ground substance present in the fascia that transports metabolic materials, probably both *Yin* and *Yang,* throughout the body. The fascia continuity from skull to toe has powerful effects on sympathetic nerve function. The fascia organ is a maze that allows travel from one end of the body to the other. Each visceral organ has carried its own fascia with it during embryonic development. All of these features share a commonality with the concepts, ancient and modern, of the *San Jiao*.

The *San Jiao* and Neuropharmacology

Starting in the mid-1980s, the modern discipline of neuropharmacology has begun to identify what are being called "informational substances." These substances include hormones, neurotransmitters, growth factors, gut peptides, interleukins, cytokines, and so on. Their commonality, in terms of function, relates to the fact that they are all messenger molecules distributing information throughout the organism. The common assumption about these informational substances is that they originate via signals in the brain. In truth, what is now known is that the brain, central and peripheral nervous system, endocrine system, and immune system are a whole-body continuum that is more than a feedback loop; it is a multidirectional communication system that is ubiquitous in the body and is part of a complex of chemical and electrical merging. In other words, information exchange happens not just as a hardwired linear nervous response but also as a dynamic interplay locally and distally, chemically and electrically, and rhythmically between many types of tissue simultaneously.[134] All of the ecosystems of the human body are in communication with one another via a climactic interlocutor that is multilinguistic.

One estimate is that less than 2% of neuronal communication actually occurs at the synapse. Peptides are the molecules of information receiving and sending information. Chemical information substances travel the extracellular fluids circulating throughout the body to reach their target receptors. These extracellular fluids are ubiquitous; the human body is 70%–80% water, just as the Earth itself is mainly water.

"Peptides serve to weave the body's organs and systems into a single web that reacts to both internal and external environmental changes with complex, subtly orchestrated responses. Peptides are the sheet music containing the notes, phrases, and rhythms that allow

the orchestra — your body — to play as an integrated entity."
(Candace Pert).

Interferons, peptides made by lymphocytes, have the job of fighting
off invading pathogens. Lymphocytes also secrete endorphin and
ACTH. These newer findings have also shown that neuropeptides are in
the immune system and immunopeptides are in the nervous system.
Many of these peptides mediate the inflammatory reactions caused by
injury, trauma, or an activated immune system. So it has turned out that
the immune system is capable of sending information to the brain and
of receiving information from the brain. This has shown that the brain,
endocrine, and immune systems communicate with all parts of the
body continuously and interactively, just as the *Wei Qi* and *Ying Qi* of
the *San Jiao* utilize its communication capacities to bring together all
aspects of life. Modern neuroscience has shown that the Great Chain
of Being exists within the ecology of our bodies and has come full circle in an unexpected way while linking modern findings based on linear thinking with the circular thinking of classical Chinese medicine.

Research done by Candice Pert and others in the mid-1980s
showed that small-cell lung cancer is not a cancer of the lung tissue
itself but rather an injury to macrophages that, year after year, had
gone to the lungs to clear debris from smoking.[135] In other words, the
cancer mutation was in the macrophages, a part of the immune system, rather than in the lung parenchyma. These findings from 1984
have never been followed up at the NCI or elsewhere, because they
were out of the mainstream regarding cancer etiology. No new conclusions have ever been drawn from these early studies. But it shows
that there is an injury prior to the injury to the lung parenchymal
tissue that is the causative factor for lung cancers. Chinese medicine
would go one step further and identify the cause of the injury to the
macrophages. Speculations by the authors of this research are that
perhaps the inappropriate production of neuropeptides released by
the immune system could promote other forms of cancer.[136] Perhaps
a cancer was part of a network receiving and sending information
that linked it to the brain and immune systems. The authors found in
future research that cancerous cells were attracted to or magnetized
by neuropeptide signals, an event called chemotaxis.

The conclusion of the researcher was, and continues to be many years later, that what was being described was a bodywide communication system, perhaps ancient in origin, that was in fact the entire body system sharing information across cellular barriers. This is the *San Jiao* as expressed many centuries ago by Chinese doctors seeking also to understand how life works.

Although this is an abbreviated rendition of this complex subject, I hope that it is enough from which to put forward a hypothesis regarding the classical *San Jiao* theory, the modern interpretations of the *San Jiao* including the lymphatic and connective tissue net surrounding bodily tissues, the linkages to *shen* and *Jing* and modern psychoneuroimmunology, plus understandings from osteopathy regarding the fascia network of the body, and Pert's research on informational substances and how and where they work in the body. Looking at these three systems of knowledge helps us to gain a deeper and more sophisticated view of cancer and its causes. It helps the discussion be less linear and microscopic. And it helps us to bring in a connection of spiritual meaning and science that is always lacking in discussions about how we got to where we are in regard to cancer. It is important to seek a broader discussion on cancer because cancer prevention happens only when we have a clear and deep understanding of what causes cancer, not just at the genetic level but in the ripples that surround and intertwine the smallest and largest physical entities.

The *San Jiao* and Cancer Etiology

The etiology of cancers according to Chinese medicine is complex and very important to understand in terms of both primary and secondary prevention. The impacts that unresolved emotions have on the energetic and physical functions of the body have been verified in conventional science through work with informational substances. The field of psychoneuroimmunology, which has continued to evolve out of this work, has identified ways in which unresolved emotions can be a causative factor in cancer etiology, especially as related to immunology and the communication pathways of growth factors, hormonal essences, interleukins, cytokines, and other peptides that regulate cell growth and apoptosis. It is possible to understand these peptide substances as connections between the immune system, *mingmen* (gate of light), and *shen* (spirit). These injuries are causative factors for cancer because when the sacred is lost from daily living, the spirit is also lost. And the result is immune deficiency as the life force declines within the individual. The ability to heal is diminished in the human and in the environment because they are one.

In osteopathy, the fascia is known to be a repository of embedded emotional memory that when treated can be discharged or released.[137] The *shen*, which has its roots in the *moving Qi between the kidneys* and is carried throughout the body via the *San Jiao*, is related to these injuries and this discussion. All of these particular scientific languages and ways of knowing (the word "science" comes from the Latin "scio" — "to know," and there are many ways of knowing) are talking about the same things based on the particular system's knowledge, language, and resultant interpretations.[138]

The fascia is ubiquitous, is in constant motion, and has a ground substance present that enables it to transport metabolic materials. Is this the material aspect of the *San Jiao*? The rhythm that moves this visible system is the cranial rhythm and is probably also a connection between the "gate of breath" and *shen* and *Jing*. The energetic and invisible aspect of the *San Jiao* may actually be the peptide informational substances that utilize the physical *San Jiao* as a means of transport throughout the body, carrying messages that are *Qi*, neural, electrical, endocrine, immune, emotional, and spiritual.

Another category of cancer pathogenesis stems from *spleen deficiencies* resulting from poor dietary habits or improper foods and from other injuries. These deficiencies result in *dampness* and *phlegm* accumulations, which act as magnets for either *latent pathogenic factors* or *toxic heat*.[139] These injuries also have a relationship to the *San Jiao* because of the close link between the *Source Qi* and energies derived from food via the *spleen* function. The *San Jiao* and the extracellular fluids are possibly part of the same system. "The *San Jiao* is the pathway of water and grain, and the place where *Qi* begins and ends. "The *San Jiao* is intimately connected with the *shen*, and often food choices are made based on emotional injuries and the comfort derived from fueling food addictions rather than on a rational or physiological process of actual functional necessity fueling the body. Comfort foods and entrenched ways of eating are those that become embedded in childhood and in the *spleen/San Jiao/shen* memory of the body. They are addictions and leave deep tracks that require a rewiring of our mental/emotional processes to unwind.[140]

The *latent pathogenic factor* theory of Chinese medicine is a category of pathogenesis that is easily explained by the example of colorectal cancer as given before. Another example is Burkitt's lymphoma in young children with chronic malarial infection. The chronic infection is an external pathogen that creates in time an immune deficiency that allows the Epstein–Barr virus to then take hold, resulting in a type of lymphoma. External pathogens can turn into *latent pathogenic factors* and, in the case of some cancers, it becomes difficult to know what to call these exposures. These exposures contact the *San Jiao* through injuries to the immune system, through injuries to water metabolism, through poor food quality or choices leading to *dampness* and *phlegm*, and are often driven by tracks of injury caused by unresolved emotional material or by public health issues that could be resolved but never are, especially in the developing world.

Toxic exposures like chemical carcinogens, ionizing radiation, food additives, cosmetics, chemicals, pesticides and herbicides, and so on lodge often in fat tissue, because they are often fat-soluble and lipophilic.[141] The greater omentum and other fatty reservoirs are sites of bioaccumulation for these fat-soluble chemicals. The fatty and greasy membranes of the *San Jiao* are target tissue for fat-soluble bioaccumulative *toxins* as well as *dampness and phlegm* accumulations from a poor diet. The personal and cultural psychic injuries — interior and exterior, modern and historical — of life may contribute to the lifestyle choices we make as individuals and as cultures. Many of these choices are embedded in the individual via the *San Jiao* and in the larger world via the loss of interconnectedness between mind, *heart*, shen, and *Jing*.

The connections of the *San Jiao* with *Jing*, the *Yuan Qi*, *mingmen*, and *shen* are profound. They impact the *heart–kidney* axis, the gate of heaven, and the *water* within *fire* that is the basis of life. They certainly must take a certain toll on these energetic relationships that stand individually and as part of the overall ecology of the *San Jiao*. And they are emblematic not only of human health issues but also of the resulting Earth health issues and vice versa. These connections are mapped out by Chinese medicine in the *Neijing Tu*, the classical image used on the cover of this book. It is a map of the human microcosm within the universal macrocosm of sacred life.

Some Conclusions

Cancer is a disease process that occurs usually over a period of time and may result from injury ultimately to the *San Jiao*, an ancient analog that is primarily fluid in nature. The type of solid tumor or hematologic cancer that occurs as a result of injury at this level depends on the arena where the weakest link is present; the injury to the *San Jiao* is magnetized and pulled in by the least functional organ. The ubiquitous nature of the *San Jiao* and the overall functions of the *San Jiao* make it a primary target for injury from dietary compromises, from immune deficiencies, from emotional injury that results in physical disease, from *latent pathogenic factors*, from aging and a decrease in *Jing, mingmen,* and the *Source Qi,* from inherited injuries to the *yuan Qi,* and from toxins over which the body currently has no means of surveillance.

The *San Jiao* may be an analog for water and the hydrology cycle of the Earth. It regulates temperature, forms climate, delivers nutrition, and is imprinted with the psychic and emotional injuries of those living within it. Prevention and treatment for all cancers must begin by rehabilitating the *San Jiao* and the ecology of life that enfolds all structures, energetic and physical, and by making whole again the connections of mind, soul, heart, spirit, and *Source*.

References

1. www.propublica.org/article/injection-wells-the-poison-beneath-us
2. www.pe.com/local-news/breaking-news-headlines/2012718-region-study-finds-hig-groundwater-contamination.ece

3. www.thetimes-tribune.com/news/dep-inspections-show-more-shale-well-cement-problems-1.1205108#%23axzz1ykbprxri

4. www.pe.com/localnews/stories/PE_news_local_D_perch15.41692e6.html

5. www.un.org/en/africarenewal/agreport/keyreps.htm

6. www.nationalgeographic.com/xpeditions/guides/physicalafricaguide.pdf

7. www.palnetearth.nerc.ac.uk/news/story.aspx?id=330&cookie-consent=A

8. Drauker S. WRI 2010 Organizational Greenhouse Gas Inventory.

9. www.globalchange.4mich.edu/globalchange2/current/lectures/deforest/deforest.html

10. www.earthpolicy.org">earthpolicyinsititue.planb3.0

11. www.articles.timesofindia.indiatimes.com/2009-07-08/India/28195425_1_drought

12. www.internationalrivers.org/big-dams-bringing-poverty-not-power-to-africa

13. Glossary of International Statistics, Studies in Methods, Series F, No. 67, United Nations, New York, 1997.

14. www.hks.harvard.edu/fs/rstavins/papers/aer_final_version_stavins_feb_2011.pdf

15. www.rinpoche.com/teachings/bnwisdom.pdf

16. Article 1, International Covenant of Civil and Political Rights (ICCPR), United Nations Covenant

17. Article 1, International Covenant on Economic, Social and Cultural Rights (ICESCA), United Nations Covenant.

18. Richardson B. (2009) *Indigenous Peoples and the Law: Comparative and Critical Perspectives.* Hart Publishing

19. www.holocausetcontroversies.blogspot.com/2009/12/denial-of-herepo-genocide.html

20. Lindvquist S. (1992) *Exterminate All the Brutes.* The New Press, New York, pp. 150–152.

21. Adèyanju CT. (2011) Colonialism and contemporary African migration: a phenomenological approach. *Black Stud.* **42(6)**: 943–967.

23. Benabed T. (2009) An indigenous holistic approach to colonial trauma and its healing. *Literary Paritantra.* 1 [1 & 2 Basant (Spring)]: 88–91.

24. Weenie A. (2000) post-colonial recovering and healing. www.jan.ucc. nau.edu/~jar/lib/lib6.html

25. Vulnerability of North African countries to climate changes. www.lisd. org/cckw/pdf/north_africa.pdf

26. Climate change and Africa: stormy weather ahead.

27. Climate and water. www.nature.com/nature/climate

28. Larre C, Rochat E. (1998) *Heart Master and Triple Heater*. Monkey.

29. Marine and Coastal Ecosystems and Human Well-being. UNEP — Division of Early Warning and Assessment. UN Environment Programs, 2006.

30. Hirsch T. (2003) Katrina damage blamed on wetlands loss. *BBC News*, Nov. 1. www.news.bbc.co.uk/2/hi/Americas/4393852.stm

31. Gulf Restoration Network. Wetlands. www.healthygulf,org/our-work/ wetlands/wetland-loss

32. Wilbur K. (2000) *A Brief History of Everything*. Shambhala.

33. Pauly D *et al.* (1998) Fishing down marine food webs. *Science*, Feb. 6, pp. 860–863.

34. Oceans without fish (1998). *Rachel's Environment and Health Weekly,* Feb. 26, 1998.

35. United Nations Environment Program. www.MAweb.org.UNEP.2006

36. Bogo J. (2000) *Brain Food*. E. Jul./Aug. p. 42.

37. The facts of fishing. *New Internationalist,* Jul. 2000.

38. Puget Sound vital signs. www.psp.wa.gov/vitalsigns/orcas.php

39. Brown L. (1996) Facing reality at the World Food Summit. Worldwatch Press release, Nov. 1.

40. UN Food and Agriculture Organization, 1997.

41. *10 Salts and Trace Elements. Soil and Water Quality: An Agenda for Agriculture.* The National Academies Press, 1993. www.nap.edu/ openbook.php?record_id=2132&page=361

42. www.agronomy.org/publications/aj/pdfs/100/3/471

43. www.cdfa.ca.gov/agvision/docs/soil_salinization.pdf

44. www.ucsusa.org/gulf.gcplacesmis.html

45. Minnesota Pollution Control Agency 2011 study. www.olsonpr.com/ white-papers/the-minnesota-river-and-drainage-tile/

46. www.treehugger.com/corporate-respnosibility/shocker-worlds-dirtiest- coastal-ecosystem

47. www.serc.carleton.edu/microbelife/topics.deadzone/index.html

48. www.news.cornell.edu/stories/march06/soil.erosion.threat.ssl.html

49. www.ipm.iastate.edu/ipm/icm/2000/7-24-2000/erosion.html

50. Smith FB. Corn-based ethanol: a case study in the law of unintended consequences. Competitive Enterprise Institute. www.cei.org/pdf/5976.pdf

51. www.rodale.com/roundup-weed-killer-0

52. Into the mouths of babes: health effects of atrazine. www.ewg.org/node/25735

53. www.docs.nrdc.org/health/files/hea_07091201b.pdf

54. Sass JB, Colangelo A. (2006) European Union bans atrazine, while the United States negotiates continued use. *Int J Occup Environ Health* **12(3)**: 260–267.

55. Environment and health fund. www.ehf.orgil/en/material/pesticides

56. Global honey bee colony disorders and other threats to insect pollinators. www.unep.org/dewa/portals/67/pdf/global_bee_colony_disorder_and_threats_insect_polinators.pdf

57. Davis D. Soil depletion and nutrition loss. *J Am Coll Nutr.* www.scientificamerican.com/article.cfm?id=Soil-depletion-and-nutrition-loss

58. Bourn D, Prescott JA. (2002) A comparison of the nutritional value sensory qualities and food safety of organically and conventionally produced foods. *Food Sci Nutr.* **42(1)**: 1–34.

59. Dangour AD *et al.* (2009) Nutritional quality of organic foods: a systematic review. *Am J Clin Nutr.* **90**: 680–685.

60. Stracke. BA. *et al.* (2009) Three-year comparison of the polyphenol contents and antioxidant capacities in organically and conventionally produced apples (*Malus domestica* dark. cultivar "golden delicious"). Agri Food Chem. **57**: 4598–4605.

61. www.ewg.org/release/organic-produce-reduces-exposure-pesticides-research-confirms

62. Study sheds new light on organic fruit and vegetables. PhysOrg.com, May 27, 2011.

Plant Sciences. Critical Reviews. From Newcastle University. School of Agriculture, Food and Rural Development review of all published research on secondary metabolites and vitamin C in fruits and vegetables produced using organic versus conventional methods.

63. Zahn SH, Blair A. (1992) Pesticides and non-Hodgkin's lymphoma. *Canc Res* **52(19 Suppl)**: 5485–5488.

64. Altieri M. (2002) *The Ecological Impacts of Industrial Farming.* From Fatal Harvest. Island Press. The Foundations for Deep Ecology, pp. 197–202.

65. World Resources Institute. Eutrophication and hypoxia. www.wri.org/ project/eutrophication/about/sources

66. Marshall P. (2002) *Tilth and Technology: The Industrial Redesign of Our Nation's Soils.* From Fatal Harvest. Island Press, pp. 221–228.

67. Fava F, Bertin L. (1999) Use of exogenous specialized bacteria in the biological detoxification of a dump site — polychlorobiphenyl-contaminated soil in slurrly ptase conditions. *Biotechnol Bioeng.* **64(2)**: 240–249.

68. Snedeker SM. (2001) Pesticides and breast cancer risk: a review of DDT, DDE, and dieldrin. *Environ Health Perspect,* **109(Suppl 1)**: 35–47.

69. Kellogg R, Nehring R, *et al.* Environmental indicators of pesticides leaching and run-off from farm fields. USDA. Natural Resources Conservation Service. www.nrcs.usda.gov/wps/portal/nrcs/detail/ national/technical/nta/rca/&cid=nrcs143_0

70. National Water Quality Inventory Report to Congress. www.water.epa. gov/lawsregs/guidance/cwa/305b/98report_index.cfm

71. Soils policy: resources conservation, land and greenhouse gas reductions. www.epa.gov/oswer/international/factsheets/201002_resource_ conservation_land_and

72. Horowitz J, Gottlieb J. (2010). The role of agriculture in reducing greenhouse gas emissions. Economic Brief No. (EB-15) Sep., p. 8. www.ers.usda.gov/publications/eb-economic-brief/eb15.aspx

73. Sayed El-Sayed, Dijken G. The southeastern Mediterranean ecosystem revisited: thirty years after the construction of the Aswan Dam. www. ocean.tamm.edu/quaretrdeck/qd3.1/elsayed/elsayed.html

74. Charles D. Here's where farms are sucking the planet dry. www.npr. org/blogs/thesalt/2012/08/08/158417396/heres-where-farms-are-sucking-planet-dry

75. Groundwater depletion. USGS. www.ga.water.usgs.gov/edu/gwdepletion.html

76. Smeets PN *et al*. The Dutch secret: how to provide safe drinking water without chlorine in the Netherlands. www.drink-water-eng-sci. net/2/1/2009/dwes-2-1-2009.

77. Murray, GE. *et al*. (1984) Effect of chlorination on antibiotic resistance profiles of sewage-related bacteria. *Appl Environ Microbiol* **48(1)**: 73–77.

78. Goetz G. Drug-resistant staph linked to animal antibiotics. *Food Safety News*. www.foodsafetynews.com/2012/02/drug-resistant-staph-linked-to-animal-antibiotics

79. Ackerman S, Gonzalez R. (2012) The contect of antibiotic overuse. *Ann Intern Med*. **157(3)**.

80. Chlorine's adverse health risks. Triangular Wave Technologies. www. triangularwave.com/f9.htm

81. Hydrogen peroxide: a real treat for well-water. Essential Water Solutions. www.essentialwatersolutions.net/support-information/ hydrogen-peroxide-a ....

82. SDWA. Safe Drinking Water Act. www.water.epa.gov/lawsregs/rules-regs/adwa/index.cfm

83. Sohn E. (2009) Plastic water bottles may pose health hazard. *Discovery News*, Apr. 28. www.dsc.discovery.om/news/2009/4/28/water-bottles-health.html

84. Diamanti-Kandarski E. *et al*. (2009) Endocrine-disrupting chemicals: an Endocrine Society scientific statement. *Endocr Rev* **30(4)**: 293–342.

85. Wastes-resource conservation — common wastes and materials. Plastics. www.epa.gov/osw/conserve/materials/plastics.htm

86. Huang K. (2011) www.plasticnews.com/headlines2.html?id=23708

87. Green living. Plastic water bottles. www.greenliving.nationalgeo-graphic.com/plastic-water-bottles

88. Coates C. (1996) *Living Energies (The Work of Viktor Schauberger)*. Gateway.

89. Kornfield J. (1989) *Living Buddhist Masters*. Wisdom.

90. TAREB. Energy in the urban environment. www.new-learn.info/pack-ages/tareb/docs/special/urbenvir.pdf

91. OECD Proceedings: Towards sustainable transportation. www.oecd. org/dataoecd/28/54/2396815.pdf

92. *State of the World 1984 Through 2006.* Other Norton/Worldwatch Books. WW Norton and Company. New York, London, 2007. www.worldwatch.org

93. Climate patterns in *south-east USA.* Alabama Cooperative Extension System. www.aces.edu/climate/variability/se-us-pattern.php

94. Benefits and uses of urban forests and trees. www.ncsu.edu/biosucceed/biomass/pdf/trees-biosucceed.pdf

95. Berger K. As it grows up Seattle boughs down. Crooscut. crosscut.com/2007/11/24/mossback/9363/as-grows-up-seattle-boughs-down

96. Zereini F, Wiseman C. (2010) Urban airborne particulate matter: origin, chemistry, fate and health impacts. Environmental Science and Engineering/Environment Science, Nov 25.

97. Rakoff-Nahoum S. (2006) Why cancer and inflammation? *Yale J Biol Med* **79(3–4)**: 123–130.

98. *Yi Jing.* Hexagram 2. *Chung Fu*/Inner Truth. *I Ching,* or *Book of Changes.* Bollingen Foundation Inc., New York. Princeton University Press. 1st ed. 1950.

99. Huise DA. (2000) *The Eastern Mysteries: An Encyclopedic Guide to the Sacred Languages.* Llewellyn Worldwide.

100. *Yi Jing.* Hexagram 2. *Kun*/The Receptive. *Op. cit.* #98.

101. Harding S. Modernity, science, and democracy. UCLA. www.zemargraphics.com/biopolitics_web/NASSPWOR.pdf

102. *Sushruta Samhita. Encyclopedia of Medicine.* Author Kaviraj Kunja Lai Bhisgratha; self-published, 1916. Atharvaveda.

103. Macciocia G. (1989) *Foundations of Chinese Medicine.* Churchill Livingstone.

104. Travis J. (2005) *Wounded Hearts: Masculinity, Law, and Literature in American Culture.* The University of North Carolina Press.

105. Miller A. (1983) *For Your Own Good.* Farrar Straus Giroux.

106. Larre C, Rochat, E. (1996) *The Seven Emotions. Psychology and Health in Ancient China.* Monkey

107. Caine G *et al.* (2002) The hypercoagulable state of malignancy: pathogenesis and current debates. *Neoplasia.* **4(6)**: 465–473.

108. Rakoff-Nahoum S. (2008) Why cancer and inflammation? *Yale J Biol Med* **79(3–4)**: 123–130.

109. Lam YC *et al.* (2009) Cancer patients attitudes towards chinese medicine: a Hong Kong survey. *Chin Med* **4**: 25.

110. EKAT Appendix 2011. Structured abstracts describing RCTs. www. JSOM.orgp/medical/ebm/erc/index.html
111. Cassileth B *et al.* (2001) Alternative medicine use worldwide: the International Union Against Cancer Survey. *Cancer* **91**: 1390–1393.
112. TCMLARS. Traditional Chinese Medical Literature Analysis and Retrieval System. www.cintcm.com/e_cintcm.version.htm
113. Lieberman A. The role of biodetoxification in overcoming illness. Center for Occupational and Environmental Medicine. Programs and Treatment Modalities. www.coem.com/programstreatment_chemical-toxicity_wearepolluted.shtml
114. Wang QR. (1998) *Yi Lin Gao* ("Essentials of Clinical Pattern Identification of Tumors"), 2nd ed. People's Medical Publishing House, Bejing.
116. Henshaw EC. (1993) The biology of cancer. In: Rubin P. (ed.), *Clinical Oncology*, 7th ed. WB Saunders, Philadelphia 26.
117. Larre C. (1996) *Lungs.* Monkey.
118. Larre C. (1989) *The Liver.* Institut Ricci, Paris.
119. Jarrett L. (1998) *Nourishing Destiny.* Spirit Path. pp. 279–290.
120. Shou ZY, Jian YL. (2004) *Treatise on the Spleen and Stomach.* A translation of *Pi Wei Lun.* Blue Poppy.
121. Clavey S. (1995) *Fluid Physiology and Pathology in Traditional Chinese Medicine.* Churchill Livingstone. London: pp. 167–168, 232–236.
122. Crouther M *et al.* (2001) Dual role of macrophages in tumor growth and angiogenesis. *J Immunol.* **130**: 800–807, 121.
123. Qin BW. Lurking pathogens. Translated by Blalock J. www.chinese-medicinedoc.com/misc.-chinese-medicine-articles/lurking-pathogens
124. Zhang JY. (1959) *Jing Yue Yuan Shu* ("The Complete Works of Jing Yue"), 1624 C.E. Shanghai Science and Technology Press.
125. Larre C, Rochat E. (1992) *Heart Master and Triple Heater.* Monkey.
126. Birch S, Matsumoto K. (1988) *Hara Diagnosis: Reflections on the Sea.* Chap. 7. Paradigm.
127. Unschuld P. (2006) *Medicine in China*: Nan-Ching, *Classic of Difficult Issues.* Paradigm.
128. Wu JN. (2002) *Ling Shu*, the Spiritual Pivot. University of Hawaii Press.
129. Unschuld P. (2003) *Huang Di Nei Jing Su Wen.* University of California Press.
130. *Op. cit.* #126. Chap. 6.

131. Hua YL. (1998) *Cultivating the Energy of Life (Hui Ming Ching)*. Shambhala.

132. Upledger J, Vredevorgd J. (1983) *Craniosacral Therapy,* Chap. 1. Eastland.

133. Neuropsychopharmacology. www.nature/npp/index.html

134. Pert C. (1997) *Molecules of Emotion,* Chap. 7. Scribner.

135. Ruff M, Pert C. (1984) Small cell carcinoma of the lung: macrophage-specific antigens suggest hemopoietic stem cell origin. *Science* **225**: 1034–1036.

136. Ruff M, Pert C. (1986) Neuropeptides are chemoattractants for human monocytes and tumor cells: a basis for mind–body communication. In: *Enkalphins and Endorphins: Stress and the Immune System.* Plotnikoff W *et al.* (eds.), Plenum, *New York.*

137. Upledger J. (1990) *Somato-emotional Release and Beyond.* UI.

138. Thondup T. (1996) *The Healing Power of Mind: Simple Meditation Exercises for Health, Well-Being and Enlightenment.* Shambhala, Boston.

139. Liu GH. (2003) *Warm Pathogen Diseases: A Clinical Guide.* Eastland.

140. Gibson F. (2006) Emotional influences on food choice: sensory, physiological and psychological pathways. *Physiol Behav* **89(1)**: 53–61.

141. Disposition of chemical compounds. www.calstatela.edu/faculty/mohen/432/disposition%20of%20chemicals.ppt

CHAPTER 2

Air — Lung Cancer

> The lesser physician treats and protects the physical form while the superior physician protects and treats the spirit.
>
> — *from the Ling Shu: Jiu Shen Shi Er Yuan*

Introduction

Epidemiology and History

Currently there are only two cancers whose incidence is decreasing in the United States: lung and cervical.[1] Cervical cancer incidence has been steadily decreasing in the developed world because of the PAP smear, which finds preinvasive CINs (cervical intraepithelial neoplasms), allowing very early interventions.[2] In the developing world, where there are limited public health delivery systems, cervical cancer is a major health problem and is ranked third in mortality for women.[3] Lung cancer incidence has decreased in the US because a grassroots-driven governmental attack on smoking, smoking in public places, and advertising targeting young people has lowered the number of people who smoke. However, lung cancer continues to kill more people than all other cancers combined worldwide.[4] The number of people who die from smoking-related deaths other than cancer compounds this data. In other parts of the world the rates of lung cancer are increasing. In fact, American tobacco growers now export a large portion of their crop to Asia and Southeast Asia.[5]

The main risk factor for lung cancer is smoking. Tobacco use is considered a risk factor for many other cancers, including esophageal, stomach, pancreatic, cervical, mouth, bladder, ureter, renal, laryngeal and pharyngeal cancers, and leukemia.[6] Smoking-related diseases are reversible much more rapidly after quitting smoking,[7] and cardiovascular disease (a smoking-related disease) in the developed world remains the main killing disease, with cancer running a close second.

There are several historical pieces of information that are important to take into account regarding the smoking of tobacco:

- The tobacco industry worked to develop a product that was more addictive than the natural form of tobacco while concurrently denying that tobacco is addictive.[8]
- The tobacco industry has done its own research on second-hand smoke and this research states that second-hand smoke is not a risk factor for lung cancer.[9,10]
- At the same time, many other researchers have shown that second-hand smoke is a risk for lung cancer; in fact, people who do not smoke and live with smokers have a 30% increased risk of lung cancer.[11]
- At the present time, after a period of decline the use of tobacco is rising in American youth.[12]

These historical facts would seem to indicate that the tobacco industry is dedicated to its own survival rather than that of its consumers. Because lung cancer can take 20–40 years to actually become symptomatic, be diagnosed, and kill someone, the industry itself has steadily refused to admit, starting in the 1950s, that the smoking of tobacco is an addictive and continuously carcinogenic event.[13] And it is convenient that addicts of tobacco can live 20–40 years before they die from the effects of the addiction. Tobacco is a perfect product.

It is important for the tobacco industry to have an ongoing pool of new smokers who become hooked for life. Hence, advertising aimed at children is an important part of getting young people addicted before they are wise enough to make better, life-affirming decisions about their own health and lifestyle. Children get hooked because they believe that smoking makes them adult and cool; Joe Camel, like a street thug and dealer, is the messenger of coolness. Manipulative advertising in the tobacco industry taps into youth themes and cutting-edge antisocial themes that drive inner city youth and suburban wannabes.[14]

Given that tobacco smoking is addictive, carcinogenic, and creates so many other health problems, costing us tremendous amounts of health care dollars, it is amazing that it is still a legal substance.[15] The history of the lobby to keep tobacco legal is long and complex but one can be assured that it is not coming from the public. It is coming from the industry and with a tremendous amount of money behind it. It remains emblematic of the overall problem of tobacco that conventional medicine does not lobby against tobacco, thus demonstrating its own addiction to treatment and not to prevention.

On the other side of the coin, some people who have smoked all of their lives are never diagnosed with lung cancer. We should be studying these people. What do they have that others do not? And why do people who have never smoked or even lived with those who do smoke die from this disease? It remains true that 10%–15% of people diagnosed with lung cancer have never smoked or shared any other currently known risk factors for lung cancer.[16,17] Beverly Sills, the Metropolitan opera diva with *lungs* the size of the Amazon forest, is an example of someone who died of lung cancer but never smoked in her their life or lived with anyone who did.

The Medium is the Messenger — Air Pollution

Like water, air is a medium. When seen through slanting light the amount of visible particles in the air makes it look like a soup through which we swim upright. This soup is now more and more contaminated with gaseous and particulate matter that causes harm to the lungs.[18,19] New research has found that the tiniest pollutants in air disrupt basic cellular functions.[20] Currently, environmental regulations try to limit particles that are 10 microns in diameter and smaller particles in the 2.5-micron range.[21] But the particles that caused the most damage in the new study are one-tenth of a micron.[22] All combustion processes release particles less than 0.1 micron. These tiny particles float in the air longer, travel farther, and are more easily inhaled than larger ones. Some are more problematic than others but the obvious truth is that the lungs are truly the "delicate organ" and cannot survive unharmed without clean pure air.

The researchers found that 0.1-micron particles accumulated inside cell structures of the deep tissue of the lungs and of macrophages.[24] The mitochondria of these cells were damaged, causing the cells to stop producing ATP, the fuel that drives cellular function, and to start producing other chemicals that lead to inflammation and cell damage. Since macrophages are part of immune surveillance, and the mitochondria drive cellular fuel, it would seem that this damage contributes to lowered surveillance and concurrent lung pathologies that are *Qi-deficient* in nature and may include injuries to the *San Jiao*. I refer you back to the previous chapter.

The World Health Organization estimates that 4.6 million people die each year from causes attributable to air pollution.[25] Worldwide, more deaths occur as a result of air pollution than automobile accidents. In 2005, 310,000 Europeans died from diseases directly caused by air pollution.[25] The direct causes include asthma, bronchitis, emphysema, lung and heart disease, and respiratory allergies. People with diabetes, heart failure, chronic obstructive pulmonary disease (COPD), and inflammatory diseases like rheumatoid arthritis (RA) are at increased risk of death when exposed to particulate air pollution for one or more years.[25]

Examples

Ground level ozone pollution is now a burgeoning health issue, made especially worse by climate change and warming at ground level. It is primarily a result of vehicle exhaust and the combustion of fuels to produce energy, as in coal burning to produce electricity. It is created when sunlight and heat react with various chemicals found in air pollution. Volatile organic compounds (VOCs) and nitrogen oxides form ozone in the presence of heat and sunlight.[26] Ground level ozone and microscopic particulates, small enough to be breathed into the lungs and sticky enough to attract pollen and other allergens, contribute to asthma and allergy attacks, and other chronic lung conditions like COPD and emphysema. The lung function is measurably decreased. And sometimes the symptoms of injury from ground-level ozone exposure occur several days or even a week after the time of initial exposure.[27]

Indoor pollution also contributes to the toxic soup in which we walk. *Formaldehyde* is a major indoor polluter. Worldwide, 46 billion pounds of formaldehyde were produced in 2004.[28] It is used as a preservative, in embalming fluid, as a sterilizer, as part of foam insulation, as an adhesive in plywood and particleboard, and in textile treatment. It is listed as a carcinogen and is known to cause nasal, lung and brain cancer and some forms of leukemia. Formaldehyde is often found in carpeting, textile materials used in furniture, and in other household items that off-breathe formaldehyde gas into the air of our homes.

Indoor pollution enters our homes in the form of many household products, like paints, varnishes, waxes, aerosols, paint strippers, adhesive removers, rugs and furniture, dry cleaning fluids on newly dry-cleaned clothes, insecticides, termiticides, rodenticides, fungicides, and disinfectants. The Environmental Protection Agency (EPA) found that levels of about a dozen common organic pollutants were 2–5 times higher inside homes than outside regardless of whether the home was in a rural or urban setting.[29] Indoor pollution floats in or is tracked in, where it then accumulates, or it originates in the building itself because of products and building materials that contribute negatively to indoor air quality by off-breathing continuously in place.

Methylene chloride[30] is used in paint strippers, adhesive removers, and aerosol spray paints. It is a known carcinogen and converts to carbon monoxide when metabolized in the human body. *Benzene*[31] is found in tobacco smoke, stored fuels and paint supplies, and in auto emissions in closed garages. It is a known carcinogen and a primary cause of leukemia. *Perchlorethylene*[32] emissions off-breathe from newly dry-cleaned materials and from dry-cleaning facilities, some of which do not have adequate facilities to collect this organic gas. It is a known carcinogen.

We are now aware that the rates of lung-related diseases suffered by the first responders to the World Trade Center catastrophe and those who worked afterward to clean up the 10 storyhigh pile of rubble inhaled a gaseous soup of all of these problematic chemicals. The result has been that those responders have suffered many lung and upper respiratory diseases and a 19% higher incidence of cancers.[33] The respiratory diseases are covered by medical insurance. But because the cancer industry remains devoted to evidence-based medicine and cannot use common sense, those responders who have been diagnosed with cancer, many of whom are now dead, have not been covered by medical insurance. They had to pay for their own health care after the worst exposure in current history. Admitting that these exposures have negative human health effects would change the way we live. Research on cancer causation, even when obvious, is a major area of concern in the developed world and is emblematic of the way in which modern science has missed the boat because it is unable to connect the dots in its devotion to reductionism.

There are alternatives to this list of carcinogens. They range from dry-cleaners that do not use perchlorethylene, to paints that do not off-breathe toxics, to solvents that remove paint without being toxic, to integrated pest management (IPM), to natural materials in home building and furnishing. They require some research in your local area or on the Internet but alternatives are becoming more and more available as people learn about the health impacts of these chemical exposures in the home. It is the consumer that is driving the change in the marketplace. Become a smart and knowledgeable consumer of products for your home. And since labeling is unregulated, learn the truth about what the labels say or do not say.

Pesticides also contribute to indoor pollution. The EPA says that 80% of most people's exposure to pesticides occurs indoors.[34] The amount of pesticides in homes appears not to be associated with recent use of that contaminant. Therefore, contaminated soil and dust is generally tracked in on shoes and left in rugs and on surfaces. Easily cleaned surfaces are a good remedy for this unavoidable exposure. For example, wood floors that can be mopped weekly with water and vinegar offer no surfaces for pesticide chemicals to accumulate. Area rugs that can be removed and cleaned once a year offer an esthetic choice. Removal of shoes upon entering your home leaves the problem at the door. Talk to your neighbors about the choices that are now available to replace harmful household and garden products.

Anything with "cide" at the end of its name means "to kill." Insecticides, termiticides (termites), rodenticides (rodents), fungicides (molds and spores), and disinfectants (microbes) come in various delivery mechanisms, like sprays, liquids, sticks, powders, crystals, balls, and foggers. Not only are the active ingredients in these products harmful (if they kill bugs, they can harm us) but the inert ingredients can also be. The National Pesticide Information Center (NPIC) offers information on all known pesticides.[35]

It is important to remember that a large number of these organic chemicals are carcinogens in either animals or humans. Some have never been studied for human health effects or environmental impacts. In general, the precautionary principle that exists in Europe[36,37] regarding chemicals and their use does not exist here in the US. We cannot rely on our government to protect us from these chemicals, and it is naive to think that it will happen unless we make it so. On average, the FDA acts only when there are claims of injury. There is no process by which new chemicals must be proven to be safe unless their use is in medicine. Our primary medical insurance remains prevention of exposure to these products through knowledge and actions that require our government — federal and state and local — to oversee old and new chemicals being used in every facet of living.

There are many alternatives to using chemicals in pest control. Often, the safest and most effective solution is the simplest and least expensive intervention. Using soap and water to reduce aphid infestations instead of pesticidal chemicals, and watering in the morning to reduce powdery mildew instead of using a fungicide are both examples of very inexpensive interventions in the garden. The amount of information available regarding safer solutions to home and garden pests is stunning. A list of resources is available to gain information about your questions and includes an extensive appendix devoted to categories of issues covered in this book.

Asbestos is a mineral fiber used in building construction materials for insulation and as a fire retardant. Several asbestos products have been banned but some are not, and manufacturers have been given leave to voluntarily limit the use of asbestos.[38] Asbestos is found in older homes and in homes built even up to 1978. It is in pipe and furnace insulation materials, asbestos shingles, millboard, textured paints, and floor tiles. Asbestos causes lung cancer, mesothelioma (a cancer of the pleura of the lungs and abdominal linings), and asbestosis.[39] Removal or moving of asbestos should be done by licensed removal experts. The tiny particles of asbestos lodge in the lungs and cannot be removed. One exposure to asbestos is all it takes to cause death, albeit a long and slow death. Asbestos is considered one of the most toxic of health hazards in older homes. Spritzing an asbestos-containing product with water before removal does not guarantee safety.

When building a new home make sure that the ventilation rate is at least 0.35 ach (air changes per hour).[41] Some houses built today are so tight in construction that they actually increase indoor air pollution. If your new house is being built on a concrete slab, make sure that a vapor barrier is used to reduce the growth of molds from the ground to and through the concrete slab.[40] These molds can then enter the house and contaminate the air quality. When using carpet buy natural fiber carpets like wool. Many carpeting products, especially wall-to-wall carpeting, are made with formaldehyde, which then off-breathes into your home. Rugs and other textiles are also treated with PBDEs as a fire retardant.[42] In some states PBDEs are now banned. Many insulation products, especially expanding foam insulations, off-breathe formaldehyde and other toxic chemicals.[43] Choose building materials and furnishings that will not contribute to indoor air pollution. Do not rely on the builder to supply you with a house that is safe.

That new car smell is not perfume and can be toxic. Seats, armrests, carpets, and dashboards shed dangerous chemicals.[44] Not only are we breathing in toxic chemicals but we are also in close contact with them through our skin. The film that collects on the interior glass of new cars is actually formed from toxic gases that off-breathe and collect all over the interior of the car. The plastics used in automobile interiors contain aldehydes, esters, ketones, acetonitrile, decanol, formaldehyde, naphthalene, carbon disulfide, PBDEs, and phthalates.[45] In fact, the level of PBDEs is significantly higher in autos than in homes. Higher temperatures and UV exposure, things that happen inside closed cars parked in the hot summer sun, can cause PBDE flame retardants to become even more dangerous.

The European Union passed legislation in 2003 requiring the phase-out of PBDEs.[46] The Ecology Center, a membership-based non-profit environmental organization based in Ann Arbor, Michigan, says that manufacturers should phase out the use of PBDEs, and phthalates in auto material parts. They also suggest that the government provide phase-out guidelines. Currently, nine states have passed laws banning two forms of PBDEs, with six more in line to come on board (as of 2008).[47] Vehicle occupants should minimize health risks by using solar reflectors, parking out of the sun, ventilating the interiors of cars with non-recirculating air conditioning, and researching their potential new automobile for these contaminants. When manufacturers become aware that the consumer does not want to buy a new car that contains and exposes them to contaminants, they will change their practices.

These are only some examples of how air pollution contributes to lung injury. It is important to remember that the *lung* in Chinese medicine theory includes the skin. The pores of the skin are "regulated" by the *lung*, and *toxins* absorbed through the skin damage the *lung*. Since it is our largest organ, the potential for increased absorption via it is great; this is especially true in heat when our pores are open as part of the breathing and cooling process of the *lungs*. Remember the *San Jiao* and the theory that cancerous hits are to that realm of human bodily functioning. Remember also that children are more susceptible to these kinds of airborne exposures, and perhaps children are another canary in the coalmine. Children live closer to the ground; their skin is in constant contact with possible contaminants. Their body weight is such that an adult exposure translates into a greater impact in a child. One of the greatest health problems we have in the world. today is asthma, especially in children, who now miss more schooldays in the US due to asthma than any other single cause.[48]

Lung Patterns and Cancer Prevention

The Lung–liver Relationship and Smoking Cessation

Although there are many impacts that relate to *lung* injury, smoking increases the impacts of all forms of airborne pollution. Smoking leads to an addiction to nicotine. The damage done by the particulates inhaled by smoking is only part of the problem, as there are many other substances inhaled in cigarette smoke that are by-products of burning the tobacco.[49] Additives are included in cigarettes for various reasons and these additives also cause injury. After people become addicted they often use smoking as a coping mechanism to manage everyday stress. When one is helping people to quit smoking it is important to address all of these mechanisms. This commonly means understanding the classical relationship of Chinese medicine between the *lung* and the *liver*. By attending to the *liver* as well as the *lung*, the problem of recidivism can be greatly improved. And, most importantly, the modern problem of lung and other cancers in smokers can be reduced dramatically. This is not meant to address only the conventional medical relationship of liver and addiction but also the Chinese medicine relationship of the ascending and extending function of *liver Qi* alongside the descending function of the *lung*.[50,51]

As a pair, the *lungs* relate to *Qi* and the *liver* relates to blood. Together they smooth and regulate all of the *Qi* and blood of the body. This is an important relationship in cancer prevention because *Qi and blood stasis* are foundations of cancer. *Metal* (*lung*) restrains *wood* (*liver*) via the *ko cycle* of *five-phase theory* included in the *Nei Jing*. *Metal* is clear and moist with down-bearing qualities, so that the *wood* does not ignite. The foot *Jueyin* has a branch to the diaphragm, which then ascends to the *lungs*. For a complete iteration of these concepts of Chinese medicine, refer to any English language book that covers the foundations of Chinese medicine.[50,52,53] All of these interrelationships between the *lungs* and the *liver* are energetically important in treatment to help a person quit smoking.

The primary dynamic of injury to the *liver* is constraint (as used in the English sense of the word) when emotional suffering causes injury, and this affects the normal diffusion and descending action of the *lung*. Sucking in smoke while smoking is a form of deep breathing and oddly works to adjust *liver* constraint. It expands the intercostals, lowers the diaphragm, and draws down *Qi*. However, depressed *liver Qi* also results in *phlegm*, and *phlegm* is the *lung's* enemy. *Phlegm* resulting from depressed *liver* function results in injury to the *lung's* diffusion and descending function. The advantages of smoking are greatly outweighed by the negatives even when the body can use the habit to temporarily adjust the *Qi* mechanism in the chest and *upper middle Jiao,* thus relieving constraint. This constraint rears its head when a person quits smoking.[54] It needs to be addressed as an important part of treatment for quitting smoking, because withdrawal symptoms of nicotine include damage to the diffusing and descending functions of the *liver–lung* relationship.

Over time depressed *liver Qi* accumulates and leads to *fire*, which then follows the channel upward and disturbs the *lung*. *Damp heat* in the *liver* and primarily *gallbladder channel* also counterflows. In both cases the *lungs* lose their diffusing and descending action. The hot particulates of tobacco smoke contribute to this *fire*. At the same time, smoking is commonly done in the company of drinking coffee. Coffee is generally the essence of *dampness and heat;* it acts as a diuretic, as does alcohol. And so this particular relationship between *liver* and *lung* is enhanced by the common coaddiction to coffee and cigarettes. People who are chronically constipated because of smoking use this relationship and the *lung–large-intestine* coupled organ relationship to move stools by having a cigarette and a cup of coffee upon rising in the morning. The *lung–large-intestine* and *lung–liver* relationships are both stimulated. Constipation in people who are quitting smoking is another necessary element of treatment.[55]

The *liver* stores the blood, and *liver stasis* causes the *lungs* to lose control of the descending and diffusing functions. Also, the *liver* is a *zang* organ of *wind and wood.* It is *Yin* in substance but *Yang* in function. *Liver Yin deficiency* and *liver blood deficiency* lead to *internal wind*. *Internal wind* counterflows and invades the *lungs*.[56]

Liver deficiency leads to *lung* illnesses.[57] A common example is the occurrence of springtime airborne allergies. The *liver* and the *lung* share the same *Source*. If the *Yin* is deficient, then the *lung* above loses moisture. Deficiency *heat* will occur internally and this will disturb the *lung*. *Liver deficiency* can also involve *Yang deficiency*. *Yang deficiency* can lead to *cold*, and *cold* causes hardness and distenstion in the subcostal region with *cold* and *heat*. The *liver Yang deficiency* and *lung cold* can lead to counterflow. This pattern can occur later in the process of aging and addiction. Intercostal chondritis may be an early symptom of this pattern.[58]

It is important to remember to address any of the above patterns present between the *lung* and the *liver* when helping someone to quit smoking. Patients who relapse may have negative coping mechanisms in place that have not been addressed. Never give up working to help them. Literally, their life may be at stake. Treating for depression, anxiety, constraint, or any combination of these is extremely important. The healthy energetic relationship between *lung* and *liver* must be re-established.

There are many protocols, especially in the acupuncture realm, that are available for practitioners to help patients quit smoking. The will not be addressed in this text, as they are easily accessible. However, there are some important pointers that may be of benefit in making the stop-smoking process easier. The use of antioxidants in higher dosages early in the withdrawal period will increase the risk of failure, because scavenging free radicals and clearing nicotine receptor sites during withdrawal increases withdrawal symptoms and craving. Withdrawal occurs more easily as a gradual process and over a period of time with support for all of the relationships between *liver* and *lung* impacted by the smoking habit. Use antioxidants after the withdrawal phase of quitting smoking.

Smoking marijuana or cocaine has been found to be carcinogenic.[59] People who do not smoke tobacco but who smoke these other substances are also at risk for lung cancer. Addressing this with patients is very important. Ingesting marijuana is not carcinogenic; smoking it is.

There is confusion as to whether or not marijuana is addictive. Obviously, cocaine is. Working with patients who are using may require a referral to others who are experts in this realm. Working alongside them is immensely valuable. At the same time, it is important to realize that tobacco smoking is more addictive than cocaine smoking and much more difficult to end. Tobacco is one of the most addictive substances known. This is another reason to question why tobacco is a legal substance.

It is also important to remember that quitting smoking is just the first step in a long recovery. It usually takes at least 15 years for a person's risk of lung cancer to go back to what it was before they had smoked.[60] The cancerization process of the lung cells begins very early in one's smoking history; the cancerization effect has been found in people who have been smoking only five years but does not become symptomatic for many more years, usually when it is too late. A long-time smoker remains at risk for lung cancer for some time even after they have stopped smoking. A large number of people diagnosed with lung cancer are people who quit smoking many years ago. Quitting is essential but only a first step. Rehabilitating the *lungs* and changing other lifestyle habits that may be negative is very important.

Vigilance is a key and involves repeat CT scans of the chest on a periodic basis. Currently these scans are not covered by medical insurance, because the insurance industry is generally not interested in prevention. This is also true because lung cancer has been stigmatized in our culture since it is the result of an addiction. The addiction is perceived to be the fault of the individual and so compassion and everything that results from compassion, like early screening tools, has been very late in coming. Remember that most people who start smoking do so when they are very young. Chest X-ray imaging is not definitive for lung cancer.

In addition to imaging of the chest, Chinese medicine can begin the work of rehabilitating the *lung*. This occurs through addressing those patterns that are present, and it may take some time to accomplish. There is also an element of "decontamination" of the *lung*, and re-establishment of the normal immune response in the *lung*, which may require an even longer time. The rest of this chapter is devoted to covering those pathologies that might occur as a result of smoking or pollution. Treating these patterns is essential to preventing the injuries that drag down the *lungs* and create an environment in which the serious illness of cancer may evolve.

Lung Pathologies

Traditionally, the *lungs* govern the *Qi*, the *kidneys* root the *Qi*, and the *spleen* is the source for the generation of *phlegm*. Wheezing, shortness of breath, asthma, cough, bronchitis, and so on are treated from the perspective of these three *zang* functional units. The *liver* plays a crucial role in the ascending and descending of the *lung Qi* because of its diffusing function. Physiologically, the *liver* oversees coursing and draining, rectifies and soothes the *Qi* dynamic, and has general control over the *Qi* dynamic of the entire body.[61]

The diffusion and descending function of the *upper Jiao* (mostly up and down), the mediation of the *middle Jiao* (mostly horizontal and circular), and the implementation of the *lower Jiao* (mostly upward and inner) all allow the interior and the exterior to communicate. The *liver* is a prime motivator in this interior–exterior communication. Therefore, if it is constrained, especially in *lung* diseases, this can influence the normal ascending and diffusing function of the *lung Qi*. This is one of the infamous vicious circles of Chinese medicine that is exquisitely ecological in nature.

The *liver* again has a powerful relationship with the *lungs* in that when its coursing and rectifying function is not normal the *waterways* via the *San Jiao* become congested, *Qi* counterflows, *phlegm* develops, and then ascends to harm the *lungs*.[62]

The *liver Qi* assists the *lungs* with its diffusing and descending function by regulating the *Qi* of all of the *zang* organs. So regulating the *Qi* of the *liver* is essential in treating wheezing, cough, asthma, or any condition of the *lungs* where the *lung Qi* is flushing upward, no matter whether it is caused by smoking, asthma, allergies, or some other condition.

Blood Stasis Patterns

The indications for *blood stasis* patterns, especially of the *lungs*, include the common signs for the tongue, masses in the chest, vascular abnormalities, cyanosis, clubbing of the nails, flaky skin, numb extremities that are not numb as a result of pharmaceutical drug therapies or nerve dysfunction, some mental conditions and forms of mania, and a pulse that is choppy, knotted, hesitant, or absent.[63]

Lung illnesses and *blood stasis* are intimately related because the *lungs* regulate the *Qi* dynamic and function to circulate the blood. *Qi* is the master of the blood, and *Qi* pertains to the *lungs*. The blood of the entire body accumulates in the *lungs* via the channels and the vessels. If the *lung* function is normal, then the exchange of blood gases is normal. If the *lung Qi* is injured, then the vessels become static, and if the blood vessels become static, the *lung* disease is exacerbated. Therefore, *lung* diseases often involve stasis. Resolving *blood stasis* will improve the exchange of blood gases, which will then promote recovery from the *lung* injury. This is one way in which cancers other than lung cancer occur. And it explains one mechanism by which the first responders at the WTC. disaster were later diagnosed with cancer after suffering for many years with other respiratory diseases.

In bronchial asthma, there is typically a dark complexion, dull cyanotic lips, a green–blue tongue body, and veins under the tongue that are distended and dark; these signs can be combined with other patterns. However, these signs require that the blood be regulated as part of treatment.[64]

In cardiopulmonary diseases, the role of *blood stasis* is also dominant. The red blood cells are the *Qi* aspect of the blood. The serum is the *Yin* aspect of the blood. The *Qi* is wrapped in *Yin* and there is a powerful relationship between *Qi* and *Yin* in the blood. This relationship is furthered by the *heart–lung* connection in driving the *Qi* and blood. When *blood stasis* is present as part of *lung* disease, this relationship becomes injured in varying degrees, depending on how longstanding and entrenched the *blood stasis* is in the *lung*. The two are inseparable.[65,66]

Yang-deficient Lung Patterns

If *Yang deficiency* is the root of a *lung* disease then usually the *kidneys* are involved. If the *kidney Yang* is deficient, it cannot absorb and accumulate the *Qi*. If the *lung* is deficient, it cannot govern the *Qi* and so it loses its regulatory and circulatory capacity, leading to congealing of fluids, which results in *phlegm*. If the *spleen* is deficient, *damp* accumulates and generates *phlegm*. If the *Yang* is deficient, fluids and blood cease to circulate normally and this leads to systemic stasis and *phlegm*. And if the *Yang* is deficient, the *Wei Qi* is not strong and pathogens penetrate. When chronic *lung* diseases like asthma persist, a scenario of serious *lung* disease and systemic *blood stasis* can occur.[64]

Asthma in children is most often the result of *Yang deficiency*.[67] The *Yang* can be constitutional or it can result from constant and long-term exposures that eventually deplete the *Yang*, especially in a young person. Recurrence is the nature of asthma and this progressively damages the *Yang*. All of the *spleen*, *kidney*, and *lung* relationships are damaged. *Yang-deficient* asthma often occurs at night, because at night the *Yin* is high and the *Yang* is low. However, these classical interpretations regarding children and asthma do not take into account modern-day exposures to air pollution and allergens. It is up to us to determine the nature of modern asthma in children in terms of Chinese medicine. Analyzing the symptom picture and signs is our key to correct diagnosis.

For many children there is an allergenic component. This allergenic component is compounded by pollution, as stated earlier by the fact that pollen and other particles attach to very small particles of pollutants that act as messengers for these allergens. Global warming is increasing and will continue to increase the earlier release of pollen by plants and thus increase the amount of pollen in the air for a longer period of time in the yearly plant cycle.[68] All of these issues are interconnected. The constant exposure to pollution in a young person with as-yet-unconsolidated *Wei Qi* and a *middle Jiao* function that is still developing, gradually injures the *lung*.[69]

Phlegm stasis is very important in the recurrent nature of this pathology. The *Yang* loses its ability to warm and move, and this leads to *phlegm stasis.*[70] Ongoing *phlegm* in the *lung* impairs the *Qi* dynamic and may eventually impair the flow of blood, leading to *blood stasis.* At the same time, ongoing *blood stasis* influences the circulation of fluids, leading to *phlegm. Phlegm* and *blood stasis* bind together and result in stasis in the collaterals of the *lung* and obstructed *lung Qi.*[71] When *spleen deficiency* underlies this process in the *lungs,* it adds to the insult. Children and adults with food allergies are at risk for asthma caused by the interrelatedness of *lung, spleen,* and *kidney Yang deficiency.* Having the markers for *blood stasis* present so early in life is a major concern.

Therefore, *Yang deficiency,* binding of *phlegm* and stasis, *lung Qi* depression, and stasis are all major pathological factors in recurrent asthma.[72] The treatment principles for this vicious circle are:

- Treat the branch by diffusing the *lungs* and transforming *phlegm;*
- Treat the root by warming the *Yang* and transforming *phlegm;*
- Treat the stasis by regulating the blood when necessary.

Yang-deficient lung patterns are recognizable because they are worse with movement. When the *Yin* is coalesced, the *Qi* is absorbed. Movement causes the *Qi* to be transformed while, at the same time, the *Yin* loses its capacity to absorb, and this combination results in panting. Difficult respiration that is aggravated by activity is due to a deficiency of *Source Qi* and the *kidneys'* inability to absorb *Qi.* Exercise–induced or play-induced asthma should be considered from this point of view.

The *lungs* govern the *Qi,* and the *kidneys* are the root of the *Qi.* The *lungs* govern the diffusions, dissemination, and circulation of the *Qi.* The *kidneys* govern the absorption of the *Qi.* Respiration is normal when the function of the *lungs* and the *kidneys* is normal. *Lung* symptoms happen as a result of:

(1) *Pathogenic Qi invading the lungs.* This is usually an excess condition and in modern times can involve many new exposures to pathogens like phthalates, formaldehyde, ground-level ozone, chemical-laden dusts and particulates, and gases never before inhaled. Symptoms should give us clues as to the nature of these

pathogens — wind–heat, wind–cold, latent pathogenic factors, damp pathogens, and so on. The symptoms and signs give us a clue as to how to treat them.

(2) *Deficiency in the lungs and kidneys.* The above pathogens to which we are exposed on a daily basis that are also cyclic can contribute to *lung* and *kidney* deficiency, and discrimination of each pattern can become blurred. In general, it is best to treat the acute phase while it is happening and the chronic underlying deficiency in between acute episodes.

In clinical practice, we have traditionally tonified the *kidneys*, drained the *lungs* by transforming *phlegm*, regulated the *Qi* of the *lungs*, and strengthened the *spleen*. Because we currently do not know the nature of the chemical pathogens to which individuals are exposed, it is difficult to know how to drain or release these chemicals from the body. We do not know if all of them stay inside the lung parenchyma and accumulate. In cigarette smoke and asbestos exposure, we know that some ingredients in the smoke, silica, and asbestos particles do remain. Since this arena of conventional science and medical research is very small, what we do know about is the nature of the damage that occurs as a result of exposure. It is up to us to analyze and evaluate what we see and then devise strategies that are *both new and old* regarding how to treat patients.

Asthma

Conventional Medicine

Asthma is defined as a paroxysmal, often-allergic disorder of respiration characterized by bronchospasm, wheezing, and difficulty in expiration, usually accompanied by a feeling of constriction in the chest. During an asthma attack the bronchial passages temporarily narrow and, when combined with excessive mucus secretions, result in impaired ventilation and increased airway resistance.[73] Asthma is the leading cause of disease in children aged. 2–17. Currently, 1 out of 40 people suffer from it in all age groups. And 65% of asthma sufferers develop symptoms before the age of 5. Children who live in homes where there is a smoker are much more likely to suffer from asthma.[74] A majority of the crews who cleaned up after the WTC disaster have been diagnosed with it.[75] The EPA stated on many occasions after the disaster that there was no reason for concern. This is emblematic of the fact that many chemical substances and combinations of these substances have human health effects that have not been studied and are not known even to this day.

Early-onset asthma (extrinsic or atrophic) begins in early childhood. It may have a genetic component. It is also often associated with eczema from birth, and there are whealing skin reactions to allergens. Allergic asthma of the anaphylactic or type 1 reaction is caused by bronchospasm due to allergic reaction because of immune hypersensitivity. Upon contact with the allergen, IgE antibodies adhere to mast cells and an anaphylactic crisis is caused by antigen–antibody reaction on the surface of mast cells in the bronchi that activates enzymes, leading to a release of histamine, serotonin, bradykinin, and prostaglandins. These cause muscle contraction, accumulation of eosinophils, bronchospasm, and epithelial damage in the late phase, which then leads to an asthma attack.[76]

Common allergens are pollen, dust, mold, animal dander, feathers, textiles, fibers, detergents, petrochemicals, air pollution, smoke of various kinds, food allergens, aspirin sensitivity, cold air, and exercise.[77] Many of these allergens are made worse by climate change. For example, pollen levels are increasing with global warming combined with a plant reaction to higher temperatures and an extended and earlier flowering period in deciduous trees and other flowering plants. We read earlier about ground-level ozone pollution increased by *heat* and sunlight. All air pollution increases in amount and density during hot weather because weather patterns in many areas tend to cause inversion layers that hold in *heat* and, therefore, pollution in the air.[78] Wherever there is drought, which currently is the Southeast, Midwest, and West of the US, there is also an increased risk of fires. These fires also contribute to air pollution throughout the summer months.

These areas of the US are also rapidly growing in population. This population density has increased the need for housing and other new construction projects that typically have reduced tree cover through removal.[79] The loss of trees across the country has contributed to warming, to low oxygen levels, and to an increase in greenhouse gases which trees and other plant materials ordinarily reduce through transpiration.[80] New construction also frequently contains many of the chemicals referred to earlier.

Late-onset asthma (intrinsic) begins later in life, has no family history connected with it, has no history of eczema, and may or may not be triggered by allergens.[81] Asthma originating in infancy is often related to food allergies or to foods inappropriately fed to infants before the *middle Jiao* has consolidated its function. Asthma beginning at ages 10–13 is commonly related to inhalants, and asthma after age 45 is most often related to infection. This is changing as air quality worsens. Summertime asthma is most commonly due to increased pollens and molds; wintertime asthma is due to increased infections; and, generally, nighttime asthma attacks are related to the emotions, especially suppressed anger and grief. About 90% of asthmatics are mouth-breathers, making it easier for dust, pollen, organisms, and cold air to enter the lungs.

There are several conventional medical tests related to *lung* function[82]:

- FEV (Forced expiratory volume);
- PEFR (Peak expiratory flow rate);
- Exercise tests;
- Histamine production tests;
- Skin tests (RAST) that show wheals on the skin in response to allergens.

Sputum and blood tests are done to rule out bronchitis, chronic bronchitis, and emphysema.

The conventional medical treatment for asthma includes[83]:

- Antiallergic drugs (Intal) to stabilize mast cells and reduce their sensitivity;
- Bronchodilators (Ventolin) to stimulate receptors in sympathetic nerves to bronchi, causing bronchodilation;
- Corticosteroids (Becotide) to reduce bronchial mucosal inflammation and hypersecretion of mucus.

Of these, Prednisone is the most common, and it produces side effects that may include fluid and electrolyte imbalances, muscle weakness, peptic ulcers, impaired wound healing, headaches, dizziness, menstrual irregularities, glaucoma, and latent diabetes.[84] Because steroids are considered a *heat* toxin in nature, they injure the *Yin*. Injury to the *Yin* can cause advancement of the *lung* pathology for which it is being used when it is withdrawn.

Determining and removing food allergens is a good first step in treating children with early-onset asthma.

Structural Signs and Acupuncture Interventions in Asthma

The Taoists say that inhalation comes *to* the *kidney* and exhalation comes *from* the Chong. In Japanese acupuncture, the following points can be used[85]:

- For difficult inhalation needle K 3 and Lu 5;
- For difficult exhalation needle Lu 5 and Sp 4;
- If both are difficult, then use K 3;
- For an autonomic nervous system imbalance, burn moxa on all reactive points on the governing vessel line between Du 7 and Du 12;
- The Hukaya bronchial/*lung* infection point is 1″ above to 1″ below Lu 5 and is found via palpation;
- Lu 5 treatment with moxa will enable *phlegm* expectoration;
- Lu 4 is for shortness of breath with *lung* and heart connections;
- Du 12 is an important point for allergies and any *lung* pathology.

Du 12 is an important point; the Chinese name for it is *Shen Zhu* meaning "pillar of the body." It is a pivot point structurally and is where kyphosis begins. Kyphosis is a common sign of *lung* deficiencies. Du 12 is also the thymus reflex point. As an immune point it works with several *gao* and *huang* points, like BL 43 and triple intestine 10 (Kiiko Matsumoto), to treat allergic hypersensitivity manifestations and other immune regulation issues.[86,87]

Bronchial asthma often manifests in the reflex line of the upper *kidney* channel. Many people with asthma will demonstrate· a response on the *kidney* channel but not at Lu 1 as would be anticipated in infectious diseases. The upper *kidney* channel is called the "bronchial reflex." And Lu 5 will release the *kidney* channel when needled toward Lu 9 with moxa applied afterward.[88]

Asthma patients will also have scapular tension on the medial border or a lump of tension above BL 17. If there is a lump in this area, place four needles into the lump, then remove and moxa the area. The lump should reduce in size. Tension around BL 43 may indicate that the muscles of breathing are somehow disturbed; these muscles of inhalation and exhalation are disturbed because of the tension around BL 43, a *gao* and *huang* point. Its name is *Gaohuangshu*. If there is a ropelike tissue texture around this point, needle into it and then moxa it. It should release and diminish.[89]

If this ropelike tension exists around BL 43, it may be a *liver* indication. Pinching the costal area along the flank can elicit a reaction, and it points to emotionally related *liver* issues that are not physical problems except in that they manifest in this way. If the pinching of the intercostals (accessory muscles in the breathing mechanism) elicits reaction and feels thick, this is a sign that treatment may be slower and that addressing the *liver* is definitely indicated.[89]

For allergic asthma use inner Nei Ting, which is found by bending the second toe to the ball of the foot, and where the tip of the second toe touches, that is Nei Ting. Apply moxa.

When needling BL 43 place the arms of the patient above the head and then needle obliquely under the scapula.

Metal points are thought to relate to the *lungs* and to the oxygen supply of the channel itself. Numbness on a channel can indicate a lack of oxygen as well as a blood sugar imbalance. Diabetic neuropathy is an example of this. "Sugar" points are at TI11 and TI12 *hua tou jia ji*. Water points involve the lymph system. And *fire* points are thought to be connected to the blood.

In chronic bronchitis with repeated sore throats, one can assume weak *lungs* and weak lymphatic function. To test for this, squeeze the lymph in the axilla. Press in three ways — on the crease, on Lu1, and above the breast on the upper outer aspect. If this palpation elicits pain, then check three *fire* points in the palm — Ht 8, P 8, and Lu 10. Disperse the most painful point by massaging it. Do not needle. Treat the metal and water points of the channel involved the most. If you tonify water there will be a 50% change in signs and symptoms. This technique tonifies the axillary lymph and will help to treat chronic or repeated bronchial infections.[90]

Liver-related respiratory conditions usually present with symptoms that are intermittent, recurrent, that last for many years, and are accompanied by flank pain, possibly a red face, and a dry and scratchy throat. It is common for this type of respiratory condition to include an underlying condition of *liver heat* but the *lung–liver* relationship is complex, as discussed earlier in the text. If *heat* or *fire* is involved, then the treatment principles are to soothe the *liver*, bring down the *fire*, stop the *lung Qi* from flushing upward, and clear *heat* from the *lungs*. Good points for addressing this condition are:

- Lv 2 or Lv 3,
- Lu 6,
- Ren 22,
- GB 34,
- Bl 13,
- Bl 18.

Classical Theory and Asthma

In the discussion of wheezing there are usually four main etiologies:

- EPI — *cold* or *wind–heat*;
- Exposure to abnormal "smells" like dust, pollen, paint, smoke;

- Improper diet — allergic foods, raw foods, salty foods, and so on;
- Emotions, exhaustion, and fatigue.

People who develop wheezing from these causes are said to have a "pathological constitution." This is in contrast to the regular types of constitution, like *Yang-deficient* or *Yin-deficient* and so on. The term refers to a constitutional type that has allowed for the development of a related pathological disorder. *Fu Yin* refers to invisible *phlegm* or invisible fluid. Invisible *phlegm* does not move, and no disorder occurs until one of the above causative factors comes into play. The factor will cause the invisible *phlegm* to move.[91] Once the invisible *phlegm* starts to move, it can cause the *lung Qi* to ascend, which then leads to wheezing. This is an example of a pathological constitution evolving into wheezing or asthma. It also explains why some children are more susceptible to pollution and allergens as causes of asthma even though other children living in the same environment are not. It may explain why some adults are diagnosed with *lung* cancer even though they have no explanatory exposures to known carcinogens for *lung* cancer.
Invisible *phlegm* can manifest in different ways:

- *Cold-type* wheezing;
- *Heat-type* wheezing;
- *Deficiency-type* wheezing.

Invisible *phlegm* will manifest according to the patient's constitution. These conditions of invisible *phlegm* are difficult to treat. Some practitioners say that there is no such thing as invisible or insubstantial *phlegm* because *phlegm* is *phlegm*. They say that the *phlegm* that we can see through expectoration is visible and this visibility is what makes it substantial. Some *phlegm* we cannot see and never see (or even hear) making it insubstantial or invisible. Invisible *phlegm* probably occurs in the *lungs*, in the epithelial tissues of the gastrointestinal tube, and in the blood vessels in the form of plaque. However, *phlegm* is spoken of in relation to epilepsy and mental disorders as well. Regardless of which type of

wheezing occurs, there are certain points from the classical literature that are commonly used in treatment[92]:

- Lu 6 must be needled so that the patient gets a needle sensation
  down to the fingertip and up to the shoulder;
- Running cupping from Bl 12 to Bl 15.

Additional points include:

- Ren 6 with moxa for deficiency-type wheezing;
- *Dingchuan* as the main stop-wheezing point;
- Bl 20 for *spleen deficiency* with *phlegm*;
- Bl 23 for *kidney Qi deficiency* and inability to grasp the *Qi*;
- Lu 3 clears the *upper Jiao* and adjusts the *lung Qi*;
- Lu 7 is the *luo* point, and circulates and regulates the *lung Qi*;
- Lu 9 is the *Source* point, and tonifies and moistens the *lungs*;
- Lu 10 cools *heat* in the *lungs*.

Blood Stasis Patterns

It has been shown that *blood stasis* is a common characteristic of
lung pathology. Therefore, regulating the blood and transforming
stasis helps to promote rehabilitation of the *lungs*. Depending on the
pattern presentation, the following herbs can be added to address
this common issue[93]:

- For unaccompanied *blood* stasis, use *tao ren, chi shao,* and *e zhu*;
- For deficiency patterns, use *dan shen* and *ji xue teng*;
- For "*men*" sensation (chest stifling) use *xiang fu, yu jin,* and *jiang
  xiang*;
- For *blood stasis* with *phlegm*, use *hong hua* and *yi mu cao*.

Tao ren regulates the blood and simultaneously diffuses the *lungs*
and suppresses *lung Qi* flushing upward. *Dan shen* transforms *blood
stasis* without damaging the *zheng Qi*. *Chi shao* regulates the blood and

also helps to resolve bronchial spasms. *E zhu* cracks the *blood,* clears *heat,* and resolves *toxins. Hong hua* and *yi mu cao* regulate the *blood* and transform *dampness. Xiang fu, yu jin,* and *jiang xiang* regulate the *blood* and *Qi,* and are helpful in treating chest pain.

There are several guiding formulas used as an underlying basis to treat bronchial asthma with *blood stasis.* They include:

- *Fu yuan huo xue tang,*
- *Tao hong si wu tang,*
- *Xue fu zhu yu tang,*
- *Tong qiao huo xue tang.*

A primary formula for treating *blood stasis* bronchial asthma is:

Shen lian zhi sou tang

Dan shen 12 g
Chuan huang lian 4 g
Fa ban xia 10 g
Chen pi 10 g
Gua lou pi 10 g
San qi 1.5 g
Gan cao 2 g

- If *blood deficiency* accompanies the presentation, then add *dang gui* and *bai shao;*
- If *Qi deficiency* accompanies the presentation, then add *dang shen* and *bai zhu;*
- If *phlegm* accompanies the presentation, then add *hai fu shi, bai quan,* and *bei mu.*

All of these formulas can be found in *Formulas and Strategies,* edited by Volker Scheid *et al.*[94]

The etiology of bronchial asthma is always *phlegm.* However, the underlying mechanism is stasis. *Phlegm* and *dampness* entangle, the *phlegm* congeals and becomes static, interrupting the *Qi* transformative dynamic, and the *Qi* becomes static and in turn causes *blood stasis.* Regulating the *blood,* which in the *lung* has such a strong intimate connection with the *Qi* and *blood* motion, becomes a primary intervention in treatment.[95]

When asthma is accompanied by a *liver Qi stasis* component, adding herbs like *chai hu, bai shao, huang qin, zhi ke,* and *di long* helps to move the *liver Qi* and free the connecting vessels. This manifestation is due to chronic depression inhibiting the *Qi* dynamic of the *liver* and transforming into fire. The fire scorches the fluids and produces *phlegm.* This creates a vicious circle of *Qi* obstruction that when chronic can lead to *blood stasis.* It is a good example of how a disease when chronic can cause emotional depression which, in turn, worsens the disease, entrenching it deeper in its tracks.[96]

A formula that treats this presentation was designed by Ru Xiao Hua as a modification of *Fu yuan huo xue tang:*

Chai hu 9 g
Dang gui 9 g
Tao ren 9 g
Hong hua 5 g
Da huang 9 g
Gan cao 5 g
Tian hua fen 9 g
Di long 18 g
Ma huang 9 g
Bai shao 12 g
Zhi ke 9 g
Cang er zi 9 g
Gua lou shi 12 g
Yu xing cao 12 g

Yang Deficiency Asthma

In a *Yang*-deficient constitution, the *lungs, spleen,* and *kidneys* will be deficient. In the *lungs* this leads to injury to their regulatory function and to congealed fluids. If the *Yang* is deficient, then the exterior defensive *Qi* is not stable and external pathogens can enter the body, particularly through the skin and *Jade Screen*. Asthma in children is most often due to *Yang deficiency*. The recurring nature of asthma due to recurring exposures progressively damages the *Yang* and leads to an ongoing and worsening cycle of injury.[97] In modern times, when children are exposed to air pollution indoors and out, it is difficult to say if the children themselves are *Yang-deficient* and this is why this is happening, or if the constant exposure to pollution causes *Yang deficiency*, or both. It is for us to determine child by child which is the root and which is the branch in each situation.

A knotting of *phlegm and stasis*, especially *blood stasis*, due to *Yang* deficiency is also part of this cycle of injury. *Stasis* that develops in the network vessels of the *lung* obstructs the *lung Qi* and causes *Qi* flushing upward. The major pathological factors in recurrent asthma are *Yang* deficiency, knotted *phlegm and blood stasis*, and *lung Qi deficiency*. Therefore, regulating the *lung Qi* and transforming *phlegm* is the branch treatment, and *Yang deficiency* and *phlegm* transformation is the root.

The following formula warms the *Yang*, regulate the *lung Qi*, transforms *phlegm*, and stops wheezing[98]:

Ma huang 5 g
Gui zhi 5 g
Xi xin 3 g
Gan jiang 5 g
Ban xia 10 g
Chi shao 10 g
Wu wei zi 10 g
Zhi gan cao 5 g
Fu zi 10 g
Tao ren 10 g
Xing ren 10 g
Lai fu zi 15 g
Su zi 10 g

When this pattern becomes chronic with a deep-lying rheum (*tan yin*), it can transform into *heat*. This kind of pattern is due to *Yang deficiency* but has signs and symptoms of *heat* as well. There is a persistent night cough, with *phlegm* stuck in the throat. There may be epistaxis and night sweats. The tongue is red, with little coating. The night wheezing suggests a root of *Yang deficiency.*

Zhi ma huang 5 g
Tao ren 10 g
Xing ren 10 g
Lai fu zi 15 g
Su zi 10 g
Sang bai pi 10 g
Ting li zi 10 g
Zhi gan cao 5 g
Yu xng cao 30 g
Fu zi 10 g
Chi shao 10 g
Bai shao 10 g
Bai mao gen 30 g

Asthma has acute and latent phases that require somewhat different treatment, depending on the phase of the patient at any given time. All of the following formulas are from Shoucun Ma. For an acute asthma with *blood stasis*, use this formula:

Hong hua 15 g
Di fu zi 20 g
Yin yang huo 20 g
Huang qi 15 g
Yu xing cao 20 g
Chuan xiong

For nonacute asthma with *blood stasis*, use:

Hong hua 15 g
Huang qi 15 g
Yin yang huo 20 g

Qi dai, one half-piece
Chuan xiong 20 g

For a *wind–cold* invasion of the *lungs* in an asthmatic with internal *phlegm stasis*, use
Xiao Qing Long Tang and add:

Di long
Chi shao
Dan shen
Dang gui wei
Qian cao gen

Add in the appropriate amounts to balance the herb quantities in the base formula of *Xiao Qing Long Tang*.

For *wind–heat* EPI of the *lungs* in an asthmatic patient with internal *phlegm stasis*, use
Ma Xing Shi Gan Tang and add:

Di long
Chi shao
Dan shen

For *liver Qi stasis* and depressed *lung Qi* and internal *phlegm stasis*, add to the first formula:

Di long
Dang gui wei

Wind Spasm as an Additional Mechanism in Asthma

Common methods for treating wheezing and asthma include clearing *heat*, regulating the *lung Qi*, helping the *kidneys* to grasp the *Qi*, harmonizing the *liver–lung* relationship, and transforming *phlegm* and *blood stasis*. Sometimes these techniques are not clinically effective. Adding techniques to diminish *wind* increases therapeutic efficacy.

Bronchospasm which leads to wheezing is a branch phenomenon that is often part of an allergic process. Antispasmodics can also be antiallergenic.[99] In acupuncture therapy, tonifying the function of the *liver/gallbladder* and nourishing the blood also increases, the efficacy of treatment. For example, by adding Lv 8 the *liver* blood is nourished to clear *wind*. And since Gb 34 rules the tendons and some other connective tissue structures, including the diaphragm and the connective tissue in the bronchioles, the addition of Gb 34 also increases efficacy. These points plus Lu 5 and Lu 7 or the xi-cleft point Lu 6 all work together to calm the *liver* and regulate the *Qi*, regulate the *lung Qi*, expel *phlegm*, and calm cough.[100]

Seven-star or plum-blossom needle tapping along the bladder channel in the upper back will open the collaterals. Tap till the skin is hot and the patient begins breathing more easily.

On the hottest day of the year, use 10 grains of moxa directly on:

*   Du 14,
*   Du 12,
*   Bl 43,
*   Bl 13.

It turns out that this approach may be useful in other *lung* conditions as well. For example, whooping cough, chronic or acute bronchitis, and radiation-induced cough all benefit form treatment according to the pattern and the addition of antispasmodic herbs.

Antispasmodics clear *wind* and include those odd insect substances like *quan xie, wu gong, di long, Jiang can*, and *tian nan xing*. These substances are especially helpful in treating allergic asthma. An allergic process causing brochospaim and asthma is a branch phenomenon, and treatment requires the use of antispasmodics with *spleen* and *kidney* function interventions.

Ma Xing Shi Gan Tang, which includes *Yin* and blood-nourishing herbs and *di long, jiang can, tian nan xing, wu gong, gua lou ren*, and *ting li zi*, is a studied formula to treat wheezing and severe asthma.

Another formula used in asthma that has been studied in modern-day China is *Tian Di Xiao Ling*:

Zhi da huang 10 g
Tao ren 10 g
E zhu 10 g
Tu bie chong 10 g
Di long 15 g
Bai shao 15 g
Zhi huang qi 20 g
Shu di 20 g
Gan cao 6 g

For *cold wheezing* these herbs were added to the above formula:

Zhi fu zi 10 g
Gan jiang 10 g

For *hot wheezing* these herbs were added:

Sheng shi gao 30 g
Sang bai pi 12 g

The formula uses blood-cracking methods to resolve gelatinous *phlegm* that obstructs the airway. It is a modification of *Da Huang Bie Chong Wan*. *Da huang* and *tu bie chong* are the chief herbs in the formula and work to drain the *lungs*, transform stasis, and dissipate binding of *phlegm*. *Tian long* and *di long* act as assistants, and regulate the blood and open the network vessels. Although there are no herbs that are antiasthmatic or *phlegm-transforming*, this formula works very well in treating bronchial asthma.[102]

Yin Fire Asthma

Yin fire is a *deficiency* pattern but is not due to *Yin deficiency*. It is due to *spleen deficiency*.[102A] The *spleen* takes fluid from the *kidney* and adds nutritional *Qi.* It then sends this body fluid to the stomach. *Spleen Yin deficiency* is caused by insufficiency of body fluid. In the process of becoming deficient, the route of body fluid that supplies nutrition shuts down. As the fluid decreases, deficiency and empty *heat* rises. The symptoms are fatigue of the whole body or fatigue of the extremities only. Empty *heat* is rising and the patient will feel a feverish discomfort and a vague sense of malaise. This discomfort is worse in the spring and summer, when the *Yang* is full and the body becomes more open, especially the pores of the skin. It can also be seen as a step in malnutrition and starvation. The empty *heat* will rise to the surface and get dispersed. In the fall and winter the patient may feel a chill, because they are deficient. This condition is also related to *liver Yang deficiency.* As it worsens, there may be muscle cramps and pain.[103]

Children who are quiet and sedate may have *spleen Yin deficiency.* Adults may appear lazy or inactive. They may have loose stools and frequent urination but a dry mouth. There may be a constitutional component to this manifestation and people who react more drastically to food poisoning or even mild overeating can react more intensely, because of a constitutional propensity. However, more commonly, this presentation is the result of an external pathogen, diet, lifestyle, and stress that leads to *spleen deficiency.* The *spleen deficiency* results in *phlegm dampness* and sinking *Qi.* It also leads to *liver blood deficiency* and *liver Qi* and *blood stasis,* which in turn contribute to *phlegm dampness* and depressive *heat.* The *Source Qi* is drawn off from all of these injuries and the ministerial fire is damaged, leading to *Yin fire.* The *Yin fire* rises to the chest.[104] This is another vicious circle.

Heat from a *taiyin* condition rises to the upper body. *Heat* from a *yangming* condition expands. The pulse of *spleen Yin deficiency* is poorly defined. The *spleen* is about boundaries, whether they are physical or emotional.[105] When it is deficient in this way, there may be joint pain as well. The theory of this presentation is that *spleen deficiency* with *dampness* and *cold* is accompanied by simultaneous *heat.*

Points that are useful in treating this somewhat rare condition in the developed world are:

- Lu 10,
- Sj 5,
- Ht 4,
- Ht 7,

- St 25,
- Ren 12,
- Sp 13,
- Bl 17, 18, 20, 21, 25.

Herbal treatment strategies include several interventions:

- Tonify the *spleen* with warming *Qi* tonic herbs;
- Lift the *Yang* to suppress *Yin fire* with sweet but cool herbs;
- Clear *heat* using bitter and cold herbs;
- Address any other patterns that may be presenting;
- Use principles of treatment whenever possible in conjunction with evaluating the priorities of patterns and their severity.

Bu Pi Wei Xie Yin Huo Sheng Yang Tang:

Huang qi
Cang zhu
Qiang huo
Sheng ma
Ren shen
Huang qin
Huang lian
Shi gao

This formula tonifies the *spleen*, supports the *Source*, lifts the *Yang*, and clears *heat*. The amounts are left out because the specific severity of symptoms and patterns must be adjusted to suit the individual patient. This approach is directed toward the *middle Jiao*. If the deficiency and *heat* are addressed, the *lung* condition should resolve.

In children, the *lung* is the last functional organ orb to consolidate prior to birth. After birth the *middle Jiao* and especially the stomach/ *spleen* consolidate continuously up to the age of 7–9 years. Food is a very important part of this consolidation and what children are fed or are allowed to eat contributes to the consolidation of their digestive function. Children are often fed inappropriately, not in concert with their constitution, too much, and with foods that they are "allergic" to at the age of 4 but would not be allergic to at the age of 10.[106] Too much sugar is a major problem for children in the West. Reactions that lead to *spleen Yin deficiency* and this type of asthma in children are most often due to dietary mistakes made by parents. When these mistakes are compounded by poor air quality and lack of exercise, the result is severe asthma.[107]

Other formulas that address this presentation include:

- *Qing Zao Tang*;
- *Yang He Tang* — especially when *blood stasis* is a primary part of presentation;
- *Sheng Yang Yi wei tang* — especially for allergic asthma with externally contracted pathogen;
- *Yi Xue Zheng Chuan* — with binding *phlegm* and *Yin fire*.

Binding Phlegm

Wheezing as a symptom is recurrent, produces a sound called rales, manifests as short and fast distressed respiration, and may include the symptom of orthopnea. *Phlegm* is part of the root of all of those manifestations. The disease is in the *lungs* but in the long term the injury is also to the *spleen* and *kidneys*.[108] The disease transformation is at the *Qi level*. It may begin as an excess condition but ends as a deficiency condition. There may be deep-lying internal *phlegm* and this precipitates a pathogen. *Damp/phlegm* acts like a magnet for EPIs. Wheezing is due to internal obstruction of the *Qi*, an externally generated and ill-timed pathogenic contraction, and the presence of sticky consolidated *phlegm* in the chest. These three factors combine to obstruct the airways and produce wheezing.[109] When the patient is asymptomatic, the *Qi* and *Yin* are becoming deficient, and so are the *lung, spleen,* and *kidney*:

- The *lung Qi* is deficient and *Qi* is not transformed, and this leads to fluid and *turbid phlegm* accumulation;
- The *spleen Qi* is deficient and the transformation and transportation function is lost, and this leads to *phlegm*;
- The *kidney Qi* is deficient and this leads to essence deficiency, which results in loss of assimilation and absorption injury, which in turn leads to *phlegm*.

Therefore, when wheezing is not present, treatment is aimed at tonifying the normal *Qi* by tonifying the *lung Qi*, the *spleen Qi*, and the *kidney Qi*. When wheezing is present, treatment is aimed at regulating and tonifying the *lung Qi*.

Cold Phlegm

When wheezing occurs because of *binding phlegm* in the chest and becomes symptomatic due to contact with *cold*, use *She Gan Ma Huang Tang*.[110] The symptom picture is wheezing, chest distension, rales, a *cold* body sensation, aversion to *cold*, cough with a thin sputum, no thirst or a desire to drink only warm fluids, a tongue coating that is white and slimy, and a pulse that is wiry and forceless or wiry and forceful. Use moxa.

Hot Phlegm

When wheezing occurs in a *lung heat* pattern, the symptom presentation includes an elevated chest, wheezing and rough inhalation, rales, a red face and sweating, profuse thick sticky *phlegm*, thirst, and a tongue that is red with a slimy yellow coating as well as slippery and rapid. At this time use *Ding Chuan Tang*.[111] In addition, use Lu 5 and moistening techniques.

Lung Qi Deficiency with Phlegm

When the *lung Qi is deficient* with *phlegm* obstruction, the symptom presentation includes a white complexion, a phlegmatic sound in the throat, cold hands and feet with sweating on exertion or clammy extremities, shortness of breath, a pale tongue with a white coating, and a deep fine slippery pulse. *Su Zi Jiang Qi Tang*[112] treats this presentation. This pattern manifests as a tendency to catch colds. *Yu Ping Feng San*[113] with *Shen Ling Bai Zhu San*[114] can be used in combination.

Lung and Kidney Qi Deficiency with Phlegm

Longstanding patterns like these can result in incapacity of the *kidney* to grasp the *Qi*. There is rapid distressed respiration, shortness of breath, hard inhalation, a white complexion, the patient running cold, sore and weak low back and knees, a tongue that is pale and swollen, and a pulse that is sunken and fine. This is the time to use *You Gui Wan*[115] combined with *Shen Jie San*.

Cough and Phlegm

Cough is a common symptom of an EPI or internal injury. Either way the *phlegm* must be treated. To clear *phlegm*[116]:

- Regulate the *lung Qi*;
- Transform *phlegm*;
- Astringe the *Qi* of both the *lung* and the *kidney*.

Phlegm is differentiated according to consistency, color, and volume[117]:

- Thin white *phlegm* is due to *cold–damp*;
- Thick yellow *phlegm* is due to *wind–heat*;
- Transparent/clear *phlegm* with little volume can be due to either *heat* or cold; one must rely on the accompanying symptoms;
- *Phlegm* that is like drool but is still difficult to expectorate is usually due to *wind–heat* or food stagnation;

- Thick *phlegm* needs to be thinned in order to facilitate expectoration, so use moistening techniques;
- Thin *phlegm* usually produces a frequent cough; thickening it will reduce its volume and thus relieve the cough; to thicken it, use warming techniques with a warming needle or moxa.

A night cough is usually due to a *heat* pathogen or upward steaming of fire into the *lung* that scorches the *lung* fluids. The *lung Qi* becomes depressed and counterflows.

Cough can also be due to gastroesophageal reflux. This is called a food cough. There is thoracic fullness, sour reflux, feverishness, a tight abdomen, and thick *phlegm*. The tongue has a white coating. To treat this condition support the *spleen* to transform *phlegm*, regulate the *Qi* of the *middle Jiao*, and regulate the *Qi* of the *lung*. The best formula for this presentation is *Er Chen Tang*.[118]

A gallbladder cough usually accompanies spitting up bile. The pulse is wiry/slippery and the tongue has a white coating. This is not necessarily a *heat* or *damp–heat* condition. It is best treated with *Zhi Sou San*[118] or with *Xiao Chai Hu Tang*.[119]

A *heart* cough is accompanied by chest pain and a lump in the throat. *Zhi Sou San*[118] plus *niu bang zi* or *Liang Ge San*[112] plus *niu bang zi* are good approaches to this presentation.

It is important to remember that these patterns and relationships of health, pathology, and injury are in varying degrees applicable to all *lung* diseases. Although patterns are given for each condition, the mechanics of this information are relevant in almost all cases.

Chronic Bronchitis, Chronic Obstructive Pulmonary Disease, and Emphysema

Chronic bronchitis is defined as the presence of chronic cough with sputum production that occurs most days of the week for at least three months a year and for more than two consecutive years in the absence of other specific causes like asthma, bronchiectasis, and cystic fibrosis. Most patients who have only chronic bronchitis do not have airflow limitation. There is usually accompanying submucosal and mucosal edema and inflammation, and an increase in the size and number of submucosal lymph glands.[120]

Emphysema is defined as a permanent, abnormal air space enlargement that occurs distal to the terminal bronchiole, and includes destruction of the alveolar parenchymal tissue. Chronic obstructive pulmonary disease (COPD) and emphysema are linked. COPD typically develops in patients who have smoked more than 20 pack years, i.e. a pack of cigarettes per day for 20 years. There is cough with sputum production, dyspnea, and exercise limitations. This is accompanied by an increased respiratory rate, an increased diameter from front to back of the thoracic cavity, use of accessory respiratory muscles, prolonged exhalation, and bronchospasm. Treatment for emphysema and COPD is usually symptomatic to promote bronchodilation, decrease airway inflammation, and improve gas exchange.[121]

In emphysema and COPD, the patterns of *lung wilt* apply.[122] The term *"fei wei"* refers to the lobes of the *lungs* atrophying and ceasing to function. Atelectasis is a probable Western analog.[123] There are two etiologies for *lung* wilt:

(1) *Lung dryness* with fluid damage causes chronic cough, deficiency *fire* leads to wasting of the *lung* parenchymal tissue (the alveolae), and pathogenic *heat* damages the fluids.
(2) *Lung Qi* deficiency can end up damaging the *Yang*. *Deficiency heat lung wilt* also damages the *Yang*. *Lung* deficiency with cold *Qi* causes a failure to transform fluids, resulting in *lung* wilt.[124]

There are three criteria for classifying a chronic condition as *lung* wilt:

- The disease is longstanding and the whole body is deficient;
- There is coughing of turbid sputum with foamy spittle;
- The pulse is rapid.

General symptoms:

(1) *Respiratory*

- Expectoration of turbid sputum with foamy spittle;
- Thin and foamy drool, or thick and gluey drool that is white or streaked;
- There may or may not be cough but activity will cause shortness of breath and panting.

(2) *Generalized symptoms*

- The complexion is pale-white or green–blue;
- The body is emaciated, the spirit is low, and the mind is unclear;
- There are intermittent fevers and chills.

In this condition, there is deficiency of *Qi* and *Yin*. The disease develops slowly, with a protracted course that injures the *zheng Qi* and the body as a whole. It is important to differentiate deficiency *heat* from deficiency *cold*. In the *heat* syndrome, the *lung* fluids are dessicated and the fire is rising. In deficiency cold, there is a deficient-type chill in the *lung* and the *Qi* is unable to transform fluids. In terms of treatment[125]:

- *Deficiency heat lung wilt* — moisten *lung dryness*, generate *lung* fluids, and clear *lung heat*.
- *Deficiency cold lung wilt* — warm the *lungs*, tonify the *Qi*, and generate fluids.

Associated symptoms:

- In the deficiency *heat* pattern, the expectoration of drool and spittle that is thick and gluey is due to *heat* scorching the fluids and generating *phlegm*;
- A cough with blood-streaked *phlegm* in deficiency *heat* is due to fire scorching the *lung* network vessels;

- Fast breathing and panting in *Yin deficiency heat* is due to fire causing a counterflow *Qi*, making the *lungs* lose their descending function;
- Loss of voice, and dry mouth and throat are due to dry *heat* damaging the *lung* fluids;
- Afternoon tidal fever is due to *Yin deficiency heat*;
- Emaciation and skin dryness are both due to fluid damage in the *lungs* and stomach.

For the above symptoms in *Yin deficiency lung wilt*, use:

Mai Men Dong Tang[126]
or Qing Zao Fei Jiu Tang[127]

In the deficiency cold pattern, the associated symptoms include:

- Expectoration of clear thin spittle and drool is due to *lung Qi* deficiency with cold;
- The absence of cough and thirst is because there is no *Yin deficiency* or *Qi* flushing upward;
- Shortness of breath and panting is due to the *lung* losing its ability to govern the *Qi*;
- Lassitude, weakness, anorexia is due to *lung Qi deficiency*;
- A pale tongue and a weak pulse is due to *lung Qi deficiency* with cold.

For the above symptoms in *lung Qi* and cold-type *lung wilt*, use:

Gan Cao Gan Jiang Tang[126]

Lung wilt can be seen in the remission phases of chronic bronchitis and some other *lung* diseases of a chronic nature. It primarily damages the *lung Yin*. Treating the presentation as an unresolved EPI will exacerbate the condition. *Lung wilt* is a chronic and enduring disease that results from uncured previous conditions. However, in some cases it may be clinically efficacious to add a few exterior-releasing herbs to *Yin*-nourishing herbs to enhance their effect.

Although *lung wilt* is mainly a disease of interior *Yin deficiency heat*, it is also a *Qi-deficient* disease, and *Qi* tonic herbs should, be added, especially those that are neutral in temperature and contain moistening properties. The turbid spittle and drool in this pattern is due to *Yin deficiency heat* and should not be treated with *Yang* and warming herbs or *phlegm*-transforming herbs. Using these methods will cause any *phlegm* to thicken and become harder to expectorate. At the same time, clear *heat* herbs for the *lungs* should be used sparingly.

The following formula for *lung wilt*, which was designed as a modern formula by Wang Hai Zang, contains the listed herbs:

Zi wan 20 g
Chuan bei mu 12 g
Jie geng 12 g
Ren shen 30 g
Fu ling 15 g
Wu wei zi 15 g
Zhi mu 15 g
E Jiao 15 g
Xing ren 12 g
Gan cao 6 g

In intractable chronic *lung* conditions like *lung wilt*, it is possible to make the formula into a honey pill form for use over the long term. It is necessary to resolve the *phlegm* component of this presentation first. The patient may expectorate for a long time *phlegm* that has been lodged in the *lungs* for years. Once this has occurred the bronchioles and alveolae can recover to the extent possible (given the nature of the disease underlying *lung wilt*). In emphysema, the damage is quite permanent but whatever functional tissue remains will function better. In pulmonary tuberculosis, another cause of *lung wilt*, the *lungs* may almost fully recover. In chronic bronchitis caused by long-term smoking, the *lungs* can also recover but, as said before, vigilance is the key to permanent recovery.

It is important to remember the relationship between the *lung* and the heart, especially in chronic *lung* diseases.[128] If the *lung Qi* is deficient and is unable to gather the *Qi* in the heart vessels, the blood circulation will be weak. This results in *blood stasis* and symptoms like palpitations. If this condition continues it may result in depletion of the *kidney Source*, so that it is unable to warm and drive the *Qi* transformation process relating to water metabolism. Water *dampness* in the interior contributes to abdominal distension with water swelling and an incessant cough. The deficiency becomes a whole-body deficiency that allows pathogens to enter. Pulmonary *heart* patients have a chronic condition with often an acute disease overlaid. When *phlegm* drool and an external pathogen bind together, a life-threatening situation may evolve.

The presentation of pulmonary heart disease is a pattern of root and branch deficiency. Treatment is aimed at expelling the pathogen in the acute phase while simultaneously supporting the *zheng Qi*. During the chronic phase, the emphasis is on supporting the *zheng Qi* while simultaneously expelling pathogens. Although this sounds the same, the focus changes during each phase.

The treatment principles of *lung wilt* include:

- Warming the *Yang* and inhibiting water;
- Quickening the blood and transforming *stasis*;
- Transforming *phlegm* and keeping the bowels open;
- Supporting the *zheng Qi* and anchoring the *Source Qi*.

Chronic bronchitis usually occurs in older patients with generalized weakness. However, it can happen in younger patients who have been exposed continuously to materials that undermine *lung* health, the most common of which is smoke from cigarette use. People who smoke marijuana and cocaine are at risk, as are those who smoke tobacco. Marijuana, if at all, is best eaten and not smoked. Cocaine is best eliminated altogether, since it has no life-giving characteristic. The *zheng Qi* becomes depleted due to these exposures and then the condition recurs, which reinjures the *zheng*

Qi. If the *lung Qi* and *Yin* is depleted, then the *lungs* lose their capacity to govern the *Qi*. If the *kidney* function is also injured, then the *kidneys* lose their capacity to absorb the *Qi*. In this way, another vicious circle of Chinese medicine evolves.

When an EPI is contracted, the *lung Qi* counterflows, resulting in cough, shortness of breath, and wheezing. The *lungs* also control the hundred vessels, and when the *lung Qi* is deficient there is no strength to move the blood. The smooth movement of the blood is lost, which results in the inhibition of *Qi* movement and then the *lung Qi* flushing upward. This manifests as cough, wheezing, shortness of breath with dull lips and tongue body, or even outright cyanosis. These symptoms are the result of stasis. This is yet again another vicious circle of injury that feeds on itself and worsens the original injury.[129]

In bronchitis, the disease is in the *lungs* but the etiology is in the *lungs* and *kidneys*. Therefore, treatment is aimed at treating the root by banking the fire of the *kidney*, opening the network vessels, and regulating the *Qi* of the *lungs* to stop cough and wheezing. With each cough and wheeze *Qi* is lost.

The *Yin* and *Yang* need to be secured and anchored. The *Yang* should reside at the *Source*. If the *Yang Qi* is not secured and is deficient, it can float to the surface. This is like a forest fire that has crowned; the fire is of the top of the trees and there is only smoldering smoke on the ground, with no fire. Unsecured *Yang* ascends and deserts the *Yin*. This is not due to *Yin deficiency* but *Yang deficiency*. The result produces asthmatic counterflow, spontaneous perspiration, or clammy skin. The pulse is floating or superficial but is not due to an EPI or *Yin* deficiency. The *Yin*, which is sinking downward, causes urinary incontinence if the *Yin* and *Yang* are both deficient.

Just as in asthma, it is common to have a chronic condition with an acute EPI on top of it. This is especially true in *Yang deficiency* and in winter, for obvious reasons. Treatment in summer is especially helpful in treating is root and preventing winter EPIs. When there is an acute condition overlying chronic bronchitis, treat the EPI primarily. To do this, rely on your evaluation of the strength of the pathogen versus the strength of the normal *Qi*. In deficiency patterns of any kind, one must rely on the normal *Qi* to push out the pathogen.

In many ways, chronic bronchitis is a precursor of *lung wilt* not caused by infectious diseases. People with chronic bronchitis should be treated with the goal of cure. Treating these conditions is very important, because they are considered to be risk factors for lung cancer.[130] These last conditions are on a continuum that has the capacity to evolve into the serious condition of cancer.

Rules of treatment[131]

- Alleviate acute symptoms or life-threatening symptoms first — treat cough, wheezing, and shortness of breath;
- In weak patients, treat the symptom picture and the root simultaneously;
- If the EPI is weak, and the patient's *zheng Qi* is also weak, tonify the *zheng Qi* to disperse the pathogen;
- If the normal *Qi* is weak and the pathogen is strong, eliminate the pathogen as best you can without harming the *zheng qi*;
- If the EPI is strong and the *zheng Qi* is also strong, disperse the pathogen;
- In chronic bronchitis or emphysema combined with an acute infection where antibiotics alone or Chinese medicine alone has proven ineffective and the condition lingers, use methods to absorb the *Qi* and boost the *kidneys* first; then use methods to eliminate the pathogen and transform *phlegm*.

The following formula for tonifying the *lungs* and *kidneys* in the treatment of chronic bronchitis is a modern intervention:

Fu zi
Rou gui
Sheng di
Shu di

Huang qi
Wu wei zi
Tao ren
Di long
Dang gui
Bai jie zi
Lai fu zi

The herb amounts are not given in the journal article by Peng Tao, from the *Beijing Journal of Chinese Medicine*, Vol. 4, p. 36 (1995). The primary methods used include tonifying the *lungs* and *kidneys*, transforming stasis, and freeing the network vessels.

There are several individual herbs that some practitioners feel are important for securing *Yin* and *Yang*. *Long gu* and *mu li* act to anchor *Yin* and *Yang* and rescue both. When these herbs are combined with *shan zhu yu*, they act to astringe the *Yin* and *Yang* and thereby help the *kidney Qi* to absorb *Qi*. The use of these mineral herbs also helps to settle flushing *stomach Qi*, which sometimes will in turn cause the *lung Qi* to flush upward. Strangely, *long gu* and *mu li* also transform *phlegm* — a great advantage in the treatment of *lung* patterns.

Conclusion

These patterns of injury can be preconditions for lung cancer. They are important to treat and be vigilant about. Usually, lung cancer sneaks up on patients when it is in a very late stage. This is partially because there are no early screening tools for lung cancer, even though it kills more people than all other cancers combined. The supposedly asymptomatic nature of lung cancer is in fact not asymptomatic; the symptoms have been present for many years but people engaged in addictive behaviors often become habituated to the negatives of that behavior. A dry throat and chronic unproductive cough are almost always present, even after smoking for only 3–5 years. Shortness of breath on exertion is also present and a loss of fitness may accompany shortness of breath. A propensity for allergic responses and asthma may signify a deeper-level lung injury that requires evaluation. A very careful and in-depth intake and evaluation must be done for any person who has ever smoked, even if it was long ago. Twenty percent of lung cancer patients have no history of smoking. The research evidence is mounting that air quality and airborne exposures are ubiquitous and are risks for lung cancer.

Patients who present with any lung symptoms, even if they are in their 30s or 40s, need to be evaluated for serious lung pathology, including cancer. And those patients diagnosed with lung cancer who have no history of risk require an in-depth evaluation all the way back to childhood to help determine possible injuries that may have contributed to their diagnosis.

The lung is a common site for metastatic spread from other primary cancers. This is especially true in breast and colorectal cancers. Younger people are being diagnosed with these cancers, and a thorough examination of their overall status is important, including referral to other providers. Patients who present with lung symptoms may actually have a primary cancer that has metastasized to the lung whose symptoms are their first indicator of a cancer. Often, patients see Chinese medicine health providers more frequently than they see their conventional medical providers. Our role can be expanded to include monitoring for more serious diseases, like cancer.

Lung cancer patients and those at risk for lung cancer should eat a low-fat, high-fiber, mostly vegetarian diet. Organic foods limit the exposures a person will encounter. Hormone-free meats and grass-fed beef are higher in omega-3s and are more healthy generally. There is an inverse relationship between vegetarian diets and cancer. Lignan and omega-3 components in fiber foods have demonstrated anticancer effects. Improving transit time for stools reduces colonic mucosa exposure to carcinogens and improves the overall health of not just the colon but also the lungs.

The EPA states that approximately 90% of fungicides, 60% of herbicides, and 30% of insecticides are potentially carcinogenic.[132]

Soy, green tea, garlic, and many mushrooms are good cancer prevention foods. Soy inhibits angiogenesis, a primary means by which tumors access a blood supply so that they can grow.[133] Green tea contains polyphenols, which, like catechin, are potent antioxidants. It inhibits chemically induced tumors of the lung, large intestine, liver, and breast.[134] Garlic inhibits lipo-oxygenase and is a free radical scavenger. It enhances macrophage activity and NK cell activity via TNF and alpha interferon.[135]

Maitake, shiitake, and reishi mushrooms are all approved therapies in Japan for cancer treatment. Many mushrooms contain high-molecular-weight polysaccharides, which stimulate immune responsiveness.[136]

Astragalus is also a major component in many lung cancer formulas in China. *Huang Qi* stimulaes NK cell activity.[137] And *Panax ginseng* has broad effects that improve *lung* function and immune activity.[138] There are many sources available for referencing in treating lung cancers with integrated conventional and Chinese medicine.

Antioxidants are very valuable for preventing lung cancer:

Vitamin C: 1000–3000 mg daily
Vitamin E: 400 IU daily
Selenium: 100 mcg daily

There are many lung conditions that are better treated with Chinese medicine than with any other form of medicine, including conventional medicine. One important reason is that these therapies do not require the use of steroidal pharmaceuticals, an approach that reduces symptomatic reactions but does not treat the cause, and does this at a cost to the immune system that is high. It is important to treat these conditions and diseases, not suppress the symptoms of these diseases. It is most important to help patients quit smoking. However, about 20% of lung cancers of all types occur in people with no smoking history or history of second-hand smoke. The contamination of our environment, outside and inside, is a major health issue. Working to treat the conditions that arise from these contaminants is as important as helping people to quit smoking. Protecting our environment from airborne contaminants is the best of all cures. This means that we must work personally and publicly to change our own behaviors, teach our patients why and how they must change theirs through driving less and shopping knowledgeably, rearranging their homes to include only items that are green, and working within our communities to change old laws, make new ones, and enforce laws that eliminate air pollution.

References

1. SEER Cancer Statistics Review 1975–2009. National Cancer Institute. www.seer.cancer.gov/csr/1975_2009_pops09/browse_csr.php
2. Mahick CG *et al*. Pap smear screening and changes in cervical cancer mortality. www.ncbi.nlm.nih.gov/pubmed/7909766
3. www.globocan.larc.tf/factsheets/cancers/cervix.asp
4. www.who.int/mediacentre/factsheets/fs297/en
5. www.nytimes.com/nytimes/healthprofessional-criticize-us-tobacco-export-policy.html
6. www.cancer.gov/cancertopics/tobacco/smoking
7. Guide to Quitting Smoking. www.cancer.org/healthy/stayawayfrom-tobacco/guidetoquittingsmoking/guide
8. www.justice.gov/tobacco2/williamfaronephdversusphilipmorris
9. Barnova J, Glantz SA. The tobacco industry and secondhand smoke: lessons from Central and South America. www.ncbi.nim.nih.gov/pubmed/13677420
10. Landman A. (2009) Deadly deception: The tobacco industry's secondhand smoke cover up. The Center for Media and Democracy's PR Watch. Jan 7.
11. National Cancer Institute. Secondhand smoke and cancer. cancer.gov/cancertopics/factsheet/tobacco/ets
12. www.cdc.gov/tobacco/youth/index.html
13. www.who.int/toh
14. CDC. Best Practices User Guide: Youth Engagement — State and Community Intervention. www.cdc.gov/tobacco
15. Tobacco Control Legal Consortium. Public Health Law Center. www.publichealthlawcenter.org/programs/tobacco-control-legal-consortium
16. Eldridge L. (2012) Lung cancer in non-smokers. About.com. Lung Cancer. Apr. 3.

17. Alberg AJ *et al.* (2005) Epidemiology of lung cancer: Looking at the future. *Clin Oncol* **23(14)**:3175–3185.

18. www.watchnews.org/2011/11/16/7406/why-americans-still-breathe-known-hazards-decades-after-clean-air-law

19. Le Coq C. Air pollution costs Europe billions — report. www.in.reuters.com/assets/print?aid-INindia-60705720111124

20. Global Atmospheric Pollution Forum. Policy Briefs. Effects on human health. www.sei-international.org/gapforum/policy/effectshuman-health.php

21. www.epa.gov/lawsregs/regulation/cleanairact

22. Finlayson-Pitts BJ *et al.* University of California at Irvine study on non-equilibrium atmospheric secondary organic aerosol formation and growth. *Proc Natl Acad Sci.* www.pnas.org/content/early/2012/01/24/1119909109

23. Sources of pollution in the ambient air. www.epa.gov/apti/course422/ap3a.html

24. Oberdorster G. (2001) Pulmonary effects of inhaled ultrafine particles. *Int Arch Occup Environ Health.* **74(1)**:1–8.

25. World Health Organization. Air quality and health. www.who.int/mediacentre/factsheets/s313/en/index.html

26. www.epa.gov/glo/basic.html

27. www.epa.gov/glo/health.html

28. www.nlm.nih.gov/medlineplus/indoorairpollution.html

29. www.epa.gov/iaq/1a-intro.html

30. www.osha.gov/publications/osha3144.html

31. www.atsdr.cdc.gov/toxfaqs/tf.asp?id=38&tid=14

32. www.epa.gov/chemfact/f_perchl.txt

33. 9/11 first responders plagued by health problems from toxic dust and debris. www.abcnews.com/health/wellness/911-responders-plaugued-cancer-asthma-pstd/

34. www.epa.gov/iaq/pesticid.html

35. www.npic.orst.edu

36. www.gdrc.org/u-gov/precaution-4.html

37. EU view of precautionary principle in food safety. www.eurunion.org/news/speeches/2003/031023tvdh.htm Tony Vanderhaegen.

38. www.epa.gov/asbestos

39. www.cancer.gov/cancertopics/factsheet/asbestos

40. Davies M *et al.* A review of evidence linking ventilation rates in dwellings and respiratory health. www.discovery.ucl.ac.uk/2256/1/Microsoft_word_a-review-of-evidence.pdf

41. Technology Fact Sheet. Whole-house ventilation systems. Improved control of air quality. www.ornl.gov/sci/roof+walls/insulation/fact%20sheets/whole%20house%20ventilation

42. Reducing your exposure to PBDEs in your home. www.ewg.org/pbdefree

43. Design for the environment. Spray polyurethane foam (SPF) home. www.epa.gov/dfe/pubs/projects/spf/spray_polyurethane_faom.html

44. Warner, J. Is that "new car smell" toxic? www.men.webmd.com/news/20120215/is-that-new-car-smell-toxic

45. Toxic at any speed: Chemicals in cars and the need for safe alternatives. Ecology Center. www.ecocenter.org/healthy-stuff/toxic-any-speed-chemicals-cars-and -need-safe-alternatives

46. Fire retardants in toddlers and their mothers: Government and industry actions to phase out PBDEs. www.ewg.org/reports/pbdesintoddlers/govermentand%20industrytophaseoutpbdes

47. PBDEs — toxic flame retardants. watoxics.org/chemicals-of-concern/toxic-flame-retardants-pbdes

48. The burden of children's asthma: What asthma costs nationally, locally, and personally. www.pediatricasthma.org/about/asthma_burden

49. Rabinoff M *et al.* (2007) Pharmacological and chemical effects of cigarette additives. *Am J Publ Health* **97(11)**:1981–1991.

50. Unschuld P. (2003) *Huang Di Nei Jing Su Wen: Complete Translation. Five Phase Theory.* University of California Press.

51. Larre C, Rochat E. (1996) *Seven Emotions.* Monkey.

52. Rochat E, Wu X. (2009) *The Five Elements in Classical Chinese Texts.* Monkey.

53. Wiseman N, Ellis A. (1997) *Fundamentals of Chinese Chinese.* Paradigm.

54. Boisoert M. Depression when you quit smoking. About.com. www.quitsmoking.com/content/quitting-smoking-causes-constipation

56. Zhao JY. (2011) *Atlas of Blood and Qi Disorders in Chinese Medicine*. Eastland.

57. Zhang ZJ. (2009) *Jing Gui Yao Lue (Essentials from the Golden Cabinet)*. Translated by Wiseman N, Wilms S, Fang Y. Paradigm.

58. Koei K. (1996–1997) Notes from lectures on Toyo Hari acupuncture training.

59. Marijuana. Science-based information for the public. University of Washington Alcohol and Drug Abuse Institute. www.adai.uw.edu/marijuana/factsheets/respiratoryeffects.htm

60. American Cancer Society. Guide to Quitting Smoking. When smokers quit — what are the benefits over time? www.cancer.org/healthy/stayawayfrotobacco/guidetoquittingsmoking/guide-to

61. Larre C, Rochat E. (1989) *Lungs*. Monkey.

62. Clavey S. (1995) *Fluid Physiology and Pathology in Traditional Chinese Medicine*. Churchill Livingstone.

63. Neeb G. (2007) *Blood Stasis: China's Classical Concept in Modern Medicine*. Churchill Livingstone.

64. Yan SL. (2012) *Pathomechanisms of the Lung*. Paradigm.

65. Becker S *et al.* (2010) *Treatment of Cardiovascular Diseases with Chinese Medicine*. Blue Poppy.

66. Yan DX. (1999) *Aging and Blood Stasis*. Blue Poppy.

67. Scott J, Barlow T. (1999) *Acupuncture in the Treatment of Children*, 3rd ed. Eastland

68. What is global-warming? Allergies. National Wildlife Federation. www.nwf.org/global-warming/what-is-global-warming/global-warming-is-causing-allergies

69. Liu WS. (2007) *COPD and Asthma*. People's Medical Publishing House.

70. *Op. cit.*, No. 62, pp. 166–169, 181.

71. *Ibid.*, p. 183.

72. Zhu CB. (1984) *Zhong Yi Tan Bing Xue (Traditional Chinese Medicine Phlegm Disease Studies)*. Hubei Science and Technology Press.

73. Asthma. Bronchial asthma; exercise-induced asthma. PubMed Health. www.ncbi.nim.nih.gov/pubmedhealth/PMH0001196

74. Asthma and Allergy Foundation of America. Asthma facts and figures. www.aafa.org/display.cfm?id-8&sub=42

75. New York City Government. 9/11 Health. What we know from the research. www.nyc.gov/html/doh/wtc/html/rescue/know.html

76. Asthma treatment. Information on asthma and asthma management. Early onset asthma. www.wordpress.healasthma.com/early-onset-asthma-and-late-onset-asthma

77. Halken S. (2004) Prevention of allergic disease in childhood: Clinical and epidemiological aspects of primary and secondary allergy prevention. *Pediatr Allergy Immunol* **15(Suppl16)**: 4–5,9–32.

78. NOAA. Understanding air quality. www.researchnoaa.gov/weather/_understanding.html

79. Simpson S. Loss of city trees costs billions. Discovery News. www.news.discovery.com/earth/us-urban-areas-losing-4-million-trees-per-year

80. National Geographic. Deforestation. www.environment.national-geographic.com/environment/global-warming/deforestation

81. Asthma and Allergy Foundation of America. Adult onset asthma. www.aafa.org/display.cfm?id=8&sub=17&cont=157

82. National Heart, Lung, Blood Institute. What are lung function tests? www.nhlbi.nih.gov/health/health-topics/topics/lft

83. WebMD. Asthma Health Center. Asthma medications. www.webmd.com/asthma/guide/medications

84. Mayo Clinic. Prednisone and other corticosteroids: Balance the risks and benefits. www.,ayoclinic.com/health/steroids/HQ01431

85. Matsumoto K. Notes from lectures.

86. Manaka Y. Shinkyu no Riron to Kangaikata.

87. Hoppenfeld S. (1976) *Physical Examination of the Spine and Extremities.* Prentice Hall.

88. Matsumto K. Notes from lectures on meridian therapy.

89. Kuahara K. Notes from lectures on Toyo Hari.

90. *Ibid.*

91. *Dan Xi Xin Fa (Teachings of Dan Xi).* 1481 C.E. Experiences in the treatment of phlegm. Private translations.

92. Zhao JY, Li XM. (1998) *Patterns and Practice in Chinese Medicine.* Eastland.

93. Maclean W *et al.* (1998) *Lung, Kidney, Liver, Heart.* Clinical Handbook of Internal Medicine Series, Vol. 1. University of Western Sydney.

94. Scheid V *et al.* (2003) *Formulas and Strategies*, 2nd ed. Eastland.

95. *Op. cit.*, No. 70, p. 183.

96. *Ibid.*, p. 193.

97. Mao H. (1982) *Han Shi Yi Tong (Comprehensive Medicine According to Master Han)*. 1522. C.E. Jiangsu Science and Technology Press.

98. Ma SC. Lecture notes on lung disorders.

99. Health scout. Health Encyclopedia. Bronchospasm. www.health-scout.com/ency/1/591/main.html

100. Kodo F. (1991) *Meridian Therapy*. Toyo Hari Medical Association.

101. Li PW. (1995–1996) Beijing From lectures notes on treating lung cancer.

102. Zhang ZJ. (2008) *Jing Gui Yao Lues (Essentials from the Golden Cabinet)*. Translated by Wisemann N, Wilms S, Fang Y. Paradigm.

102A. Kuahara, K. Notes on spleen patterns.

103. Kuahara K. (2001) From lecture notes on Toyo Hari: spleen and lung relationships.

104. Yan SL. (2011) *Pathomechanisms of the Lung*. Paradigm.

105. Larre C, Rochat E. (1990) *Spleen and Stomach*. Monkey.

106. Scott J. (1990) *Natural Medicine for Children*. Harper.

107. Science News. Imbalanced diet and inadequate exercise may underlie asthma in children. *Science Daily*, Sep. 19, 2010. www.sciencedaily.com/releases/2010/09/10091612134.htm

108. Clavey S. (1995) *Fluid Physiology and Pathology in Traditional Chinese Medicine*. Churchill Livingstone, pp. 193–194.

109. Zhu CB. (1984) *Zhong Yi Tan Bing Xue (Study of TCM Phlegm Disease)*. Hubei Science and Technology Press.

110. *Op. cit.* No. 102.

111. Wu M. (1990) *Fu Shou Jing Fang (Exquisite Formulas for Fostering Longevity)*. 1530 C.E. In *Formulas and Strategies*. Eastland, p. 300.

112. Chen SW ed. *Tai Ping Hui Min He Ji Ju Tang (Imperial Grace Formulary of the Tai Ping Era)*. 1107 C.E. In *Formulas and Strategies*. Eastland, p. 299.

113. Zhu DX (1985) *Dan Xi Xin Fa (Teachings of Zhu Dan Xi)*. 1481 C.E. *Essentials from the Teachings of Zhu Dan Xi*. Shandong Science and Technology Press.

114. Wang A. (1981) *Xi Fang Ji Jie (Analytic Collection of Medical Formulas)*. 1682 C.E. *Essentials from the Analytic Collection of Formulas*, Hu YJ, ed. Chao Ren.

115. Zhang JY. (1959) *Jing Yue Guan Shu (Collected Treatises of Zhang Jing Yue)*. 1624 C.E. Shanghai Science and Technology Press.

116. Wiseman N, Ellis A. (1995) *Fundamentals of Chinese Medicine.* Paradigm.

117. MS. Lecture notes.

117B. *Op. cit.*, No. 112, p. 432.

118. Cheng GP. (1982) *Yi Xue Xin Wu (Medical Revelations)*. 1732 C.E. People's Health Publishing, Beijing, p. 446,

119. Zhang ZJ. *Shang Han Za Bing Lun (Treatise on Injury by Cold)*. 210 C.E. Many translations available.

120. PubMed Health. COPD. www.ncbi.nim.nih.gov/pubmedhealth/ PMH0001153

121. www.nhlbi.nih.gov/health/health-topics/copd

122. Wiseman N. (1998) *A Practical Dictionary of Chinese Medicine.* Paradigm, p. 379.

123. Medline Plus. Atelectasis. www. nlm.nih.gov/medlineplus/ency/ article.000065.htm

124. Liu WS. (2007) *COPD and Asthma*. People's Medical Publishing House.

125. Ma SC. Lecture notes.

126. *Op. cit.*, No. 102.

127. Yu C. (1983) *Yi Men Fa Lu (Precepts for Physicians)*. 1658 C.E. Shanghai Science and Technology Press.

128. Hou JL, (ed.). (1995) *Traditional Chinese Treatment for Cardiovascular Diseases*. Academy Press.

129. Huang FM, Shou ZY. (1994) *Jia Yi Fang (Systematic Classic of Acupuncture and Moxibustion)*, 1st ed. Blue Poppy.

130. Koshiol J *et al.* COPD and altered risk of lung cancer in a population-based control study www.dceq.cancer.gov

131. Ma SC. Lecture notes.

132. Pesticides: Health and safety. www.epa.gov/pesticides/health/ human.htm

133. Su SJ *et al.* (2005) The novel targets for anti-angiogenesis of genistein on human cancer cells. *Biochem Pharmacol* **69(2)**: 307–318.

134. Yang C.S. and Wang, X. Green tea and cancer prevention. *Nutr Cancer* 2010;**62(7)**:931–937.
135. National Cancer Institute. Garlic and cancer prevention. www.cancer.gov/cancertopics/factsheet/prevention/garlic-and-cancer-prevention
136. Burchers AJ *et al.* (2004) Mushrooms, tumors, and immunity: An update. *Exp Biol Med* **229(5)**: 393–406.
137. Mandy MY *et al.* Astragalus saponins induce growth inhibition and apoptosis in human colon cancer cells and tumor xenograft. www.carcin.oxfordjournals.org/content/28/6/1347.full
138. Shin HR *et al.* (2000) The cancer-preventive potential of *Panax ginseng*: A review of human and experimental evidence. *Canc Causes Contr* **11(6)**:565–576.

CHAPTER 3

Earth — Colorectal Cancer

> An agrarian economy rises up from the fields, woods, and streams — from the complex of soils, slopes, weathers, connections, influences, and exchanges that we mean when we speak, for example, of the local community or the local watershed. The agrarian mind is therefore not regional or national, let alone global, but local. It must know on intimate terms the local plants and animals and local soils; it must know local possibilities and impossibilities, opportunities and hazards. It depends and insists on knowing very particular local histories and biographies.
>
> *Wendell Berry — "The Whole Horse"* (included in The Art of the Commonplace: The Agrarian Essays of Wendell Berry).

Introduction

Food, shelter, clean air and water, and community are considered basics of human life. These essentials contain in cellular memory a primary emotion that really has no descriptive. Without these basic needs met, peace, within and outside of us, is not possible. In the 20th century, 250 wars were fought on our planet; and food, clean water, shelter, and community were the subjects of those wars or were lost for those people who were or remain victims of them. It is usually women and children who die and suffer the most from this strife. According to the United Nations, 80% of all deaths in wars occur in women and children; 90% of all refugees are women; and women are signatories to peace treaties only 3% of the time.[1]

It would seem that we are in a global crisis of masculinity. Wars, after all, have been mainly masculine-driven events. And they are usually about resources, beliefs, power, and control. The disenfranchised males of our world, especially young men, are at war with poverty and the loss of the right to a fulfilled life and the positive power that comes from it. Rage seems to be the primary content on the ground driving many of these wars. Rage over past wrongs, killing for revenge and for killing's sake, raping and pillaging, and rioting are all extreme acts of anger, rage, and powerlessness. Poison to treat poison.

For those who are in power, wars remain a means of maintaining and increasing that power, selling a way of life, and accruing more resources to control life. Who is going to be at the top of the heap and, therefore, have the most right to live? The affluent controllers of power and resources are also expressing the crisis in masculinity through short-sighted, greed-driven, violent acts of narcissism against others and the natural world; abuse of wealth, corruption, economic enslavement, noncompassion, and insecurity are all manifestations of a split between heart and mind, between the wisdom of truth and linear one-sided knowledge that has no relationship to anything but itself.

These blood-spilling wars are blunt and obvious wars pitting starvation against gluttony, and poverty against power. But there are other "blood-spilling" wars that are taking place concurrently and are deeply connected with activities of human life. They are also making the news in the form of global climate change, loss of species, epidemics like AIDS, the crumbling of sub-Saharan Africa, globalization based only on the rights of corporations, the ownership of knowledge, even the ownership of the blueprint of life. Even the weapons of war have been extended, through chemical inputs, into the war against nature commonly called agribusiness and corporate individualism. All of these wars are in part crises of masculinity. But the reference is not to maleness or men. It is to the loss of true fulfilled masculinity and the male expression of initiative within all of us, of the clear and bright *Yang* nature of hope-filled initiative, to the south side of the mountain and the sun, to ethics and what is right, to the ability and capacity to see the larger picture and the future and, most importantly, care about it.[2] This crisis affects men but is not limited to men. It is a crisis for all of us and is not about gender. It is about a balance based on living not from our minds as the first source of truth but from our hearts as the foundation for true living that causes no harm to us or to any generations to come, including the generations of flora and fauna — and what has become known, in the face of the largest cultural psychic split known to date, as the natural world.[3] It is about the balance between *Yin* and *Yang*.

In our world, the tremendous loss of habitat for species other than our own is a silent war mirrored by loss of diversity.[4-6] This loss is expressed even in our food crops and occurs for the same reasons that wars do. Something is being stolen, sold, destroyed, overlooked, or eliminated because of the beliefs and actions of usually a small group of people who will benefit but who are encouraged by a larger community in denial. It may seem odd to juxtapose the loss of humanity through war with the loss of plants and food crops but the basis and mindset for this loss is the same — power and greed. Although we have more food availability, we simultaneously have fewer choices than 100 years ago.

The loss of food crops immensely affects human life. Changes in agriculture and the resulting food crops that are now being produced are having an effect on the quality of human and environmental health through loss of topsoil, loss of groundwater, loss of biodiversity, contamination of soils, air and water, and poorer quality foods and pseudofoods with lower or no nutritional value.[7-9] This says nothing about the loss of the Commons — for everyone and for indigenous peoples who have lived from the land and as part of the land for millennia.[10] And if we think of the Commons in terms of air, water, Earth, and biodiversity, then all of us suffer from the loss of the Commons as a free and clean environment. We have lost a part of ourselves.

In terms of modern processed foods, the Western world today is relegated by monocultural industrial agriculture to corn, wheat, rice, and potatoes and the foods made from these crops; and the varieties of these four food crops are far more limited than they were at the turn of the last century.[11,12] Modern wheat contains about 4% protein. The wheat found in the tombs of the pharaohs contains 18% protein.[13] The onslaught of genetically engineered food crops, like Roundup Ready corn and soy, uses the land as a holding area for huge acreages of the same crop grown not by healthy living soil but by synthetic inputs, most of which are petroleum-based. These changes in agriculture and the resulting food crops[14] that come from it are having an effect on the quality of human and environmental health[15] not unlike the changes caused by the ravages of wars, albeit more long-term and more subtle.

For more than 12,000 years, farmers have selected seeds from better-performing crops, thus encouraging the development of thousands of individual seed varieties in different ecosystems and geographies throughout the world. These diverse seeds have special critical characteristics that confer pest and disease resistance, drought tolerance, and nutrient content.[16] The local farmers of areas around the world know how to foster a healthy and diverse world of edible plants specific to their area. These seed stocks and the people who embody the knowledge of them are no longer valued, respected, or treasured, not because they are no longer necessary but because we have been misinformed.

After World War II, distribution of hybrid seeds with their accompanying reliance on fertilizers, pesticides, herbicides, and more water than indigenous crops, all exports of the West, became a worldwide phenomenon as a result of global interests, mainly from the United States, forcing the industrial way of farming onto our own and other nations' farmers. Using struggling governmental entities in the Third World as a driving force, farmers were given no choice in this burgeoning of new technology. Traditional farming practices gave way to monoculture and mechanization, what is known as agribusiness or industrial farming, because governments were duped into thinking that this way of growing food was "progress."[17,18] This way of farming, along with other factors, has forced many people from their land because the hybrid seed is expensive and must be bought on a yearly basis, unlike the seeds they have traditionally saved from year to year, because the required irrigation water is too expensive to buy, because the necessary petroleum-based fertilizers and other inputs to grow this seed are too expensive to buy, and because the land they once either owned or farmed as a part of centuries of family practice in the Commons is now owned by "larger interests."[19] This has left more and more corporations on the land in developing and developed countries as opposed to the farmers who had farmed that land for centuries — a new form of imperialism.[20,21,22] The story of the European way of life and colonization of the world with this way of life continues now into the 21st century.

A related form of colonialism is the phenomenon of biopiracy through which Western corporations are stealing centuries of collective knowledge and innovation evolved by primarily Third World peoples.[23] It is now ubiquitous across the world. Basmati rice is an example. A US corporation called RiceTec has claimed that basmati rice is "an instant invention of a novel rice line" developed by them. In fact, basmati rice has been cultivated and developed in India for centuries by women farmers who view this effort to patent centuries of communal work as theft.[24] The stealing and patenting of the pesticide and fungicide uses of the neem tree by WR Grace Company is another good example.[25] RiceTec lost their bid to patent basmati rice. The Indian farmers with the Indian government behind them fought back and won. WR Grace lost a similar patent battle.

Women have been the seed-keepers and seed-breeders over millennia. The basmati is just one among 100,000 varieties of rice evolved by Indian women farmers. Diversity and a perennial nature in all natural societies is the culture of the seed.[26] And worldwide annual festivals rejuvenate the duty of saving and sharing seed among farming communities. This establishes partnership among farmers and with the Earth. Intellectual property rights (IPR), however, are criminalizing this duty to the Earth and to each other by making seed saving and seed exchange illegal through patenting the seed under IPR law.[27,28] And it is not only IPR that is attempting to prevent farmers from saving seed but also new genetic engineering technologies. Monsanto and the USDA have established a new partnership through a jointly held patent to seed which has been genetically engineered to ensure that it does not germinate on harvest, thus forcing farmers to buy seed at each planting season.[29] Termination of germination is a means of capital accumulation and market expansion. As abundance in nature and for farmers shrinks, markets grow for Monsanto.

The most widespread application of genetic engineering (GE) in agriculture is herbicide resistance. Monsanto's Roundup Ready soya and cotton are examples. These applications to soy and cotton have led to an increased use of agrichemicals, thus increasing environmental problems.[30] This GE also destroys the biodiversity that is the sustenance and livelihood base of many Third World rural women, because what are weeds for Monsanto are food, fodder, and medicine for Third World women. The spread of Roundup Ready crops would destroy diversity.[31] It would also undermine the soil conservation functions of cover crops and crop mixtures, thus leading to soil erosion.

The biotech industry states that without GE, the world cannot be fed. However, while biotechnology is projected to increase food production by four times the current levels, small ecological farms have productivity hundreds of times higher than that of large industrial farms.[32] And the costs of industrial agriculture when "external costs" are included far exceed those of sustainable and ecological farming because of increased use of water, petroleum-based inputs, pollution, contamination of the soil and water and air, costs of shipping to distant markets, and reduced quality of the food produced leading to less healthy foods, just to name a few.[33–35]

In the Third World, women provide the basis of food security, and they provide food security in partnership with other species. The partnership between women and biodiversity has kept the world fed through history and in present times, and will feed the world in the future.[36] It is this partnership that needs to be preserved and promoted to ensure food safety. Agriculture based on diversity, decentralization, and improving small-farm productivity through ecological methods is human-centered and nature-friendly agriculture. Knowledge is shared, other species and plants are kin, not property, and sustainability is based on renewal of the Earth's fertility and on renewal and regeneration of biodiversity and species richness on farms in order to provide internal (not external) inputs. There is no place for monocultures of genetically engineered crops and IPR monopolies on seeds.

These monocultures and monopolies symbolize a masculinization of agriculture,[37] especially in the Third World and down through history where farming is and has been traditionally women's work. The masculine war mentality underlying military–industrial agriculture is evident from the names given to herbicides. Monsanto's herbicides are called "Round up," "Machete," "Lasso," "Pentagon," "Prowl," "Squadron," "Avenge." This is the language of war and not of sustainability. Sustainability is based on peace with the Earth. These monocultures and monopolies are emblematic of the split between mind and heart, science and meaning, male and female, and the split of humanity from nature — the loss of the *Yin* and receptive in all of us.

The violence intrinsic to methods and metaphors used by the global agribusiness and biotechnology corporations is violence against nature's biodiversity and women's expertise and productivity in the First and the Third World. Any violence toward women is violence toward the natural world and vice versa. This violence toward women including the receptivity of the natural world is perhaps the final injury that must be transformed and healed in the 21st century. The violence intrinsic to the destruction of diversity through monocultures and the destruction of the freedom to save and exchange seeds through IPR monopolies is inconsistent with women's and the diverse nonviolent ways of knowing nature and providing food security. This diversity of food systems and production systems is the way forward. GE and IPR rob the world of creativity, innovation, and decision-making power in agriculture. This in turn robs us all of the right to eat real food, the right to a clean environment, and the right to biodiversity on the Earth.

While the small farmer has been losing land, many wild and heritage species of food plants are also being lost. From 1903 to 1983, 80.6% of all tomato varieties were lost.[38] Extinction of wild varieties of tomatoes could ultimately mean the disappearance of the entire plant species of tomatoes, because hybrid tomatoes do not have resistance to many plant diseases, and if the wild varieties become extinct there will be no gene pool to draw from to confer resistance ensuring the ongoing availability of tomatoes. The varieties of lettuce lost during this same time period equal 92.8%.[39] When it comes to field corn varieties, 90.8% have been lost, and 96.1% of sweet corn varieties have been lost in the last century.[40] Corn is an open-pollinated crop and, as a result of biotechnology, there has been a massive biological contamination of nonengineered corn seed by gene-altered varieties. One bioengineered variety, called Starlink, was a mass contaminant. It has not been approved for human use and entered the human food stream through contamination of nonengineered corn, causing one of the largest mass recalls ever done.[41]

From 1903 to 1983, 86.2% of all apple varieties were lost.[42] And worldwide there are 5000+ varieties of potatoes. The major commercial varieties of potatoes that are now grown number four.[43] The potato famine in Ireland has taught us that monocultures are very risky.[44] But industrial agriculture continues on the same road toward possible famine. Luther Burbank invented the netted gem, or the russet baking potato. Monsanto has recently engineered the netted gem so that it contains a pesticide gene — *Bacillus thuringensis* (BT) — in every one of its cells. These potatoes are not labeled and you have no way of knowing if you are eating them or not. No one knows if this engineering has human health effects. Public outcry against the GE potato led to farmers discontinuing the use of BT potatoes. The number of ways that the human race is participating in a noncontrolled study of one kind or another is huge. Fortunately, there are a growing number of farmers across the world who are part of an expanding movement to save what are now known as heritage foods for future generations. These heritage foods are grown primarily by organic farmers and hold more than our past food history in them.[45] They are generally higher in nutrition and more sustainable than their modern hybrids, which have been designed purely for marketing purposes — like ease of travel from farm to market, long shelf life, their ability to be packaged easily, and color — but not for taste or nutritional content.

There are many insults that are happening to our world through modern agricultural practices. These same insults, as they enter the food chain and our drinking water and the soil, have an impact on the internal environment of our bodies: the soil of the human body — the Earth phase of Chinese medicine. There truly is not a separation between the outside world and the inside world, because it is one and the same. The natural world is all around us, even in our food, in our homes, and on our streets. Because we live primarily in our heads and not in our bodies, the split between mind and body, interior environment and exterior environment, nature and humanity allows these insults to continue. We are either not aware or we are in denial. Modern agribusiness is the result of a linear form of thinking that reduces the outcome from the means. This split has allowed us to continue on this path of destruction mentioned so many years ago by Rachel Carson in *Silent Spring*. We may not notice that peaches, one of the most contaminated fruits grown in an agribusiness setting, do not taste like they used to, but the injuries incurred to the environment, and to many cultures of peoples who live close to the land, are now exacting a price from their and our health. With a century filled with war after war, with a global environment that is now changing so dramatically, the price is now one we can actually see and feel. It is not only what we eat but the quality of the food that we eat and how it was grown that is contributing to the modern epidemic of cancer in the developed world.

Colorectal Cancer

Good-quality, clean, and nutrition-filled foods are essential to all life. The changes in the last century to food nutritional quality and the changes in the actual foods we eat have resulted from changes in how we grow our food, how we use the land, and the industrialization of food. Industrial agriculture and the methods used for growing vast amounts of food crops have contributed to a lowering of the nutrient value of many foods we traditionally eat and destruction of the soil community in which we grow food.[46] The designing of vegetable and fruit crops for a long shelf life rather than improved nutrition and taste means that those foods no longer have the same nutritional value that they once did. Although many fruits are traditionally round in shape, many have become more square than round, allowing easier packing. This long shelf life and necessity for packing is required in industrial farming, not take place hundreds and even thousands of miles from the consumer.

When was the last time you saw or ate an Empire apple, or a Liberty, or a Criterion, or an Aroma? When was the last time you ate an Ozette potato, or a Caribe, or a Butterfinger, or Penta? When was the last time you used a variety of corn called Gehu, or Purple Dent, or Tennessee Red Cob, or Hickory King? And when was the last time you saw or even heard of a lettuce called Cosmo, or Winter Density, or Perilla, or Lollo Rossa, or Kaluba? And let us not talk about tomatoes, or squashes, or beans. We have an illusion of choice at our local supermarkets but the reality is that we have lost hundreds of fruits, vegetables, tubers, legumes, and squashes in the last century because marketing and growing choices were made for us by industrial agriculture and food processing based on criteria that have to do with profitability and not nutrition. No wonder not only children but also adults no longer eat their vegetables. Vegetables have become boring and tasteless.

The gastrointestinal tube — the body's garden or soil, if you will — is exposed to many of the additives that are used to get a crop of vegetables or fruits, meats or dairy to the market. The constant exposure to nitrates and nitrites, pesticides, herbicides, solvents, chemical additives to preserve a food, food dyes, and other chemicals cannot help but add to the incidence of gastrointestinal cancers. There are few statistics on the subject, because no one seems to be watching. The USDA is interested in quantity but not quality. However, the Environmental Working Group's website[47] is one of the best in terms of monitoring the amount of contaminants used in specific crops and the resulting levels of pesticides and herbicides that are coming through our food chain and that are therefore also in our drinking water. Visiting that website will allow you to analyze those foods that should absolutely be bought as organic and those that can be purchased as nonorganic based on the predictable levels of residue left on or in the plant.

The Environmental Working Group has also analyzed the public water supplies of 29 Midwestern cities along the major rivers from

Minnesota to Mississippi. They found that of the 29 cities whose water was tested, 28 had unacceptable levels of atrazine, the most common herbicide used in agriculture. Atrazides have been banned in Europe and Israel, because these chemicals have endocrine-disrupting capacities and have been implicated in the causation of several cancers.[48] Just the possibility of carcinogenicity was enough to remove this chemical from the market in these countries. In fact, in Israel the use of atrazine has been phased out and in ten years the rate of breast cancer was reduced by 30%.[49,50] Atrazine is just now being studied for any human health effects in the United States. It is unknown if other injuries occur as a result of the use of atrazine in industrial farming. However, the primary means of movement of atrazine is via water. Since water is an essential need and we drink it many times per day, and since very few except for the Environmental Working Group have looked at herbicides in water, it seems fair to assume that it may be found in many water supplies and implicated in other diseases as well.

In 2003, 145,000 new cases of colorectal cancer (CRC) were diagnosed in the US.[51] CRC ranks second only to lung cancer in mortality, and approximately 60,000 deaths per year in the US are attributed to it. The highest rates of incidence are in the US, the UK, Canada, New Zealand, Australia, Denmark, and Sweden. The lowest rates of incidence are in Colombia, Japan, India, South Africa, Israel, Finland, Poland, and Puerto Rico.[52] The main differences between these two groups are diet and the means by which food crops are grown.

CRC is an almost completely avoidable cancer except in people who carry a genetic predisposition or have familial polyposis syndrome (FAP) or Lynch syndrome types I and II. CRC incidence due to these genetic factors is less than 5%. The evolution of CRC occurs over a period of about ten years through a multistage process where loss of normal controls and balances leads to a mutational activation that results in enhanced cell growth of enterocytes (the building blocks of colon tissue), the knocking-out of tumor suppressor genes that would run surveillance against malignant cells, and disorganization of the DNA.[53]

This happens through environmental, nutritional, genetic, and familial factors. Diets high in saturated fats, especially animal fats, and low in fiber and low in calcium, along with a lack of exercise, all contribute to CRC. Low-meat diets that are high in vegetable, fruit, and whole-grain intake are protective against CRC, and people who eat these diets have a lowered risk of this cancer.[54] The risk of colon cancer for women who eat red meat daily compared to those who eat it less than once a month is 250% greater.[55] The risk of CRC for people who eat red meat once a week compared to those who do not eat any red meat is 38% greater.[56] The risk of CRC for people who eat poultry once a week compared to those who do not eat poultry is 200% greater.[57] People who eat beans, peas, or lentils at least twice a week have a 50% lower risk of CRC compared to people who do not eat these foods. The ratio of CRC for white South Africans compared to black South Africans is 17 to 1.[58] It may be that this is one case where being poor is actually a benefit to health.

Mechanisms of CRC

Animal fat and protein lead to increased bile acids, which foster the growth of certain anaerobic bacteria. These bacteria release enzymes that are carcinogenic and cause colon cancer.[59,60] It is not only a problem of animal fat but also of the protein itself. However, there are no studies on people who eat a diet of grass-fed red meats, like grass-fed beef, which is higher in omega-3s than even fish.[61] These omega-3s are protective against cancer and are often supplemented in the form of fish oils. So it may be that eating red meat is not the primary problem in CRC but rather how the red meat or beef is raised.

Several world trials found that a diet high in fiber from fruits and vegetables was more beneficial than fiber from cereals.[62,63] Fiber decreases fecal transit time through the bowels, resulting in decreased exposure of the bowel wall to fecal carcinogens, reduced carcinogenic microflora in the bowels, decreased pH with a consequent decrease in bacterial enzymatic activity, and diluted carcinogens via an increase in stool bulk.

Sucrose increases the fecal concentration of both total and secondary bile acids. And insulin resistance and the associated changes in insulin and insulin growth factor (IGF) promote colon tumor growth.[64] Therefore, a high-fat, high-sugar, low-fiber diet results in the promotion of CRC. Today's corn crops are used primarily for animal feed, ethanol production, and prepared foods containing high-fructose corn syrup — in other words, for foods found in the center aisles of your grocery store. The truth is that the bovine species does not have a digestive tract with the capacity to digest grain or corn; many grain-fed animals, especially beef cattle, have to be treated for resulting complications of this diet and many die before they are ready for market.[65]

Ethanol production uses a tremendous amount of the groundwater from the Ogalalla aquifer; in fact this aquifer, the largest in the United States, is being drained at an astonishing rate for growing corn, soy, and wheat in the plains states, where those crops require irrigation. And high-fructose corn syrup in prepared foods is a major cause of this overuse of water, and of diabetes and hyperinsulinemia, or insulin-resistant diabetes.[66] Both of these conditions are primary causes of cardiovascular diseases and contribute to the evolution of cancers. Stevia is a viable substitute for these types of sugars that contribute to human disease. It does not raise blood sugar levels and is not metabolized in the same way as cane sugar.[67] The sugar and sugar substitute lobbies in Washington, DC have stopped stevia from being used or becoming a healthy substitute for sugar in the US since the 1940s. Only recently has it begun to be sold outside of health food stores.

All of these problems are connected; and their connectedness undermines quality of life in many ways and on many levels. "Five to ten percent of all cancers are caused by inherited genetic mutations. By contrast, 70 to 80 percent have been linked to diet and other behavioral factors," states Karen Emmons, MD, Dana-Farber Cancer Institute, Boston. On the other hand, *The Beef-Eater's Guide* to *Modern Meat* states, "The associations between cancer and meat-eating are overblown. Genetics are more important than diet." Why would such a statement, an outright lie based on no science whatsoever, be acceptable or even tolerated legally? Why is the sugar and sugar sub-stitute issue not addressed since insulin-resistant diabetes is epidemic in the US? Why are cigarettes still sold when the damage they cause in terms of heart disease and many cancers is a major health disaster in the US? All of the issues mentioned here, when combined, are responsible for the health crisis in which we now find ourselves. And this health crisis contributes to the economic downturn as more and more people require health care from a broken system. These are examples of skirmishes in a silent war in which we are participating without our knowledge — a war for which we are paying with our own health and lives. We are spilt in so very many ways.

Some solutions

Knowing the very particular environment of our local selves helps heal the split between mind and body and gives clues as to how one is doing physically. We must live *in* our body and within our local communities in order to know it. Although we live in our body, we are not our body. We are also not our mind. We are a spirit having a human experience. Living in our mind cuts us off from the rest of our body and the small symptoms and ongoing conversations it contin-ues to have with us no matter if we are consciously listening or not. Nowhere is this more pertinent and applicable than in the arena of the digestive system. Our digestive system is like the soil of the Earth. When Chinese medicine speaks of the element Earth, it is speaking of the entire process of assimilating energy from food.[68] It is a living entity made up of layers of actions that break down and recycle all food materials to provide the active energy to repair and grow new life that supports every species on the Earth, including our own.

Since we eat on a daily basis, continual clues are available to us as to how the digestive tract is receiving and assimilating the foods that we have chosen to eat. Stools allow us to actually observe the end results of our digestion and absorption. We should be able to assess the capacity of our own bodies to digest and assimilate certain foods through their impacts. The "local possibilities and impossibili-ties, hazards and opportunities" for our own bodies should be made clear by comfort or discomfort of our digestion, the quality of our stools, and the energy specific foods give us or take from us.

As practitioners, one of our quests in helping patients to retain health and prevent cancer is to teach how to live in one's body and listen to the ongoing feedback that the body gives[69] — to live as an ecological system. We must also teach how to live in the larger ecosystem of our local and distant world, listening and adjusting to its feedback. A touchstone for many people is the memory of how they felt as children living and reveling in their own bodies, and reveling in all of the fauna and flora of home. As we age, there are many phases through which we go — physically, emotionally, spiritually; and how we experience our own living changes. But we should be able to retain the energy and gusto, albeit balanced *Yang* and *Yin*, we had as children. Living within our bodies and in our local world was always part of the glory of being young. And if we returned to our homes of childhood, would we find it as we left it with all of those species we knew then still intact? To a large extent, I think, there are ongoing and persistent cultural themes embedded in our experiences — experiences of emotional trauma, of competition, of gender identity in a culture, of the split between science and spirituality, of reductionism, all of which have taught us gradually to separate from our bodies and our neighborhood ecosystem, driving through it rather than living in it. This separation becomes a door for diseases — diseases of the spirit and, over time, the resulting physical diseases.

Many eating habits are the result of cultural and familial habits that relate to the climate and growing conditions of geographical areas. Inuit people have traditionally eaten meat and blubber from cold water animals and fish. With almost no vegetables and virtually no fruit, they have survived for 15,000 years in the polar regions of the Earth with very little CRC or ischemic heart disease.[70] Inhabitants of India tend toward vegetarianism combined with many spices and rice. Basmati rice is, in fact, a culturally driven evolutionary gift from India. This diet of rice, legumes, vegetables, and certain spices has protected Indians from CRC, and these people continue to have one of the lowest rates of CRC in the world. It is remarkable that Monsanto (RiceTec) tried to patent basmati rice based on the length of the grain, the fragrance, and other characteristics. It is equally remarkable that the Indian farmers and government rose up and fought Monsanto in this outrageous power grab to patent a food crop developed over centuries by the Indian farmer that would have given Monsanto control over all of the seed for basmati rice grown in the world. Food is part of the Commons and should remain so.

The modern eating habits of the West, particularly the US, are not based on what is geographically available or grown according to the local natural conditions that would foster that plant food. Modern Western eating habits are based on marketing and cheap production, which usually ends up being very expensive in long-term and external costs. The externalized costs of food production are ones that we never pay for when purchasing that food. They are paid for through government subsidies given to farmers who grow wheat, corn, and soy but not to farmers who grow vegetables and fruits, the very foods that we need to remain free of CRC. The corn and soy are used in making feed grains for cattle, dairy cows, and poultry. Many of our eating habits are based on a scarcity theme from old Europe — meat and potatoes. We eat diets that are high in animal fat, highly refined foods, highly refined sugar; no fiber, and no vegetables and fruits. Our own government supports this diet by subsidizing foods that are implicated in cancer causation and by not supporting farmers who grow foods that are preventive of cancer. We have no innate sense anymore about what our bodies need. Nor do we have a sense that we have choices, and the meaning of those choices when it comes to food and how it is grown.

Changing food and eating habits is a major and long-term project for any individual. Neuropeptides are ubiquitous and are found not only in the brain but also in the gut.[71] There is very much a brain chemistry and emotional connection between endorphins and food.[72] These become almost hardwired into our habituated responses to the foods we grew up eating and our sense of wellbeing. Breaking this connection to Mom's cherry pie can be as hard as breaking an addiction, and may actually be breaking an addiction. Giving patients information about this connection and the reasons many foods available to us now are not serving our health helps them make better choices and gradually overcome the cravings until a new template is programmed into the body. The global community has enabled many peoples, especially in the West, to learn about new dietary habits, many of which are better for us, especially those from the East. Unfortunately, the export of American fast food does not contribute to Asian health in the same healthy way as the Asian diet has contributed to Western heath.

A diet high in animal fat and protein and low in complex carbohydrates and vegetables is not the only cause of CRC. Many prepared foods, especially processed meats, contain carcinogenic additions used as preservatives. Nitrites and nitrates are carcinogens used to preserve bacon, ham, cold cuts, and other foods.[73] When these meats and foods are eaten on a daily or even a weekly basis, the result is not just the *excess* bile acids that lead to anaerobic bacteria and their carcinogenic enzymes but is also a direct chemical assault on the large intestine. Other examples include the use of calcium channel blockers to treat hypertension in patients who eat the same diet. Calcium channel blockers reduce the inhibitory effects of vitamin D on the proliferation of CRC.[74] Vitamin D and calcium work synergistically in combination. Low levels of many vitamins and minerals may be risk factors for CRC, especially when combined with a high-fat, high-sugar, low-fiber diet. In fact, the risks of cardiovascular diseases are very similar to those of CRC, and conventional treatments for cardiovascular diseases often contribute to CRC. The use of calcium channel blockers in conventional medicine is an example of how linear thinking that results in treating one symptom with one drug leads to ecological injury in a living system.

Calcium-rich foods decrease colon cell turnover rates and reduce the colon-cancer-promoting effects of bile and fatty acids. Calcium inhibits proliferation of human colonic cells, and low calcium results in proliferation and diminished differentiation.[75] Selenium, vitamins C, D, and E indoles, and betacarotenoids also reduce CRC.[76] Glutathione protects DNA and the p53 tumor suppressor gene. In CRC, 50%–75% of patients have lost the function of both alleles of the p53 gene. Selenium reduces the formation of new adenomatous polyps in 44% of patients. Several studies showed that there was a 61% reduction in

CRC in those who took supplemented selenium. Vitamin E arrests tumor cells in the G1 phase and leads to apoptosis. When it was combined with omega-3 fatty acids, the survival time in terminal patients with any kind of cancer was significantly increased. Although supplementation is one way to get these vitamins and minerals, foods should be considered the primary means of meeting our nutritional needs. High-quality foods, especially vegetables, fruits, and legumes grown in sustainable and clean ways, can provide all of our daily requirements. It is when we do not eat *living* foods that supplementation is required to prevent disease.

It should not be assumed that these statistics about the incidence of CRC and supplement levels are identifying a deficiency in supplementation, but rather that the best source of these vitamins and minerals, one's diet, is deficient. Food sources for most of these vitamins and minerals are fruits and vegetables. This is one way in which a diet high in vegetables and fruits is protective against colorectal cancer. And diets consisting primarily of organically grown fruits and vegetables, as noted before, have higher levels of these valuable micronutrients.

People living in the Third World who live closer to the land, know generally where their food is coming from, and eat far less meat than their affluent cousins in the developed world. They know the huge costs of raising meat for food.[77,78] And they are more likely to die from starvation than from cancer unless they live in a contaminated area. Many Third World peoples are forced to leave their farms and land in Latin America because of the pressures placed on them (and on the land that they have lived on for centuries) by powerful interests seeking to clear the land to raise beef.[79] The human costs of a cheap McDonald's burger are greater than the costs borne by the consumers of such a poor diet but also include the influx from Latin America into the US of displaced peoples from the burger wars. When land is fought over by affluent peoples who are usurping poorer peoples' land and way of life, the affluent always win.[80,81]

Chinese Medicine

The colon and rectum constitute the distal end of the gastrointestinal tube. They are part of the *fu* aspect of the *zang–fu*. This hollow tube is within the body but its interior is actually outside of the body and acts as a conduit for the reception and extraction of nutrition from foods and water (outside). The *lung and large intestine* are coupled organs perhaps because they are the only two organs in the body that have such an interaction between the outside and the inside. As a result, they both must have a tissue type that allows the exchange of life-giving substances, oxygen (lung) and nutrition in the form of chyme (GI tube), between a mucosal barrier and the blood. This makes them at once delicate and strong. Protection against outside pathogens through *Wei* (protective) *Qi* and especially through *Ying* (nutritive) *Qi* is built into these organs and their relationship to the *San Jiao*, and is part of their commonality.

The colon is easily exposed to pathogenic factors. Some of these are endogenous, like bile acids formed from the breakdown of fats.[82] Some are exogenous and include the microflora that the human body lives with over a lifetime beginning in early life as part of the natural and healthy exposures to certain bacteria that aid in digestion and constitute the maturation of the digestion in a young child around the age of 7–9.[83]

In terms of pathogenic unhealthy exposures to the colon, *damp–heat* and *wind* are the two main ones. *Damp–heat* can be synonymous with a diet high in animal fats, sugars, and refined foods that lead to *spleen*/pancreas injury, which can result in lower *Jiao damp* accumulations. Colonic polyps are a material form of *dampness*. They are like little mushrooms growing on the rainforest floor. Excessive mucus in the stools is another material form of *dampness*. It is a precursor to polyps and can occur alongside them. *Wind pathogens* refer to the anaerobic bacteria that evolve from the same diet. They also refer to chemical exposures that generally enter like a spreading fog as part of the food chain in contaminated food. Nitrites and nitrates are examples but there are many others, including food dyes, sugar substitutes like saccharin and aspartame, pesticides, and many of those things on labels that are unreadable chemical constituents. These exposures are modern analogs for the classical Chinese medicine concept of *dampness* and *heat* and *wind* belonging to the *external pernicious influences* (*EPIs*). See any *Huang Di Neijing Su Wen* for in-depth and classical explanations of these concepts.

In CRC these pathogens evolve into two manifestations: *organ toxin (zang du)* and *intestinal wind (chang feng)*. *Du* refers to poison and to many other things, including *toxic heat*, pathogenic *damp–heat, inverted fire, wind–heat*, and *latent pathogenic factors*.[84] The *toxins* that enter the digestion from contaminated foods and water are all a form of external *toxin* exposure. In the case of the promoting factors for CRC, *toxins* can also form endogenously through an improper diet that leads to *excess* bile acids, which foster the growth of anaerobic bacteria.[85] Promoting factors are those things we do that create an environment that is conducive to the evolution and proliferation of cancers. Diet is one of the primary promoting factors, and the most common result is *damp phlegm stasis*.

Chang feng refers to the accumulation of *wind–heat* or the constant exposure to *wind–heat* in the intestines, where it forms toxins. The evolution of colon cancer usually takes about 8–10 years. This constant exposure is key to the injuries that accumulate over time in CRC. *Wind–heat* is primarily an external exposure from contaminated food but anaerobic bacteria may also be considered a form of *wind–heat*, and so the two are related. As well, the promoting factor for *spleen deficiency* is related to both of these manifestations, because *spleen deficiency* allows a greater insult to take place from external and internal pathogenic processes, partly through deficient *Ying Qi*, which in modern medicine equates to the IGg and IGm immune capacity of the mucosal lining of the gut, and partly through *deficient* function of the *spleen*'s charge of transportation and transformation. *Spleen deficiency*, also leads to *blood dryness*, then *blood deficiency* and then *blood stasis*. And *blood stasis* is a terrain on which *heat* and *toxin* evolve. The inflammation from these injuries has a direct relationship to the evolution of cancers and, in this case, to the evolution of CRC.

The *spleen/pancreas* is the middle and the mother of the body. It is the Earth. It expresses the twofold meaning of simultaneously receiving and giving. The functions of the *middle Jiao* and *spleen* are most easily injured by neglect. Neglect is something in which parents engage, and every human being must first learn proper parenting of themselves. If the *spleen* function is weak, the *liver* can overact in a *transverse rebellion* that becomes stronger and more symptomatic over time. A vicious circle is begun where the injured *spleen* fails to nourish the *liver blood*, which then causes restraint and a stronger *transverse rebellion* that weakens the *spleen* even more. These stresses can lead to *spleen Yin deficiency*, a precursor of *spleen Yang deficiency*, and a sign that body fluids are *deficient*. This can be amplified by *liver blood* and *Yin deficiency*. A *transverse rebellion* also contributes to *spleen* weakness and the loss of transforming and transporting functions, which result in *dampness* and then *phlegm*.[86] Therefore, the *dampness* and *phlegm* come from two sources — *spleen deficiency* and *spleen deficiency* leading to a *transverse rebellion* from *liver* constraint. A *stomach* and *gallbladder transverse rebellion* can also evolve from this terrain. The result is acid reflux disorder, which is typically treated with antiacids. Antiacids lower the body's ability to absorb calcium, and lowered calcium absorption can contribute to CRC.[87]

Spleen deficiency patterns manifest in signs and symptoms below the navel and in *sinking spleen Qi*. *Damp accumulations* are a form of sinking *Qi*. Polyps are a material form of *dampness accumulation* that is partly the result of *dampness pouring down* and partly a result of sinking *spleen Qi*. Intermittent stools are a manifestation of *sinking spleen Qi* and are a characteristic precursor of CRC.[88] The diarrhea or loose stool aspect is due to *Qi deficiency* in the *spleen* and a failure to extract the right amount of water via the digestion. The constipation aspect is due to *spleen Qi deficiency* failing to support the *Qi*-transporting function of peristalsis. Diets high in sugar are an addictive expression of a poor diet. However, sugar is also a *spleen* tonic and is considered a Chinese herb. Many *middle Jiao* tonic herbs are high in polysaccharides and natural sugars. Eating a diet high in refined sugar is a poor attempt at righting a *spleen* imbalance and actually worsens it. It is part of a vicious circle.

In *transverse rebellion* the symptoms will manifest as combinations of *excess and deficiency*. Irregular and inadequate or excessive food intake, as in anorexia and bulimia, or in going too long between meals (more than 4–5 h during the day), sporadic eating and then binge eating because of low blood sugar — all of these are especially hard on the *middle Jiao* and the *spleen*. They are examples of how the *liver–spleen* relationship is injured. In these vicious circles it is often difficult to determine what is the chicken and what is the egg. The extremes cause serious injury to assimilative processes that may lead to food allergies, chronic constipation and/or loose stools, low *digestive fire*, *Qi* and *blood deficiency*, *kidney Yang deficiency*, and issues of water metabolism. All of these contribute to more and more extreme *spleen deficiencies*, *damp accumulation*, *stasis*, and then *heat*. These are all underlying concepts of Chinese medical theory that are foundational to cancers.[89] A recipe for cancer is born over time.

Adenomatous polyps are a form of *damp/phlegm stasis*, a possible *latent pathogenic factor*, that act as a magnet for *toxins* and for *wind–heat* drawing these exposures deeper into the body.[90,91]. Therefore, the internal and external contributions to the pathogenesis of CRC are intertwined and complex. The inhibition of the immune and surveillance system of the mucosal lining of the gastrointestinal tract is also due to *spleen deficiency* and injury to both the *Ying* and *Wei* aspects of immunity, since the *spleen* has a direct relationship to both of these aspects of the immune system according to Chinese medicine.[92] Because of the *spleen*'s orb of function to transform food and fluids, *spleen deficiency* allows pathogenic accumulations like polyps, anaerobic bacteria, and increased bile acids from foods, and these in turn cause further *spleen deficiency*. The bowel's ability to separate the pure from the impure is damaged and signs like intermittent diarrhea and constipation, mucus in the stool, hemorrhoids, and *blood stasis* occur. All of these problems either expose the intestinal wall to constant pathogens or scrape away the mucosal lining (in the case of diarrhea), lowering immunity and protection from these pathogens. The mucosal lining is lessened and rebuilt with every bowel movement and one or two stools per day is adequate in a proper diet that conserves the *spleen Qi*. Frequent diarrhea damages the mucosal lining and depletes the *spleen* function as it tries to repair its orb of action. This depletes the *Ying Qi*. Accumulations of *dampness*, *phlegm*, *phlegm heat*, and *toxins* injure the *Qi*, and enter the *blood level* and cause *stasis*, leading to malignancy.[93]

Besides the diet leading to these conditions, there are other risk factors for CRC. Lynch syndrome types I and II both have a markedly higher incidence of CRC.[94] Familial polyposis, where multiple adenomatous polyps after the age of 10 years can literally carpet the colon wall, is a risk factor. A previous history of polyps in the colon demonstrates that an underl*ying* environment has not been addressed and polyps can continue to form because of this lack of dietary and lifestyle change. People who suffer from inflammatory bowel disease (IBD), ulcerative colitis, or ileitis (Crohn's disease) have a greatly increased risk of CRC.[95] In ulcerative colitis the risk is 20 times the average.

Other risk factors for CRC include high consumption of charbroiled foods.[96] The charbroiling of foods and especially animal fats changes normal fats/oils into carcinogens through exposure to high *heat*. These carcinogens are *wind–heat toxins*. Chronic constipation is also a risk factor, because the longer the transit time for the stools, the longer the exposure of the bowel wall to *toxins* of various kinds, depending on one's diet. Asbestos is also a known cause of CRC and is probably a *wind–heat* pathogen.

The evolution to CRC usually takes about 10–15 years[97] but can take even longer in these cases. Early symptoms of digestive imbalance require an in-depth intake and evaluation. Patients need to be taught how to parent their own body by eating a proper diet. Explaining what a proper diet is within the traditional framework of the individual patient is one of the most important interventions in which a practitioner can engage. Teaching patients how and where to buy food and how to cook are baseline actions for providers. All of the early symptoms of digestive imbalance are immensely important to pay attention to because some of them can evolve into conditions that place an individual at greater risk for CRC.

Spleen Patterns in Detail[98]

Spleen-Yin deficiency

The *spleen* takes fluid from the *kidney* and adds nutrition. It then sends body fluid to the *stomach* along with directives about how to use it. We could say that these directives are in the form of enzymes. *Spleen Yin deficiency* is caused by insufficiency of body fluid. As the *spleen* becomes *deficient*, the route of body fluid that supplies nutrition shuts down. As the fluid decreases, the whole becomes insufficient and *empty heat* rises. The cause of this condition is overwork, insufficient sleep, and a poor diet. The whole body becomes fatigued; the patient may feel discomfort from low-grade fever or a sense of malaise. This is especially true in spring or summer, when the natural environment is filled with *Yang* and the human body is open. The experience is one of feverishness and malaise. The empty *heat* rises to the surface and gets dispersed. In the fall and winter, the experience is the opposite and the patient with this pattern may easily feel chilled because they are *deficient.*

As this pattern deepens, cramping or pain in the muscles can result, because body fluids are low. Some forms of fibromyalgia are due to this condition. The *spleen* is unable to deliver body fluids to the muscles along with, one would think, calcium. Adults may appear lazy or inactive, there is little appetite, the stools are loose, urine is more frequent, and the mouth is dry. The patient will crave water in the summer, partly because they are not eating. Overeating or mild food poisoning can also produce these symptoms. In a typical American setting, it is probably the combination of overworking and worry to make ends meet, improper eating and eating of foods that are truly pseudofoods, plus food contamination, that leads to this condition. It may also be seen in some patients with chronic conditions related to cancer therapies.

This condition becomes more prominent in the *stomach* and *large intestine. Heat* can stagnate in these organs. When an *EPI* invades, in the first stage there is chill and fever. When it does not resolve and progresses, it invades the *yangming* channel, resulting in fever and dry throat and dryness in the eyes and nose. There may be diarrhea and vomiting. If antipyretics are given to lower the fever or laxatives are given to move the stools, the *heat* will be drastically reduced. However, even more body fluid will be lost, exacerbating the condition of *spleen Yin deficiency.*

In *spleen deficiency* the pulse is not well defined. It is easier to say what it is not. It is soft and amorphous without proper boundaries. Tonifying fire points like Sp 3, P 7, Sp 2, and P 8 can help to provide the *spleen* with *Qi* in order to lend definition to the pulse so as to enable a clear diagnosis.

Spleen Yin deficiency with heat in the bladder

Heat in the bladder is difficult to determine via the pulse. However, the abdomen over the bladder organ will be hot to palpation. The patient will also feel pressure pain in this area. The pattern is caused by febrile disease, like a bladder infection, or is due to incorrect treatment of a febrile disease.

When a patient is having fever, they may feel extreme thirst but cannot urinate. The *heat* is restrained in the back *taiyin* and goes into *the fu organ — the urinary bladder. Yin* Earth cannot control *Yang* water. Treatment concentrates on returning urinary function. Steamed green onions over the lower abdomen combined with acupuncture points will work. This pattern has been seen in prostate cancer patients who have been treated with brachytherapy and/or external beam radiation.

Stomach Yang deficiency with heat in the chest

A *cold stomach* is often caused by pharmaceutical drugs and by improper eating habits. This results in *middle and lower burner cold. Heat* stagnates in the *upper Jiao,* because the *heat* exchange mechanism at the diaphragm is not functioning. The symptoms include substernal tightness, borborygmus, unrelenting hiccups, belching, and irregular appetite. Appetite is regulated when there is circulation between the *upper and lower burners.* When the harmony is broken, the appetite becomes irregular. There is underlying *spleen deficiency* with loose stools and incomplete evacuation. At the same time, there are ulcers in the mouth or tongue, or canker in the corner of the mouth. There also may be sinusitis, because of *upper burner lung heat* and insomnia. This is a very common presentation of patients undergoing cancer treatment, especially with chemotherapy. The oral ulcers can be assumed to be present in much of the gastrointestinal tract lining. That lining is within the purview of the *spleen.*

Stomach Yang deficiency with water stagnation

"Swallowing *phlegm* disease" occurs in patients with *spleen Yang deficiency*. Water easily becomes stagnant in this pattern. Wrong treatment, constitution, and diet all contribute. The symptoms are vomiting, diarrhea, dysuria, headache, dizziness, palpitations, substernal pain, poor appetite, and *cold* extremities. There is no thirst. Very commonly there will be a prolapsed *stomach* and this is why the water is stagnating. The prolapse may be due to a hiatal hernia. It is the *heat* rising from stagnation that causes the headache. Treatment consists of Si 4, Sp 3, P 7, Sp 4, and Bl 39 (*he-sea* point of the *San Jiao*). For prolapse use St 36 and the extra point for prolapse medial to St 39 against the tibia.

Spleen Yang deficiency with severe spleen Yin deficiency

Spleen Yin deficiency deteriorates into *spleen Yang deficiency*. As body fluids decrease, *empty heat* becomes static in the *stomach*. When deficient body fluids are severe, the *stomach* becomes completely chilled. Body fluids are interpreted as blood and, therefore, this condition is considered serious.

The causes are childbirth, abdominal surgery like a Whipple procedure, constant worry, and loss of a very close relative. Insomnia is the primary symptom. *Blood deficiency* insomnia has the characteristic of never actually falling asleep. There is a tendency to bleed from the nose, anus, uterus, and intestines. It is not due to platelet deficiency. There is no appetite. The *stomach* has stopped functioning.

Severe deficiency creates a *small heat* that leads to low-grade fever in the late afternoon or evening. There is no fever in the morning. This pattern is difficult to recover from. Strong treatment will cause deterioration. Often the pulse is big and floating. As *Yin* and *Yang* are tonified, the pulse will shrink and sink. This is an improvement. This pattern is not uncommon in later-stage cancers where many treatments have been given over time. Even though the chemotherapy is given by intravenous infusion, its impacts are still systemic and include damage to the *middle Jiao*. Over time, the *middle Jiao* damage becomes severe.

Spleen deficiency and liver excess

Pathogenic Qi goes through stages and can affect any organ with fever or *heat*. It begins with a weak *spleen* and therefore it tends to show in the *liver or pericardium*. The main symptom is fever that rises and falls. With *pathogenic heat* in the *liver* there will be hepatitis. *Heat* in the abdomen can manifest as constipation, lack of appetite, or a bitter taste in the mouth. When this condition is present, *heat can easily enter the lung* or kidney. *Pathogenic heat* in the *lung* presents with wheezing cough and pneumonia. In the *kidney* the presentation is dysuria, edema, or nephritis.

Kidney *pathogenic heat* shows with an *excess* pulse but the practitioner may have to rely on the symptoms for diagnosis. When a patient has a problem with the *zang* organs, it is often safe to guess that it is coming originally from the *spleen*. The root cause of the acute condition is in reality a chronic condition.

Spleen deficiency with liver excess and blood stasis

Blood stasis comes from chronic patterns. It is a common gynecological problem but it is also seen in HIV masses and tumors and other static blood conditions like Kaposi's sarcoma. Hardness around the navel is indicative of *blood stasis*. Cupping the navel will give information about the level of *blood stasis*. Common moving points for this condition are Sp 3, P 7 and dispersing Lv 14 and Lv 8, Sp 10 and Sp 6. Use moxa on Bl 17. Bloodletting on *jing-well* points and vascular spiders is also helpful. Movement is one of the very best mechanisms for treating *blood stasis*.

Spleen deficiency with lung excess

Symptoms of pneumonia will have *pathogenic heat* that has entered the *liver*, creating a *spleen* deficiency and *liver excess* condition that enters the *lung* via the *ko cycle*. The chest is painful with pressure. There is a high fever and constipation.

Spleen deficiency with kidney Yang deficiency

If the *Yang Qi* has collapsed, *ming men fire* weakens and the kidneys are weakened also. When there is *spleen Yin and Yang deficiency*, this is called *kidney Yang* deficiency. The symptoms are dribbling urine and diarrhea. The treatment is to tonify Sp 6, K 3, Sp 9, Bl 58, and Bl 59. If the back *shu* are tonified, care must be given not to leak *Qi* or deplete the *Yang Qi* of the *taiyang channel*.

Irritable bowel syndrome; inflammatory bowel disease, ulcerative colitis, crohn's disease

Gastrointestinal diseases are divided into two categories: structural and functional. IBS and IBD are gut motility disorders that are functional in nature; no pathophysiological mechanism in conventional medicine has been identified for IBS.[99] IBS has been known as nervous dyspepsia, spastic colon, irritable colitis, nervous colitis, or intestinal neurosis. Although it can occur at any age, its incidence tends to be concentrated in the 20–40-year age group. The incidence of CRC is far higher in patients who have an ongoing history of IBD, ulcerative colitis, and Crohn's disease. Many people diagnosed with IBS recall suffering from similar symptoms during childhood and adolescence. Women are three times more likely to suffer from the chronic symptoms of IBS. However, since men do not seek medical advice as frequently as women, it may be underreported in men. Patients with IBS make approximately 2.5–3.5 million physician visits annually.

Mixing and propulsive contractions constitute the movement in the bowel.[100] Normally, chyme stretches the intestinal wall, promoting a series of regularly spaced concentric contractions called segmentations. Chyme is the semiliquid acid mass that is the form in which food passes from the *stomach* through the small intestine. It is the result of the rotting and ripening function of the upper digestive tract.

As each segment relaxes, a new one begins chopping the chyme into sections at about 8–12 turns per minute, thoroughly mixing food with intestinal secretions, depending on whether one is in the upper, middle, or lower digestive tract. The combined contraction of smooth and longitudinal muscle in the colon causes portions of the large intestine to bulge outward into balloon-like sacs called haustrations. Colonic slow-wave contractions are normally measured at a cycle of six per minute in the sigmoid and rectum. But, in IBS patients, this cycle occurs only three times per minute, regardless of whether the patient is experiencing symptoms. This is why IBS has been designated an intestinal motor function or motility alteration. IBS patients who are fasting experience no increase in contractile activity during the fasting phase. However, when they eat there are spikes in the myoelectric activity that coincide with episodes of cramping abdominal pain.

Colonic symptoms of IBS include:[101]

- Diarrhea — frequent, loose, and watery, mostly in the morning;
- Constipation — consisting of small pellet-like stools (goat turds), or bowel movements less than three times per week;
- Stool urgency;
- A feeling of incomplete evacuation;
- Intestinal spasms;
- Acute abdominal pain — usually cramping in the left lower quadrant; may be worsened by eating and temporarily relieved by bowel movement or passing gas;
- Bloating and flatulence — usually mildest in the morning but worsening as the day progresses; bloating may be severe enough to force the patient to loosen their clothing;
- Thick, pasty stools that are difficult to eliminate and have a foul odor;
- Hypersecretion of colonic mucus.

Noncolonic symptoms of IBS include:

- Heartburn;
- Acid regurgitation;
- Dysphagia;

- Back and thigh pain;
- Urinary frequency and urgency;
- Nausea and loss of appetite;
- Fatigue;
- Headaches;
- A general feeling of weakness;
- Varying degrees of anxiety or depression;
- Dyspareunia — painful or difficult sexual intercourse for a woman;
- Fibromyalgia.

The classical symptom triad consists of abdominal pain, distension, and altered bowel movements. However, almost 50% of IBS patients feel that the noncolonic symptoms are more intrusive.

The triggers may include antibiotic or other drug use, infection, abdominal surgery, food intolerances, stressful or emotional situations, and sleep deprivation. Some researchers characterize IBS as a purely psychological disorder. And it is true that IBS patients have a significantly higher prevalence of major depression and generalized anxiety, panic disorder, as well as childhood rape or molestation. It is difficult to determine if these disorders are ones of cause, effect, or coincidence. However, these symptoms resemble posttraumatic stress disorder (PTSD).

There are some conditions that may mimic IBS. These include:

- Cancer;
- Disturbed bacterial microflora as a result of antibiotic use;
- Diverticular disease;
- Infectious diarrhea like giardiasis;
- Inflammatory bowel disease;
- Intestinal candidiasis;
- Lactose intolerance;
- Laxative abuse;
- Malabsorption diseases like celiac disease;
- Mechanical diseases like fecal impaction;
- Metabolic disorders like diabetes, hyperthyroidism, or adrenal insufficiency;

- Response to dietary factors that interfere with digestion, like excessive coffee, carbonated drinks, or simple sugars in *excess.*

IBS is often classified according to those symptoms that are most frequent:[102]

- Constipation with abdominal pain;
- Functional diarrhea;
- Foregut dysmotility — bloating and discomfort after eating;
- Extrabowel manifestations like lethargy, migraine, or urinary symptoms.

Diagnosis

The key to diagnosis, if not already done by another provider, is effective history-taking. This is often a diagnosis of exclusion and is based upon characteristic bowel patterns, time and character of pain, physical exam and palpation including of the *hara,*[103] and routine diagnostic procedures that rule out other causes (may need to be done by a different provider). The typical laboratory tests that are done are an ESR to rule out inflammatory problems, a CBC, stool examinations for parasites, fecal occult blood (cancer), WBCs which can suggest infection, food allergy testing (which can be done through an elimination diet rather than RAST or a blood test), a barium enema, and sigmoidoscopy. It is important to remember that when ruling out colon cancer, only a colonoscopy is completely definitive because only colonoscopy looks at the entire colon.[104]

Elimination of aggravating factors that then reduce symptoms may be one way of diagnosing IBS when all other factors and risks have been ruled out. The things that aggravate the condition include:

- Sugar;
- Caffeine;
- Gluten foods — wheat, oats, barley, and rye;

- Foods one is allergic to — most common are wheat, corn, and milk;
- Check the stools for candidiasis and treat with lactobacillus except in Crohn's disease.

The elimination of aggravating factors is sometimes combined with treatment to heal the GI mucosa in holistic medicine. The following have been found to be useful in this healing[105]:

- Some liquid food products of high quality, e.g. Metagenics;
- Glutamine at 500 mg–1000 mg;
- Cabbage juice (avoid brassicas in Crohn's);
- Gentian;
- Robert's formula;
- Quercitin — a bioflavonoid;
- Some antispasmodics, like peppermint oil in enteric caps 200 mg bid;
- Chamomile tea;
- Increase fiber;
- Rice bran;
- Psyllium seed powder — 1 tbsp. daily in 8 oz. water;
- Fenugreek seed crushed in tea;
- Decrease stress through counseling, biofeedback, yoga, or meditation;

The diagnosis according to pain qualities:[106]

- *Nature of the pain*
    Qi stasis — distension and bloating;
    Blood stasis — stabbing, fixed pain;
    Empty conditions — stuffiness.

- *Reaction to pressure*
    Aggravated by pressure — *excess* and full conditions;
    Better with pressure — deficiency conditions.

- *Palpation*
    Hard abdomen — *excess*;
    Soft abdomen — *deficient.*

- *Reaction to activity/rest*
    Better with moderate exercise — *stasis*;
    Better with rest — deficiency.

- *Reaction to bowel movement*
    Better with passing of stools — a "substantive pain," — due to blood and *food stasis.*
    No change with passing of stools — a "nonsubstantive pain," due to *dampness, Qi stasis, cold.*

Following are varying and overlapping diagnostic patterns for what are commonly called IBS, colitis, or Crohn's disease in Western terminology. IBD and Crohn's disease are considered high-risk factors for CRC.

Irritable Bowel Syndrome Treatment[107]

(1) *Transverse rebellion with spleen deficiency and an overcontrolling liver*

- Recurrent borborygmus;
- Abdominal pain;
- Diarrhea with pain that is better after passing stools;
- Tongue — a thin white coating;
- Pulse — wiry moderate or wiry thin.

The pain is caused by a *transverse rebellion* of *liver Qi*; this depletes the *spleen* and impacts the motility of the peristalsis of the intestines. The diarrhea is caused by a collapse of *spleen Qi* leading to a loss of the *spleen*'s ability to transport nutrients upward, with a concurrent descending *turbidity.*

Dampness is a component of the weak *spleen* function but the tongue does not demonstrate this because all of the *dampness* is going down and does not affect the tongue coating. If the diarrhea were a result of *damp excess* and *turbidity* accumulating in the intestines, then the tongue would have a thick white coating. This is one way to differentiate this type of diarrhea and helps in the understanding of treatment options.

In this presentation the treatment principles are to spread the *liver Qi* and to tonify the *spleen*. The main formula is:

Tong xiao yao tang[108]

(2)   *Dry intestines due to injury from a warm febrile disease*

- Constipation that is dry, with stools that are difficult to pass;
- Thirst and dry mouth;
- Little appetite;
- Abdominal pain not better with passing of stools;
- Tongue — dry and red;
- Pulse — thin and rapid or weak and forceless.

When there is a history of a *warm febrile disease* or chronic symptoms over a long time in a patient with constitutional *Yin deficiency*, *heat* will clump in the *yangming*. This depletes fluids, especially in the large intestine, where the final extraction of water occurs in the body. This leads to dry hard stools that are difficult to pass.

The treatment principles are to generate fluids, moisten dryness, and unblock the bowels.

(3)   *Middle Jiao Yang deficiency*

- Diarrhea with watery stools;
- May have nausea or queasiness;
- No thirst;
- Little appetite;
- Abdominal pain;
- Tongue — pale;
- Pulse — submerged and thin.

If the *spleen* is *deficient*, the clear *Yang* cannot rise, and this causes diarrhea and watery stools. If the *stomach* loses its ability to make the *turbid Yin* descend then the *stomach Qi* will flush upward and nausea will result. Low appetite indicates *spleen deficiency*. *Cold* in the abdomen causes contraction and, therefore, pain. *Cold* is also an indicator of no thirst and of the tongue color and submerged pulse.

The treatment principles are to warm the *middle Jiao* and to strengthen the function of the *spleen–stomach* axis.

The main formula for this presentation is:

Wen pi tang[109]

(4) *Spleen Qi deficiency*
   - Pale complexion;
   - Low and soft voice;
   - Low appetite;
   - Loose stools;
   - Possible abdominal pain around the umbilicus;
   - Weak limbs;
   - Tongue — pale;
   - Pulse — thin and weak or moderate.

Improper eating habits, overwork, obsessive thinking, and worry all damage the *spleen/pancreas*. The transformation of food into *blood* and *Qi* is impaired. This makes the voice low and the complexion pale, and reduces the appetite and the ability to digest foods because of loss of transport through the *stomach* (formation of chyme). This results in unformed stools. And since the *spleen* governs the muscle tissue and some forms of connective tissue, weakness in the extremities is a common complaint. This is garden variety *spleen/pancreas deficiency* that can take on so many different manifestations.

The treatment principles are to tonify the *zheng Qi* and especially the *spleen Qi*.

The main formula could be:

Xiang Sha Liu Jun Zi Tang[110]

As is true with all of these presentations, there are many herbal formula possibilities.

(5) *The liver invading the spleen or transverse rebellion*

- Alternating constipation and diarrhea or loose stools;
- Abdominal and epigastric distension;
- Borborygmus;
- Poor appetite;
- Flatulence;
- All worse with tiredness or depression;
- All worse with anger or worry;
- Tongue — pale, possibly dark, greasy white coating;
- Pulse — wiry and slippery but forceless.

This is a very common presentation, especially for women (who are more likely to be diagnosed with any of these conditions). A *transverse rebellion* occurs when the *spleen* is weak or the *liver Qi* is stagnant. There is not necessarily a way to say which came first. If the *spleen* fails to nourish the *blood*, then the *liver blood* is *deficient* and fails to nourish the *liver*. This can lead to *liver Qi stasis* and *constraint*. *Constraint* itself can cause the *liver Qi* to rebel transversely and injure the *spleen* function, causing it to fail to transform and transport. Thus, a vicious circle evolves that gets worse and deeper wearing tracks of injury in the body, causing widespread harm.

Depression, anger, frustration, lack of self-esteem, and lack or loss of one's vision for life can cause *liver Qi* damage. Constant worry and obsessive thinking over what could have been or what could be or might happen cause *spleen/pancreas* damage. Because the liver/*gallbladder* and *stomach/spleen* are part of the up-and-down, horizontal, and circular flows of the *middle Jiao*, injury to any of these for whatever reason can upset the apple cart, so to speak. It may be one reason why IBS has been considered to be a psychiatric disorder. And certainly various stress reduction, biofeedback, and meditation techniques have helped in recovery from IBS. IBS is very much emblematic of the mind–body connection.

The treatment principles for this pattern are to tonify and uplift the *spleen*, smooth the *liver Qi* and nourish the *liver blood*.

The common formulas for this pattern:
Xiao yao san and Tong xie yao Fang[111]

Colitis

The symptoms and patterns can be similar to those for item No.1 under "Irritable Bowel Syndrome Treatment." However, they also include:

- Anemia;
- Fatigue;
- Fever;
- Nausea;
- Weight loss;
- Anorexia;
- Rectal bleeding;
- Loss of bodily fluids and nutrients;
- Skin lesions;
- Growth failure in children.

These signs and symptoms characterize an inflammatory disease that is much more serious than IBS. It is the inflammation that makes colitis or IBD a high-risk factor for CRC.
Possible diagnostic patterns:

(1) *Externally contracted wind–cold with concurrent internal injury due to stagnation*

- Nonspecific acute colitis;
- Fever and chills;
- Headache;
- A "*men*" sensation, i.e. chest stifling;
- Epigastric and abdominal pain;
- Nausea and perhaps vomiting;
- Loss of taste sensation;
- Diarrhea;

- Tongue — a white and greasy coating;
- Pulse — moderate or soggy.

An *EPI* that is *wind–cold* constricts the *Wei Qi*, producing chills, and battles with the normal *Qi*, producing fever. The *taiyang channels* that traverse the head at the *Yang* point will be affected by *cold* and cause headache. The internal stagnation obstructs the *Qi* mechanism in the *middle Jiao*, leading to a "*men*" sensation. It also disrupts the normal ascending and descending functions of the *middle jiao*, causing abdominal pain, nausea, vomiting, borborygmus, and diarrhea. Internal stagnation of damp causes loss of taste and also the presenting tongue and pulse.

Although this is presented here as an acute condition, *wind* and *cold* pathogens can be extended to include some allergic foods and some chemical exposures to which many people are exposed on a daily basis. Remember that the interior of the gastrointestinal tract is an inside/outside phenomenon and the same types of pathogens that attack the *lung* and *taiyang* can attack the intestines. The route of entry is somewhat different but the impacts are similar in manifestation — cramping pain, mucus production, diarrhea (almost like the equivalent of sneezing), and so on. Because many of these impacts are new and without an historical basis from which to derive a pattern category, it is up to us to determine the characteristics of the impact and then from them find the pattern diagnosis for determining treatment options.

The treatment principles in this presentation are to release the exterior, transform *dampness*, regulate the *Qi*, and harmonize the *middle Jiao*. Does this sound familiar?

(2) *Spleen and kidney Yang deficiency*

- *Wu gen xie*; cock's crow diarrhea;
- No appetite;
- Undigested food in the stools;
- A weak and aching low back that is chronic;
- Fatigue;
- Lethargy;

- Cannot eat many foods, because they cause upsets, or cannot be fully digested;
- Abdominal pain that is chronic but worse with some foods;
- Tongue — pale, may show tooth marks, may have little coating;
- Pulse — submerged and slow.

Diarrhea that occurs at 5 a.m. every day happens because when the *Yin* is at its peak and the *Yang* is just starting to rise, fluids prevail. If the *kidney Yang* is weak, the *Yang* will not properly rise and the *Yin* will suddenly descend, causing diarrhea especially at that crucial moment of *Yin–Yang* exchange. *Spleen* and *kidney Yang deficiency* manifest as a lack of interest in food; the *digestive fire* is low but hopefully not out. An inability to "cook" internally what is eaten results in undigested food in the stools. There is no fire on which to cook the food. Pain results from *cold* contracting the abdomen or musculature of the bowel wall, causing spasm. The food allergies are due to the *spleen*'s inability to transform and transport. The fatigue and lethargy are typical signs of *Yang deficiency* but are also possibly due to malnutrition and resulting anemia. The tongue and pulse are both from *spleen* and *kidney Yang deficiency*. The tongue is pale from *Qi* and *blood deficiency*, because the *spleen* is not transforming food to *Qi* and *blood*. *Cold* may contribute to that. The tooth marks are due to *spleen* deficiency failing to transform fluids. *Kidney Yang deficiency* may contribute to that although upper body edema is primarily a sign of *spleen deficiency*. The little tongue coating indicates that the *spleen* has not the *Qi* to give a normal white coating to the tongue. The submerged pulse indicates *Yang deficiency* and *cold*, and the slowness indicates *cold*.

The treatment principles are to warm the *middle Jiao* and to benefit the *Yang* of the *kidneys*.

A typical formula for this presentation is *Zhen Wu Tang*,[112] or even *Si Shen Wan*.[113]

The above pattern can sometimes be seen in patients who have suffered chronic dysenteric disorders that have never been resolved. We rarely see this in the West but it can be seen in Africa and other countries where parasitic infestations, especially in children, are more common. The dysenteric disorder was originally a *damp–heat pattern* but over time the *spleen* and *stomach*, and possibly even the *kidney Yang*, are injured and the condition transforms into one of *cold* from deficiency and loss of fluids. In the West, some of these more severe presentations can be seen in HIV/AIDS patients and sometimes as a result of multiple drug therapies over years of treatment or as a result of an undetected parasitic infection — most commonly giardiasis or cryptosporidiosis.

The treatment principles in these cases can be to warm the *middle Jiao*, return the *Yang* to the *Source*, and bind up the bowels, which means to astringe intestinal fluids, while discharging the pathogen. In stronger patients, where parasites are present, a two-stage process is undertaken that first expels the parasites and then rehabilitates any function that was injured by their presence and by the process of expulsion. In weaker patients, the use of cathartics is contraindicated and a slower approach that concurrently drains and tonifies is employed.

Crohn's disease

The symptoms and patterns are similar to those for colitis and include the following specifically for Crohn's:
Food stagnation

- Reduced appetite;
- Difficult digestion;
- Bloating and focal distention of the epigastrum and lower abdomen;
- Loose and watery diarrhea;
- Tongue — yellow greasy coating;
- Pulse — frail.

The digestive symptoms in this picture come from *stomach/spleen deficiency* that leads to *food stagnation*. Even though there are excess symptoms in this presentation, the main treatment is to tonify the *spleen* so as to harmonize the *stomach/spleen* and resolve *food stagnation* and diarrhea. Although this sounds more simple than any of the other pattern strategies presented here, treating Crohn's disease is a long term process. There are degrees of *spleen deficiency*, and the degree of *spleen deficiency* in Crohn's is severe. Some patients end up having portions or all of their colons surgically resected.

All the Chinese medicine pattern diagnoses may be relevant to any of the Western diagnoses presented here. The main points in diagnosis are to identify the abnormal flows of *Qi*, to rule in or out parasitic infestations, to understand the nature of the patient's diet and eating habits including conditions under which they eat or do not eat, surrounding symptoms like *heat* or *Qi* flushing up, *turbidity* sinking downwards and to assess the general strength of the upper and middle digestive tract.

General considerations in treatment

If we look at the traditional functions of the *spleen*/pancreas in Chinese medicine, we see elements of many conventional medicine body systems. The anatomical spleen is a part of the immune and lymphatic system; one suggestion is that — since the Chinese medicine concept of the *spleen* includes the production of the *Ying Qi* — the mucosal lining of the entire GI tract, the IgE and IgM aspects of intestinal immunity, and possibly many aspects of the lymphatic system of the abdomen along the GI tract are part of the *spleen* terrain. This area contains more lymph than any other part of the body. The mesenterium and greater and lesser omentum are also aspects of immune organs that speak to the *spleen's* relationship with the *Ying*, the *San Jiao*, and water metabolism.[114]

The *spleen* also plays a major part in food metabolism. The rotting and ripening function of the *stomach*, gastric enzymes and acids, pancreatic enzymes and sugar metabolism, and the ultimate formation of chyme can be attributed to the *spleen/stomach/pancreas*. Fat metabolism and, therefore, the *gallbladder* may be considered to be a part of this major body axis. And water distribution and absorption, much of which takes place in the upper small intestine (jejunum), is considered classically to be a part of *spleen* function.[117B] When looked at from this anatomical perspective, it becomes obvious why the *spleen* is considered the center of the body. It has a very large charge in overall body health. Metabolic disorders fall into this realm. The Chinese historical and metaphorical concepts regarding the *middle Jiao* and the *spleen/pancreas* axis are emblematic of the land, of farming, irrigation, and food storage. In other words, the microcosm of the body is an expression of the macrocosm of the Earth/Earth and its ecosystems. These concepts are depicted in the Taoist map of the human microcosm and the universal macrocosm. How healthy we are inside is indicative of how healthy our world is outside and vice versa.

There are many dietary and food recommendations that can be made regarding the *middle Jiao* and overall health. One main consideration is that the establishment of regular bowel habits is central to health. In fact, traditionally Chinese medicine has said that there are ultimately two necessary foundations for good health — regular stools and good sleep. Part of establishing regular bowel habits is to get adequate fiber, especially vegetable fiber, and drink at least half your body weight translated into ounces of water daily. Many of the fluids we drink are diuretic and a large percentage of people are chronically mildly dehydrated. This, of course, contributes to irregular stools and also to poor sleep from *Yin deficiency*, among other things.

Another aspect of recovering from IBS, IBD, colitis, or Crohn's disease is to steam vegetables in order to break or soften the cellulose wall of vegetable cells. This enables chewing to do much of the breakdown of the nutrients within the cells before absorption. Generally, humans are unable to chew enough and break down plant materials in an efficient way when eating only raw foods. *Digestive fire* is used to warm the raw food to body temperature, then more *Qi* is used to break down the cellulose wall of the food, and finally the actual assimilation and absorption can begin utilizing more *Qi*. Two additional steps are added to a raw foods diet. In summer raw foods are more easily digested. However, for people suffering from the above conditions with injury to the *middle Jiao* and *spleen* function, it is best to lightly steam vegetables before eating them. The Chinese also add ginger slices to tonify and warm the *spleen* and help it break down vegetables.

Root vegetables are high in polysaccharides and are easily digested while providing good food quality and nutrients. Squashes, yams, carrots, turnips, and rutabagas are all excellent foods for *spleen* deficiency. These foods are yellow or orange in color; they contain natural and complex sugars that are not contraindicated and do not break down in the same way as refined cane or corn sugars. Elimination of refined sugars is essential to CRC prevention and to re-establishment of a healthy GI tract. Refined sugars tend to paralyze the motility of the duodenum and jejunum and they contribute to the growth in the small intestine of nonbeneficial bacteria.[115] These are the same bacteria that produce enzymes that are carcinogenic. Refined sugars "swamp" the *spleen* and all of its manifestations. Complex carbohydrates help to maintain a consistent blood sugar level over time and, therefore, help to curb sugar cravings. Again, sugar cravings are a sign of *spleen deficiency* from a poor diet. The habit of sugar includes injury to the *spleen*, just as the habit of nicotine includes injury to the lung, or the habit of alcohol includes injury to the *liver*.

Diets that are simple do not stress the *stomach–spleen* axis, and patients with IBS or other intestinal chronic conditions do worse with a complex diet where many foods are eaten at one sitting. Avoiding spicy foods with these conditions eliminates the irritation caused by them. If a patient complains that they cannot eat these food items without GI tract pain, then they should not. The modern use of antacids like Tagamet and Prilosec is not contributing to health. The need for these agents is due to eating foods that cause either hyperacidity or hypoacidity. They are symptomatic treatment and do not address the cause. The treatment goal in digestive functional disorders is to rebuild the gastrointestinal function through giving the digestion a rest and through food choices.

The use of Tums or other antacids in order to get one's daily calcium dose is a mistake, even though many doctors recommend it. Calcium is absorbed best in an acidic environment. Tums reduces *stomach* acid, and therefore absorption of calcium is poor. Reducing *stomach* acid also leads to hypoacidity and poorer digestion of proteins.

Meeting calcium requirements by using supplements that are often synergistically combined, like calcium and magnesium and vitamin D, is a much more functional approach. Many people who use antacids are actually low in stomach acid and either have caused this problem, are treating a misdiagnosed problem improperly, or are worsening their problem by lowering stomach acid through the use of antacids. Calcium is a major contributor to colon health, among other things, and good absorption requires *digestive fire* including adequate *stomach* acids.

Type II diabetes

Type II diabetes, or hyperinsulinemia, is a condition in which sugar metabolism is imbalanced. In diabetes mellitus, the pancreas fails to produce effective and sufficient insulin, resulting in hyperglycemia. In type II diabetes, the pancreas produces adequate insulin but the peripheral uptake of insulin is inadequate due to insulin resistance. This can be measured through blood glucose levels, which, during the fasting state, should be below 100 but above 70. In juvenile onset diabetes, the insulin-producing aspect of the pancreas (beta cells) is damaged for varying and sometimes controversial reasons (vaccinations) and not enough insulin is produced. However, in adult onset diabetes, called type II, enough insulin is produced, but, insulin utilization is blocked and the maintenance of blood sugar in the cells is inefficient. Too much sugar enters the blood, and the *kidneys* excrete it along with fluids. This causes a common symptom of diabetes — frequent urination. The loss of body fluids results in thirst, inflammations, infections, and other deficiency signs and symptoms.[116]

A high-fat diet also causes *liver stasis*. The *spleen/pancreas* is damaged by a high-fat diet, and deficiency and *dampness* can result; *spleen* deficiency leads to *dampness*, and *liver blood deficiency* leads to *liver stasis* and also *transverse rebellion* which further injures the *spleen/pancreas*.[117] In the early writings of Chinese medicine, the same character was used to denote the anatomical organs the *spleen* and *pancreas*. It is unclear if the difference in function of these two anatomically close organs was defined. In modern writings, the *spleen* has come to be considered anatomically and functionally as a composite of the *spleen* and *pancreas* and is usually called the *spleen*. The *spleen's* attributed functions include a close relationship with the *San Jiao*. Its functions also include many aspects of food metabolism that are commonly attributed to the pancreas and other digestive organs in conventional medicine. Since it is related to water metabolism, the *spleen* must also include at least part of the small intestine, where the majority of water absorption occurs. There are other aspects of *spleen* function that have been spoken of earlier in the text.[117B]

From a conventional point of view, the pancreatic function of regulating blood sugar is indispensable to the liver (in Western medicine) because the liver transforms sugars into glycogen for storage. From this same point of view, there are several causes for hyperglycemia:[118]

- Adrenal *excess* which stimulates the production of sugar by the *liver* while simultaneously slowing down the production of insulin by the pancreas;
- An *excess* of pituitary gland secretions which stimulate the adrenals;
- Insufficiency of the breakdown of sugar in the tissues (glycolysis), usually from a lack of exercise;
- Sympathetic system *excess* which stimulates the *kidneys* and adrenals;
- Slowing of the blood flow through the *liver*, with the blood taking up more and more sugar;
- Insufficiency of the small intestine, which stimulates the pancreas with its secretion, or an *excess* which causes inflammation.

All of these interrelationships speak to the large realm of function of the *middle Jiao* and the *spleen*.[119] The condition of sugar in the urine has traditionally been called *tang niao bing*. There are three varieties — upper, middle, lower — or *san xiao*. The *san xiao* Do not have the same symptoms.[120]

- *Xiao pi* is a shrinking *spleen* (*pancreas*) with emptiness of the *stomach Qi*; a raging appetite is the characteristic;
- *Xiao zhong* is a shrinking center; raging thirst is the characteristic;
- *Xiao shen* is a shrinking *kidney*; having sex that does not fulfill the desire is the characteristic.

In the *upper Jiao* the *heat* affects respiratory functions. The heart and lungs are dry and agitated, the tongue is scarlet, the lips red, the appetite small. In the *middle Jiao* there is perpetual hunger, with little urine or stools. The *heat* invades the *middle Jiao*, making the urine red and copious. When the *kidneys* become involved, the urine is thick and the *heat* dominates the *lower Jiao*. Thirst causes the patient to drink, and this leads to excessive urination but the urine is difficult to pass because of signs of *heat* manifesting as urethritis and other urinary problems. The thighs and knees can atrophy and the face becomes grayish–black. The ears are red and thin. Patients become thinner day by day. This is difficult to treat or cure. Protect the *lungs*, appease the *kidneys*; then the *spleen/pancreas* will move by itself. The root is in the *kidneys* (adrenals). Feed the *spleen*, and the fluids will be produced by themselves. This traditional take on diabetes is paraphrased from the *Yi Xue Ru Men* (*Introduction to Medicine*), by Li Chan, 1575 ACE.[121] This is an analysis for diabetes mellitus and not necessarily for type II diabetes, which did not exist during the 16th century. Still, there are overlaps in symptoms and signs and, therefore, in patterns and treatments.

The diagnostic patterns that are possible for diabetes mellitus include:

(1) *Blazing heat in the yangming channel*

This is the *yangming* stage of the *six* stages or the *Qi level* of the *four levels*. The *yangming* channel contains a high level of *Qi* and blood. When a strong pathogenic influence attacks the *yangming* channel in a healthy person, it can result in the "*four greats*" — high thirst, high fever, profuse sweating, and a flooding pulse. The fever is due to *interior heat*. And this condition is considered interior but at the upper level of interior. Therefore, the *heat* affects the upper body and forces the fluids out in the form of sweating. *Stomach fire* can result, leading to thirst, irritability, and labored breathing. This is considered an acute presentation and can be seen in juvenile diabetes or in uncontrolled type II diabetes. When severe, this is an urgent-to-emergent condition. When less severe, it is a serious condition that may not yet have been diagnosed. It is estimated that 80% of diabetic patients do not know that they are diabetic. This presentation may be the final episode that forces people to seek attention.

(2) *Wasting and thirsting disorder due to Yin deficiency*

The *kidneys* are *deficient*, the *stomach* is dry, and the *Qi* is weak and cannot spread fluids. Persistent thirst is due to *Qi deficiency* which prevents the proper spreading of fluids, and to *stomach dryness* which depletes the fluids. The *kidneys* have lost their power to grasp the *Qi*, and the *spleen* cannot hold substances in their place. This causes the fluids to flow into the *bladder*, producing turbid and copious urine. Fatigue, shortness of breath, and a *deficient* pulse all reflect *Qi deficiency*. The thinness of the pulse reflects *Yin deficiency*.

(3) *Deficient spleen*

Spleen deficiency is most commonly caused by improper eating habits, obsessive thinking and worry, and overwork. The transformation of food into blood and *Qi* is impaired. *Spleen deficiency* also leads to a loss of transportive functions and a lack of transport through the *stomach*. This manifests as reduced appetite, unformed stools, and weakness in the extremities. The tongue is pale, and perhaps swollen with tooth marks. The pulse is weak or moderate.

(4) *Kidney and liver Yin deficiency*

When the *kidneys* are weak, the *marrow* becomes depleted, resulting in general weakness of the musculoskeletal structure, especially the low back and knees. The *kidney essence* and the *liver blood* are not flourishing and are unable to nourish the upper parts of the body, especially the sensory orifices. The eyes are nourished by the *liver blood*. When the *liver blood* is *deficient*, this can end in diabetic retinopathy. The ears are nourished by the *kidney Yin* and *essence*, and when *deficient* this can lead to tinnitus or labyrinthitis. If the *Yin* is *deficient*, it cannot retain substances especially during the night, causing night sweats. *Yin* deficiency and internally generated *heat* are reflected in a red tongue with a dry coating and in a rapid and tin pulse.

(5) *Steaming bone disorder*

This is due to upwardrising of *fire* due to *liver* and *kidney Yin* deficiency. Internally generated *heat* leads to tidal fevers, night sweats, irritability, *heat* and pain in the knees and legs, a red tongue with no coating, and a rapid and forceful pulse that is more forceful in the medial position (intense *heat* in the kidneys). *Heat* rising to the *lungs* may cause cough with blood. *Heat* rising to the *stomach* can cause constant hunger.

(6) *Liver and kidney Yin deficiency with concurrent Qi stasis*

The above pattern with fire is also caused by constraint. Hypochondrium pain, chest pain, epigastric and abdominal distension, dry mouth and throat, and acid eructation can combine with the presentation of item No. 5 to manifest this pattern of diabetes.

(7) *Kidney Yang deficiency with insufficient fire at the mingmen*

Essence transforms into *Qi*, and this is called *kidney Qi*. This is also known as *kidney* or *Source Yang Qi* and is the *Source* of *Yang* for the whole body. It is the *Source* of the motivating force for all functions. When the *kidney Yang* is *deficient*, it manifests as lower-body weakness and a *cold* sensation in the lower half of the body. Fluids become stagnant. The *kidney Yang* drives the functional transformation and movement of water in the body, directing the pure upward and the turbid downward. Urinary difficulty can manifest when this directive force is impaired. Edema may result, especially of the lower extremity. Water and *Qi* may also rebel upward, causing panting and irritability.

(8)   *Heart and kidney disconnect*

When the *kidneys* are *deficient*, they are unable to store properly and this leads to frequent urination. Gray and cloudy urine may result. Deficiency of heart *Qi* leads to disorientation. This is an extension to a more serious presentation with deeper and broader injuries than item No. 7.

In the early stage, diabetes is asymptomatic and a great many people do not know they have the condition. It is appropriate to run tests on patients who are candidates for diabetes based on their weight, dietary habits, and sedentary lifestyle. A fasting blood glucose test would be the first step in determining a diagnosis and the severity of the diagnosis. For early-stage diabetic patients, diet and exercise — the primary causes of the condition — can be used to manage the disease and return pancreatic and insulin function to normal. In many cases this is considered a cure. Even in insulin-dependent or pharmaceutical-drug-dependent diabetes, diet and exercise are extremely important to treatment.

Treatment

(1)   *The upper type of diabetes, marked by fluid deficiency due to lung heat*

Symptoms: polydipsia, dry mouth and tongue, frequent urination with profuse urine, a red tongue with a thin and yellow coating, and a rapid, slippery and full pulse.

The lung and *stomach* are both suffering from *dryness* and *heat*. This leads to a failure of water to be transformed into the *Jin Ye*, and its downward flow will cause frequent urination. *Heat* in the *stomach* will result in polyphagia. The tongue and pulse follow suit.

Formula: *Xiao Ke Fang*, from Zhu Dan Xi's *Experimental Therapy*.

(2)   *The middle type of diabetes, marked by excessive stomach fire*

Symptoms: polyphagia, polydipsia, emaciation, dry stools, frequent urination with sugar in the urine, a dry tongue with a yellow coating, and a full and forceful pulse.

The *stomach* receives food, and polyphagia results from *stomach* fire. Dry *heat* in the gastrointestinal tract impairs body fluids, and polydipsia results. *Heat* in the *yangming* consumes *Jin ye* and blood, and this results in emaciation. *Stomach heat* fails to moisten the stools, causing dry constipation. *Kidney Yin* deficiency leads to hyperactive *kidney Yang* and a lack of consolidation of the *kidney Qi* which drives the *Qi* transformative process of urination, and so there is polyuria. The tongue and pulse in particular indicate *stomach* fire.

Formula: *Yu nu Jian*,[122] from *Jinggue's Complete Medical Books*; *Zeng Ye Cheng Qi Tang*,[123] from *Treatise on Differentiation and Treatment of Epidemic Febrile Diseases*.

(3)   *The lower type of diabetes, marked by deficiency of kidney Yin and deficiency of both Yin and Yang*

(a)   *Yin-deficient type*

Symptoms: frequent urination with large amounts of turbid gray urine with sugar in it, polydipsia, weak and sore knees and low back, dry mouth and lips, *five-center heat*, a red tongue, abd a deep, thready and rapid pulse.

The *deficient kidney Yin* is failing to control urination and this results in polyuria. Lack of consolidation of the *kidney Qi* results in food *essence* flowing downward and this causes turbid urine with sugar in it. *Five-center heat* is a manifestation of *Yin* deficiency and *interior heat* that results in polydipsia. *Kidney deficiency* results in a failure to nourish the areas of charge of the *kidneys* — the lumbar area and the knees. *Kidney Yin* deficiency accounts for the rest of the symptoms and the tongue and pulse.

Formula: *Liu wei di huang wan*,[124] from *Key to Therapeutics of Children's Diseases*; or *Zuo Gui Yin*,[125] from *Jinggue's Complete Medical Books*.

(b)   *Deficiency of both the Yin and the Yang type*

Symptoms: frequent urination with clear watery urine or turbid urine, thirst but no desire to drink, urinating twice as much as drinking, a dark lusterless withered face, dry ears, sore and weak low back and knees, aversion to *cold, cold* limbs, edema, diarrhea at dawn, impotence, a pale tongue with a white and slippery coating, and a deep thready forceless pulse.

Long deficiency of the *kidney Yin* affects the *Yang* and leads to decline of the astringing and consolidating function of the *kidney*, sinking of the *kidney Qi*, and impairment of the *kidney Yang*. This causes clear water-like urine. Sinking of the *kidney Qi* is responsible for the turbid urine. Decline of the *mingmen* and deficiency of *kidney Yin* lead to failure of the fire to steam upward and also of the clear water to go upward. This causes *lung dryness* marked by thirst but little desire to drink because the fire is not so excessive or exuberant. The *deficient kidney Qi* fails to control the urine and results in frequent urination and the urination output being twice the input. Loss of downward flow of food *essence* leads to a failure of the whole body to be nourished; this causes the dark lusterless face. Decline of the *mingmen* ends in impotence. *Mingmen fire* and *kidney Yang deficiency* both end in *cold* and *cold* extremities. The pale tongue and deep thready forceless pulse indicate *Yin* and *Yang deficiency*.

Formula: *Jing gui sheng qi wan*,[126] from *Synopsis of the Prescriptions of the Golden Chamber*.

The lower type of diabetes is the most serious, with various competing conditions. We rarely see this stage of chronic diabetes in the West. We see patients who are undiagnosed with early-stage disease who require diagnosis and perhaps early intervention with pharmaceutical drugs, and for whom Chinese medicine coupled with dietary and lifestyle changes can be curative.

Hypoglycemia[127]

Low blood sugar is considered a precursor of diabetes and develops from the same dietary habits as diabetes. The pancreas is impaired by a diet of high-fat and highly refined foods, losing its ability to produce sufficient or effective insulin. Hypoglycemia often precedes the onset of diabetes.

The symptoms of hypoglycemia include:

Insomnia	Pale skin
Sweating	Headache
Flushing	Low blood pressure
Photophobia	Sweet cravings
Tinnitus	Clamminess
Dry mouth	Shortness of breath
Worry and anxiety	Loss of appetite or constant hunger
Dizziness	Blurred vision
Restlessness	Depression
Inability to concentrate	Crying easily
Hyperactivity	
Cold hands and feet	Impotence (ED)
Irritability	Swollen feet

Resolving hypoglycemia requires controlling insulin production. The avoidance of refined foods is essential to controlling insulin. Complex carbohydrates are digested more slowly and they still retain essential minerals and vitamins that are nutrients which the body needs for the making of blood, hormones, and other fluids that cool and moisten. The hypoglycemic body robs its own tissues of these needed minerals losing the reserves that stabilize it during dietary extremes and stressors in general.[128]

Grains, vegetables, and legumes take time to break down and metabolize. They also contain nutrients that regulate insulin production. Thorough chewing, small frequent meals, and simple food combining all treat diabetes and hypoglycemia.[129] Cheese, nuts, and seeds in small quantities can be added for people who are not overweight or obese, and are a necessary component. Good fats can be derived from these foods and are not contraindicated.

Salt reduces blood sugar and should be used very sparingly in a good diet. Seaweeds have a salty flavor, are rich in protein and mineral content, and have many anticancer properties. They are an excellent substitute for salt.[130]

Juices are very concentrated in simple sugars and lack fiber. Overuse of even whole fruit can precipitate extreme fluctuations in blood sugar. Citrus fruits lower blood sugar quickly and should be avoided in those who are diabetic or hypoglycemic. Sweeteners like honey, barley malt, rice syrup, and real molasses can be used in moderation. As stated before, stevia does not impact blood sugar and is an excellent substitute for sugars.[131]

Hypoglycemic patients are generally mineral-*deficient* and also lack essential fatty acids (EFAs). Dry hair and skin, low body weight, poor glandular function, and *liver* deficiency can manifest as irritability, depression, anxiety, and insomnia. *Cold*-pressed oil like flax oil is a good supplement.

The conditions of diabetes and hypoglycemia are usually emblematic of a long history of dietary abuses that then cause what looks like an addiction to those very same foods, especially sugar and refined carbohydrates. Treating these conditions requires patience and constancy on the part of the patient as well as the practitioner.[132] Overcoming this cycle of eating habits requires ongoing fresh insights, treatment prods in the right direction, and inspiration to change.

Changing these food habits will change not only the inner world but also the outer world in which industrial farming is destroying the land, and the food industry makes its primary profits from the center aisles of grocery stores. Farming that is sustainable is the *Source* of and equivalent to a *middle Jiao* that is high in digestive *fire*. Industrial farming depends on our addictions to poor-quality foods and sugar, which diminish our palates and alter our ability to perceive good and living foods. It is linked to market-driven decisions that have nothing to do with human or animal health. It is only consumer demand that is driving the organics market in the US Organics and sustainability, when combined, mean that the best choices are made from seed to land to market — choices that help us live better and support the Earth which feeds us. These choices are part of our inherent task in preventing cancers. And seeing all of them as connected is step No. 1.

Calorie restriction

Calorie restriction (CR) is a technique that is currently being studied by nutritional and other researchers in aging and the prevention of chronic disease and cancer.[133] It refers to the reduction of caloric intake on a daily and long-term basis. The Surgeon General's Office provides daily caloric requirements for various ages and body types; CR falls outside these daily requirements and is often far below. Whereas the Surgeon General's recommendation may be 2000 calories per day for a 5′ 5″ woman, in CR the daily recommendation may be 1200 calories per day, depending on activity levels. CR is not fasting, nor is it an eating disorder. People who use it to manage their health are typically thinner than most other people of their height but they are not anorexic or unhealthy.

The goal is to achieve a point that is 10%–25% below the set point for body weight. The set point is that weight point to which one's body naturally drifts and stabilizes. Therefore, the aim is to lose 10%–25% of one's lean baseline weight in order to live more healthly. This diet requires a nutrient-dense diet of low-calorie foods and constant monitoring to ensure that one does not become malnourished. The approach is not about weight loss but about the number of calories one consumes per day based on one's own set point and body type.

The concept of CR evolved from studies done on two monkeys which were the same age but fed over 25 years a high-calorie and a low-calorie diet, respectively. The monkey fed the low-calorie diet remained more active and healthy and appeared to age significantly more slowly than the monkey fed the high-calorie diet. Studies were done on other animals and finally on humans. These later studies show that over 6 months there was a weight loss of 10%–14%. They also showed that fasting insulin levels were significantly lowered, and that the core body temperature was reduced. The 24 h energy expenditure decreased while CR was utilized. And DNA damage was significantly reduced from baseline.[134]

There are two main biomarkers for overall health — fasting insulin and body temperature as a marker for inflammation. Both of these were significantly reduced by CR. Higher insulin levels have been found in patients with CRC and breast cancer, the only two conditions studied to date. These higher insulin levels were found to have a relationship with the proliferation of tumor cells.[135] Fluctuating blood sugar levels cause spikes in insulin that may play a role in the cancerization process. It may be that, although sugar is the preferred substrate for tumor cells, the role of insulin is more important in proliferation and prognosis.

Alternate day fasting and chronic disease prevention have also been studied. In people who fasted every other day, there was a low diabetes incidence, lower fasting glucose, and lower insulin concentrations. Also, the total cholesterol level was lowered and the HDL cholesterol levels were raised. The heart and blood pressure in these people was also decreased.[136] When it came to cancers, there was a decrease in lymphoma incidence, longer survival in patients with any cancer, and lower rates of proliferation of several cancer cell types.[137]

CR requires a break in our addictions to food and a change in our relationship to food that many find difficult. Ultimately, it would seem somewhat obvious that many people overeat on a regular basis, and overeat many foods that are promoting factors. Most people do not overeat vegetables. And yet this is exactly what a CR diet is — a mostly vegetable diet with some fruit and primarily protein derived from grains and legumes.

Fasting

Fasting and purification seem to be a part of every perennial tradition that has ever been studied.[138] Even in prehistoric cultures, seasonal cycles often imposed a time of scarcity in terms of food. The foods that were available in the down time of the cycle were often roots, new spring shoots, and other plant materials which probably played a role in cleansing as part of an annual process. Those early fasts may have limited people to only one food or no food, and they may have lasted for a period of days or weeks.

The word "fast" refers to a speeding-up of the cleansing process by slowing down the regular digestive routine. This cleansing involves the detoxification of the products of oxidative stress, residues left over from a high-protein and refined diet, and toxins, some of which are normal and some abnormal, resulting from environmental contamination. In the earlier days of humankind and even in many countries in modern times, especially countries of Asia, the diet is partially one of building foods and partially one of cleansing foods — usually in the same meal. Building foods are usually heavier foods and include protein, grains, beans, nuts and, in our culture, overrich foods. Cleansing foods are fruits and vegetables. It would be typical for building foods to be used and even required during winter, and for cleansing foods (which are lighter) to be used in summer, when cleansing is more appropriate because fewer calories are needed to run the body.[139]

Fasting helps not only to detoxify but also to alkalinize the body. The residues from many foods are most often acidic, high-fat, or mucus-forming. The body performs best when it is slightly alkaline.[140] Alkaline foods include fruits and vegetables — plants. Acidic foods are dairy, meats, poultry, refined sugars and grains, and chemicals. You can see from the list that acidic foods are exactly those foods that contribute to a cancer environment. There is controversy on this subject. It is left to you to determine what your diet should be for health. Certainly, there is ample evidence that eating a largely plant-based diet promotes health.

There are many precancerous signs that the body manifests in an effort to discharge impurities and toxins. Abnormal discharge occurs through diarrhea, frequent urination, imbalanced emotions, and chronic restlessness. The skin is a macrocosm for observation of ineffective discharge of chronic exposures. Some of these skin signs are:

- Skin tags that are seen to be manifestations of blood and *phlegm stasis*;

- White points (usually on the face) that are seen to be *phlegm stasis* caused usually by an inability to properly digest dairy products;
- Brown skin markings that are seen as manifestations of highly refined carbohydrate and sugar consumption.

Accumulations like these represent the body's inability to discharge through normal functioning. Chronic sinus discharges, middle ear discharges, cysts, fatty organs, *kidney* stones, chronic noninfectious vaginal discharges, and benign swellings are all signs of localized accumulations that demonstrate an imbalance and the body's inability to handle what is being put into it. Some of these accumulations act as magnets for *latent pathogenic factors —* especially damp accumulations. *Latent pathogenic factors* can transform into toxins and, therefore, a scene for possible malignancy is set.

There are several signs of a possible precancerous environment. They include:

- Calcified deposits that show up on conventional scans and indicate *blood stasis*;
- Cysts anywhere in the body, which can indicate *phlegm* and *blood stasis*;
- Mucus and fat accumulations around centrally located organs, which indicate *phlegm stasis*;
- Skin tags anywhere but especially on the naso and muno areas, which indicate *blood stasis*;
- Cupping at the navel for 3 min that results in a dark color of long duration, which can indicate systemic *blood stasis*;
- Tongue areas that are dark or veins that are dark and swollen, which can indicate *blood stasis*;
- All of the blood and/or *phlegm stasis* pulses;
- Spider veins or angiomas, especially on the trunk, which can indicate *blood stasis* underneath.

These latent and asymptomatic manifestations of a struggling body mechanism are signs that the practitioner can use to combine with the overall intake to determine a patient's risk factors for cancer or a precancerous body ecology. Almost all of them are usually due to diet and lack of exercise. The intake should include a diet diary and intensive questioning about, and careful evaluation of, the patient's diet and lifestyle routines. These routines may be unconscious or conscious but knowledge of them enables the practitioner (and the patient) to truly facilitate change and empower patients to live well and live long, usually without disease and without cancer of any kind. Fasting may be an initial and important part of recovery of health.

Our cells, weak and congested with cell-generated wastes, are overtaxed and unable to detoxify. According to *wen bing* theory, the resulting internal environments — *dampness, liver Qi stasis, spleen deficiency, Yin deficiency* — magnetize *latent pathogenic factors* and create an environment where more and more waste accumulates, marking the cells as aged. The symptoms of many autoimmune diseases can be reversed or at least improved if cellular detoxification through CR and fasting is implemented to reduce the load of metabolic wastes and toxins, thereby allowing these cells to return to normal.

When the beneficial effects of fasting were investigated within the parameters of conventional medicine and science, substantial improvements were seen in the autonomic nervous system, the endocrine system, and adrenal function after the fast. Fasting and CR have a powerful effect on the modulation of free radical production, repairing free radical damage, and facilitating removal or detoxification of the products of free radical damage, for example through oxidative stress.[141] CR and fasting also decrease the rate of free radical generation by reducing the rate of electron transport and oxygen utilization. This may be the conventional science language for the concept of how damp *phlegm* knotted with toxin impedes the overall function of the *Wei Qi* and the *San Jiao*. Fasting may help reset the *San Jiao* and all of its interrelationships, from water metabolism to the *Source Qi*, to the *shen*, to the *Wei Qi*.

Conclusion

All of these issues, from agriculture and where our food comes from to the diseases created by the food habits we foster and the issue of food scarcity in the world at large, are interconnected. The physical and internal environment of the human body includes our mind and spirit, and as such is sacred. At the same time, our mind and spirit live on in the exterior environment that we have made. There is no separation of inside from outside on this globe. Who we are, what we think, and what we eat are interconnected. Who we are and what we eat are based upon who we decide to be and know ourselves to be as expressed in all of those actions that bring our food to our tables. Wisdom regarding who we are, who we become, and what we eat and how we produce our food comes from inner dialogue and from listening — listening within ourselves and listening outside of ourselves and to the larger wisdom known as the Sacred. Our health and the health of our world is rooted in listening for the truth. We must live a life of connectedness to ourselves and to our world. It is from here that we must listen. We are what we eat, and what we eat comes from our decisions. We are what we hear in our hearts.

References

1. United Nations. Mortality. unstats.un.org/unsd/demographic/scon-cerns/mortality/mort2.htm
2. Rochat E. (2012) Phythm at the heart of the world. Chap. 5 of the *Nei Jing Su Wen.* Monkey.
3. Kilborne B. (1999) When trauma strikes the soul: shame, splitting, and psychic pain. Am J Psychoanal **59(4):** 385–402.
4. Luoto M *et al.* (2003) Loss of plant species richness and habitat connectivity in grasslands associated with agricultural change in Finland. Ambio **32(7):** 447–52.
5. Discovery Channel. Lost animals of the 20th century. 1990s documentary series.
6. Third Global Biodiversity Outlook Report. United Nations Environment Programme. www.guardian.co.uk/science/2010/may/10/un-report-economic-impact-biodiversity-loss
7. Sustainable table. Biodiversity. www.sustainabletable.org/issues/biodiversity
8. SwissAid. Securing biodiversity. www.swissaid.ch/en/biodiversity
9. FAO Corporate Document Repository. What is happening to agrobio-diversity? www.fao.org/docrep/007/ys609e/y5609e02.htm

10. Hardin G. Tragedy of the Commons. www.econlib.org/library/enc/tragedyofthecommons.html

11. UN News Centre. Conserving plant genetic diversity crucial for future food security. www.un.org/apps/news/story.asp?newsid=3654#.ucy-daUbUes0

12. Thrupp L. (2000) Linking agricultural biodiversity and food security: the valuable role of agrobiodiversity for sustainable agricultre. Int Aff **76(2)**: 265–281.

13. Shewry P R. W*heat.* J Exp Bot. www.xb.oxfordjournals.org/content/60/6/1537.full

14. Dimitri C *et al.* The 20th Century transformation of the US Agriculture and Farm Policy. USDA. www.ers.usda.gov/publications/eib-economic-information-bulletin/eib3.aspx

15. Harrigan L *et al.* Environmental health perspectives. www.ncbi.nlm.nih.gov/pmc/articles.PMC1240832

16. Gutierre D. (2011) Natural News. Global food security at risk as crop biodiversity is lost. Jan. 29. Naturalnews.com

17. Global Exchange. Food security, farming, and the WTO and CAFTA. www.globalexchange.org/resources/wto/agriculture

18. Carino J. Poverty and well-being. Chap. 1. www.org/ese/socdev/unfil/documents/SOWIP_chapter1.pdf

19. ETC Group. Biotech activists oppose the terminator technology. New patent aims to prevent farmers from saving seed. www.unv.etcgroup.org/content/biotech-activists-oppose-terminator-technology

20. Grain. Why are the FAO and the EBRD promoting the destruction of peasant and family farming? www.grain.org/article/entries.4572-why-are-the-FAO-and-the-EBRD/

21. Grain. Land grabbing and food sovereignty in West and Central Africa. Ibid.

22. Hubbard K. (2009). Out of hand. Dec. Farmers trace the consequences of a consolidated seed industry. www.farmertofarmercampaign.com/out%20of%20hand.fullreport.pdf

23. Gadban R M, Gwynn R E. (1988) *Intellectual Porperty Rights. Global Consensus, Global Conflict?* Westview, Boulder, CO.

24. Rai S. (2001) India–US fight on basmati rice is mostly settled. *The Newyork Times* Technology. Aug 25.

25. Hoggan K. (2000) Neem tree patent revoked. BBC News. May 10.

26. Navdanya, to Dr. Vandana Shiva's blog. www.navdanya.org

27. Shiva V. The Indian Seed Act and Patent Act sowing the seeds of dictator-ship. CounterCurrents.org. www.countercurrents.org/gl-shiva150205.htm

28. Patented GM crops: making seed saving illegal? Technology. The African Executive. www.africanexecutive.com/modules/magazine/articles.php?article=766

29. Shand H. Rural Advancement Foundation International. Avalanche of public opposition to Monsanto's suicide seeds. www.greens.org/s-r/19/19-03.html

30. Benbrook C. (2009) Impacts of Genetically-engineered crops on pesti-cide use: the first thirteen years. Nov 2009. GM Watch. www.gmwatch.org/index.php?options=com_content&vIew=article&id=11696.cherry-

31. Klinkenburg V. The folly of big agriculture: why nature always wins. Environment 360. Yale Environment 360. www.e360.yale.edu

32. Vasilokiotis C. UC Berkeley. Can organic farming "feed the world"? www.agroeco.org/doc/organic_feed_world.pdf

33. Land degradation in the developing world: issues and policy options for 2020. www.ifpri.org/2020/briefs/number44.htm

34. Acidification form fertilizer use linked to soil aging. www.news.cals.wisc.edu

35. Pretty J N *et al.* An assessment of the total external costs of UK agriculture. www.essex.ac.uk/ces/research/externalities/agsysttotalextcostukagri.shtm

36. Shiva V. Monocultures, monopolies, myths and the masculinization of agriculture. Gifts of Speech. www.gos.sbc.edu/s/shiva2.html

37. *Ibid.*

38. *Fatal harvest. The Foundation for Deep Ecology.* Island, 2002, p. 73.

39. *Ibid.*, p. 75.

40. *Ibid.*, p. 77.

41. Starlink corn regulatory history. Pesticides: regulating pesticides. www.epa.gov/oppbppd1/biopesticides/pips/starlink_corn.htm

42. *Op. cit.*, No. 38, p. 79.

43. *Ibid.*, p. 81.

44. Monoculture and the Irish potato famine: cases of missing genetic variation. Understand Evolution. www.evolution.berkeley.edu/evoli-brary/article/agriculture_02

45. Heritage and heirloom foods. Sustainable table. www.sustainabletable.org/issues/heritage

46. Long C. Industrial farming is giving us less nutritious food. Mother Jones News. www.motherjonesnews.com/sustainable-farming/nutrient-decline

47. www.ewg.org

48. Philpott T. Mother Jones. Independent Panel: EPA underestimates atrazines cancer risk. www.motherjones.com/tom-philpott/2011/11/atrazine-cancer-epa

49. Pesticides. Knowledge Center. Environment and Health Fund. www.ehf.org/IL.en/interim/pesticides

50. Pesticides and breast cancer. www.nan.pow-uk.org/pestnews/issue/pn22/pn22p3,htm

51. Colorectal cancer. www.cdc.gov/vitalsigns/cancerscreening/

52. Colorectal cancer incidence and mortality worldwide in 2008 summary. Globocan 2008. www.globocan.larc.fr/factsheets/cancers/colorectal.asp

53. Colrectal cancer overview. American Cancer Society. www.cancer.org/cancer/colonandrectumcancer

54. *Ibid.*

55. Signh P N *et al.* (1998) Dietary risk factors for colon cancer in a low-risk population. *Am J Epidemiol* **148**: 761–74.

56. *Op.cit.*

57. *Op.cit.*

58. O'Keefe S J *et al.* (1999) Rarity of colon cancer in Africans is associated with low animal product consumption, not fiber. *Am J Gastroenterol* **94**: 1373–82

59. Bruce W R, Garcia A. (2000) Possible mechanisms relating diet and risk of colon cancer. *Cancer Epidemiol Biomarkers Prev* **9(12)**: 1271–79.

60. Jones S. *et al.* Comparative lesion sequencing provides insights into tumor evolution. www.ped.fas.harvard.edu/people/faculty/publications_nowak/jones_pnas08.pdf

61. Ponwampalam E N *et al.* (2006) Effect of feeding systems on omega-3 fatty acids conjugated linoleic acid and trans fatty acids in Australian beef cuts: potential impact on human health. *Asia Pac J Clin Nutr* **15(1)**: 21–29.

62. Negri E *et al.* (1998) Fiber intake and risk of colorectal cancer. *Cancer Epidemiol Biomarkers Prev* **7(8)**: 667–71.

63. Doheny K. Hig-fiber diet linked to lower colon cancer risk. CRC Health Center. WebMD. www.webmd.com/colorectal-cancers/news/20111110/high-fiber

64. *Op. cit.*, No. 60.

65. What about grass-fed beef? John Robbins, 2010. www.johnrobbins.info/blog/grass-fed-beef

66. Parker H. A sweet problem: Princeton researchers find that high fructose corn syrup prompts more weight gain. www.princeton.edu/main/news/archive/S26/91/22k07

67. Dunsinger M. Diabetes Health Center. Is stevia a good subsitute for sugar? WebMD. www.diabetes.webmd.com/features/stevia-good-subsitute-sugar

68. Rochat E, Wu X. (2009) *The Five Elements in Classical Chinese Texts*. Monkey.

69. Dossey L. (1999) *Reinventing Medicine*. Harper One.

70. Denally E *et al.* (2001) n-3 fatty acids and cardiovascular disease risk factors among the Inuit of Nunavik1'2'3'. *Am Soc Clin Nutr.* Abstract 464.

71. Polak J M *et al.* (1979) Neuropeptides of the gut: a newly discovered major control system. Springerlink. *World J Surg* **3(4)**: 393–405

72. The Science of food addiction. www.foodaddiction.com/publications/sciencepage5.html

73. Swann P F. (1977) Carcinogenic risk from nitrite, nitrate and n-nitrosamines in food. *Proc R Soc Med* **70(2)**: 113–115.

74. Vitamin D. www.bidmo.org/yourhealth/holistichealth/functionalfoods.asp

75. Colorectal cancer: causes, risk factors, and prevention topics. American Cancer Society. www.cancer.org/cancer/colonandrectumcancer/detailedguide.colorectal

76. Cancer prevention (reducing the risk). NYU Langone Medical Center. www.med.nyu.edu/content?chawk/id=32264

77. Robbins J. (2001) *The Food Revolution*, Conari. Chap. 11: Misery on the menu.

78. Schulbach H *et al.* (1978) *Soil Water* **38**(Fall).

79. Myers N. Conversion of tropical moist forests: a report prepared for the Committee on Research Priorities in Tropical Biology of the National Research Council. National Academy of Sciences Washington, D.C.

80. Durning and Brough. Taking stock. P. 31.

81. De Walt B. (1983) The cattle are eating the forest. *Bull Atom Scientists.* **39(1):** 22.

82. Bernstein C. Bile acids link high fat diet to colon cancer. *J Arch Toxicol.* Reviewed at www.uanews.org/node/37770

83. Kiani L. Microflora in the intestinal tract. www.csa.com/dbcouryguides/probiotic/review2.[php

84. Zhang ZJ. (1987) *Shang Han Za Bin Lun (Discussion of Cold-induced Disorders).* 210 C.E. People's Health.

85. Kirby D, Dudrick S. (1994) *Practical Handbook of Nutrition in Clinical Practice.* CRC.

86. Macciocia G. (1989) *The Foundations of Chinese Medicine.* Churchill Livingstone, pp. 108–109, 227–228.

87. Di Roda A. Antacids may spell trouble for some. City of Hope. www.cityofhope.org/about/publications/chtome/2009_vol8_num_5_may_28

88. Seattle Cancer Care Alliance. Colon cancer. signs and symptoms. www.seattlecca.org/dispasb/colon-cancer-sign-symptoms.cfm

89. Li PW. (2003) *Management of Cancer with Chinese Medicine.* Donica. Chap. 2, *Etiology, Pathology, Diagnosis and Treatment of Tumors in Traditional Chinese Medicine,* pp.17–47.

90. Jian MW, Seifert G. (2000) *Warm Disease Theory. Wen Bing Xue.* Paradigm.

91. Ma SC. Lecture notes on *wen bing xue* and the concept of latent pathogenic factors.

92. Macciocia G. (1995) *The Foundations of Chinese Medicine.* Churchill Livingstone, p. 45. From the *Su Wen,* Chap. 43.

93. *Op. cit.,* No. 89, pp. 23–24.

94. FAP, Lynch syndrome and other hereditary colorectal cancers. Memorial Sloan-Kettering Cancer Center. www.maskcc.org/cancer-care/adult/colorectal/fap-lynch-syndrome-other-hereditary/

95. Tresca A. Colon cancer and IBD. www.ibdcrohns.about.com/cs/colorectalcancer/&/ibdcrohns.htm

96. Haberman T. (ed.). (2006) *Mayo Clinic Internal Medicine Review*, 7th ed. CRC.

97. Michor F *et al.* (2005) Dynamics of colorectal cancer. *Sem Canc Biol* **15:** 484–493.

98. Kuahara K. Notes from lectures on *toyo hari.*

99. Inflammatory Bowel Disease. The difference between IBD and IBS. www.ibdcrohns.about.com/cs/ibs/a/diffibsibd.htm

100. Digestive Disorders Health Center. WebMD. www.webmd.com/digestive-disorders/picture-of-the-intestines

101. Irritable bowel syndrome. National Digestive Diseases Information Clearighouse (NDDIC). www.digestive.niddk.nih.gov/ddiseases/pubs/ibs

102. Ulcerative Colitis. www.digestive.niddk.nih.gov/ddiseases.pubs.colitis/index.aspx#symptoms

103. Birch S, Matsumoto K. (1998) *Hara Diagnosis: Reflections on the Sea.* Paradigm.

104. NIH study finds sigmoidoscopy reduces colorectal cancer rates. www.nih.gov/news/health/may2012

105. Murray M. (1999) *Encyclopedia of Natural Medicine*, 2nd ed. Little Brown.

106. Sun PL (ed.). (2002). *The Treatment of Pain with Chinese Herbs and Acupuncture.* Churchill Livingstone. Chap. 5.

107. Hou JL, Zhao X, (ed.). (1995) *Treatment of Gastrointestinal Diseases in TCM.* Academy.

108. Bensky D, and Barolet R. (1990) *Formulas and Strategies.* 1st ed. Eastland, p. 149.

109. *Ibid.,* p. 127.

110. *Ibid.,* p. 238.

111. *Ibid.,* p. 147.

112. *Ibid.,* p. 197.

113. *Ibid.,* p. 359.

114. *Op. cit.,* No. 103, Chap. 8.

115. Murray M *et al.* (2005) *The Encyclopedia of Healing Foods.* Atria.

116. Diabetes basics. Type 2. American Diabetes Association. www.diabetes.org/diabetes-basics/type-2/

117. Feng WB. (2009) *Diabetes and Obesity.* People's Medical Publishing House.

117B. Li DY. (1993) *Treatise on the Spleen and Stomach: A Translation of the Pi Wei Lun*. Translators *Yang* SZ, Li JY. Blue Poppy.

118. Hyperglycemia (high blood sugar). American Diabetes Association. www.diabetes.org/living-with-diabetes/treatment-and-care/blood-glucose

119. Unschuld P. (2011) *Huang di Nei Jing Su Wen. Su Wen (Basic Questions)*. University of California Press, Chap. 5.

120. *Op. cit.*, No. 117.

121. Li C. (1575) *Yi Xue Ru Men (Introduction to Medicine)*.

122. *Op. cit.*, No. 108, p. 94.

123. *Ibid.*, p. 118.

124. *Ibid.*, p. 263.

125. *Ibid.*, p. 266.

126. *Ibid.*, p. 277.

127. Hypoglycemia. PubMed. Health. www.ncbi.nl nih.govpubmedhealth/PMH0001423

128. Hypoglycemia. Diabetes Resource Center, Inc. Center for Nutritional Medicine. www.diabetesresourcecenter.org/index.html

129. Diet for hypoglycemia without diabetes. www.Livestrong.com.article370022

130. Min SK *et al.* (2008) Effects of seaweed supplementation on blood glucose concentration, lipid profile, and antioxidant enzyme activities in patients with type 2 diabetes mellitus. *Nutr Res Pract* **2(2)**: 62–67.

131. Find a vitamin or supplement. Stevia. WebMD. www.webmd.com/vitamins-supplements/ingredientmono682-stevia

132. Obesity and Food Addiction Summit. Food addiction. www.foodaddictionsummit.org/foodaddiction.htm

133. NIH Study finds calorie restriction does not affect survival. NIH News. Aug. 29, 2012. www.nih.govnews/health/aug2012/nia-29.htm

134. Calorie restriction leads scientists to molecular pathways the slow aging, improve health. *Science*, Apr. 16, 2010. www.sciencedaily.com/releaeses/2010/04/10041541123.htm

135. Giovanucci E *et al.* Diabetes and cancer. A consensus report. American Diabetes Association. www.care.diabetesjournals.org/content/33/7/1674.long

136. *Op. cit.*, No. 108, p. 134.

137. *Op. cit.*, No. 108, p. 135.

138. McKnight S. (2009) *Fasting: The Ancient Practices.* Thomas Nelson.
139. Pitchford P. (1993) *Healing With Whole Foods: Oriental Traditions and Modern Nutrition.* North Atlantic.
140. The ph Nutrition Guide to Acid/Alkaline Balance. Naturalnews.com
141. Gredilla R. *et al.* Calorie restriction decreases mitochondrial free radical generation at complex levels and lowers oxidative damage to mitochondrial DNA in the rat heart. FASEB J **15(9)**: 1589–91.

CHAPTER 4

Yin and *Qi* — Breast Cancer

There is no one but us.
There is no one to send,
not a clean hand nor a pure heart
on the face of the Earth, nor in the Earth,
but only us,
a generation comforting ourselves
with the notion that we have come to an awkward time,
that our innocent fathers are all dead
— as if innocence had ever been —
and our children busy and troubled,
and ourselves unfit, not yet ready,
having each of us chosen wrongly,
made a false start, failed,
yielded to impulse and the tangled comfort of pleasures,
and grown exhausted, unable to seek the thread, weak,
and involved.
But there is no one but us.
There never has been.

— *Annie Dillard*, Holy the Firm

Introduction

There is a prophetic saying that when the grandmothers speak the Earth will heal.[1] It is not clear from which tradition this saying came but it may have come from a matriarchal society or one in which women were coequals and were treasured. One of the greatest gaps of inclusion made by the founders of the United States was the omission from the knowledge they gained from the Iroquois Confederacy that it was the grandmothers of the clan who appointed the chiefs.[2]

Unfortunately, it was not until 1920 that women were able to gain the vote in this country. In the present day and only 90 years after achieving the vote, women are caught in the thing that we call the "war on cancer." And nowhere is this war more visible in the United States than in the skirmishes with breast cancer. Mothers, daughters, and grandmothers are all caught in these battles. And although women have rallied around one another in this war, we still await the grandmothers speaking the truth about breast cancer. Since Rachel Carson died of breast cancer shortly after *Silent Spring* came out in 1962, we are still waiting for the connection between culture, the environment, and breast cancer to be voiced.

If men were more inclined to form circles of support like women do when stressed, we would learn that the rates of prostate cancer and breast cancer are about the same: one in six men are diagnosed with prostate cancer and one in eight women with breast cancer.[3] But many men remain quiet, accepting their fates and going down — more men die from prostate cancer than women do from breast cancer — alone and silent.[4] Some reasons for this will be covered in the next chapter. Women, on the other hand, form groups and brew a pot of tea. Women circle the wagons and hold a summit meeting. We should all, men and women and children and animals and the entire circle of life, be doing this, because we are all at risk.

This particular chapter happens to be about breast cancer and the specific healing that is required. Although mainly pertinent to women, it is more importantly about the broader realities of the receptive[5] and nurturance, the Yin side of nature that is part of us all, no matter our gender. In the last chapter, the crisis of masculinity came up, and it will come up again, even as part of the discussion of femininity. But, in this chapter, what is needed is to speak about the crisis of femininity, the crisis regarding the receptive in life, of water and the fecund dark side of the mountain that holds the seeds for all future life, the side of listening for truth, of receiving the message, of hope through giving, of caution, of carrying the responsibility for hope and healing through love, and of the positive power of darkness. Truly, masculinity and femininity are of the same mountain but femininity is on the north side. And one cannot exist without the other.

The Problem

Women, and therefore men, have been at a crossroads for some time now: one that poses the confusing question of how to live a life that expresses the need for an individual and creative life of self-fulfillment juxtaposed with the needs imposed upon all of us, but especially upon those of us of the female gender, for family and child-rearing, for nurturing the society of humanity. The questions are about giving, receiving, and sometimes taking. And they are about individuality and community, service and self-fulfillment. They include the apparent conflict between the driving force of individuality and the inherent right to do anything with one's life and property, and the inherent need to work for the general good, protecting resources that are communal and the need to forego some things for the larger good and the future. These questions seem clearly and simply put. However, the conundrum is far more complex, and the world outside and inside of the family imposes constraints especially upon women that make both parts of the question an impossible maze of contradiction that provides in our current world no clear choice or answer for women and, therefore, for the receptive side of life and nature.

As we all try to move beyond the traditional roles that women, and therefore men, have been caught in for the last few thousand years, the primary motivator and carrier of the burden of discovery has been women. Perhaps it is always the downtrodden, the slaves, the underclass, the powerless, and the poor who move a revolution. Many religious paths speak of how the meek shall inherit the Earth, and the great shall be made small and the small shall be made great. It is a very old theme — perhaps even an Abrahamic patriarchal theme that keeps us all going even in the midst of little change. This particular revolution is an immense task because it touches every aspect of life as we know it: societal roles, gender roles, work, poverty, how we own and use the land, science versus religion, and so on. And women seem to be trying to accomplish it alone. The question always is: Can women have it all? That is, if you are wealthy enough to have the choice to ask. The very question comes out of the issue of women struggling to make this change often by themselves. We do not ask if men can have it all,

·

or if children can have it all, or if Mother Nature can have it all. But the problem is bilateral, multitudinous, all-encompassing, male and female, concerning reproduction, the old and the young, the environment and sustainability. And it is multicultural. It involves all of the world's populations.

This question is about the human race and how we live on the Earth. It remains a question about the problem of the split between mind and heart, the receptive and the initiatory, the *Yin* and the *Yang*, the powerful and the powerless, humanity and nature, science and religion. We are in the throes of it now as we strive as the indigenous peoples of the Earth for a new consciousness that is the next step in our evolution.

Some Examples

It is astounding, the number of women who live out several identities within the context of one lifetime. Women are asked to bear and provide care for children while simultaneously being a spouse, a lover, the manager of the household, the caregiver for aging parents, and a breadwinner with an evolving career. The job/career is often out of necessity, and frequently is also an effort by a woman to have a professional and adult life, a career out of which some external contribution to life is made. It is an effort to be a creative coequal in life.[6] ·

In the context of the usual accepted roles of women at home and with caretaking, career and work is often seen as a personal choice and not as a human right, a right and a freedom. Women are not supported for these decisions even though they contribute to the home, the culture, the marketplace, the community, and the family.[7] If women are supported to work, it is for pragmatic reasons, usually involving income. Women who are mothers who work (versus women who work who are mothers — an important distinction not applied to men in the workforce) are usually not supported in ways that would enable them to work *and* parent.[8] And men frequently do not see coparenting as a full-time task, nor is any part of the workplace structured around them doing so. The fact is that many women now work out of necessity, and for those who do work out of

·

necessity, the work of caregiving and family is also their full-time work. Although men certainly have their own set of issues living in the complex modern world, they do not usually live these particular schizophrenic lives. We do not see politicians speaking to the needs of soccer dads. We rarely speak of men as caregivers. The word "caregiver" is a sort of second-class word depicting a particular station in life that does not require compensation or, at best, is worthy of only a lower compensation.[9]

Women put their own health on the line every day in order to provide security and stability regarding reproduction and child-rearing. Disrupting the reproductive cycle either through hormones or through mechanical means carries risks.[10] The questions regarding these issues are not considered to be male questions. The separation of status regarding work and career, child-rearing and home, and the management of reproduction is silently degrading, partly *because* these are not considered to be male issues. Women get pregnant but men do not and couples do not. Only women get pregnant. What really makes it degrading is the fact that women make these decisions and carry the resulting burdens alone. It is only in the few equitable relationships that a man will say "we are pregnant." Teenage girls get pregnant but not the boys who were also part of the pregnancy. The latter are almost always completely let off the hook before (contraception), during (equality in sexual activities), and after (pregnancy responsibility).

The last time anyone checked, it takes a male and a female donation to procreate another human being. Almost all of the issues and questions that revolve around contraception, parenting, and rearing another human being are placed on women.[11] This reality is emblematic of the status of women and, therefore, children in our society, who are primarily the charges of women. When women are low in the pecking order, children are even lower. And Mother Nature, the natural world, comes last. To not cherish and respect women means equally to not cherish and respect children, to not cherish the receptive in life, to not cherish the natural world of which we are part. Even though we say that we cherish women, children, and the Earth, our actions do not demonstrate this.

Children are seen as the future but they are not treasured by society. If they were, then adequate time and flexibility would be given to caregivers — usually women — to properly care for children. There really is no time left to spend with children teaching the basics of honesty, loving mindfulness, trust, how to live a true life as a true human being. Primary education has been languishing for years in the US because of a lack of priority that would demand the necessary funds to provide a good education for our children. It is mainly women who are our teachers. Our teachers are some of the lowest-paid professionals in the job market.[12,13]

The education of children is often seen as the preparation of the next generation's workforce. Governance and capitalism are dominated by upper-class men and, therefore, educating children becomes philosophically driven by a male-oriented class and value system, one that is remarkably profit-driven, teaches linear thinking, and has little to do with self-discovery and creativity. Although women do most of the teaching to our children, most often men determine what will be taught. Children often remain unclaimed treasures except by women who take the time to know them as creative beings. This is especially true if they grow up in poverty. And for those women who are forced to raise their children in poverty and as single parents, it is amazing that so much has been accomplished with so little.

The main thrust of child-rearing has been placed on women, no matter if they work or not. Because women are being lost in the shuffle, men live split lives, having lost touch with their receptive selves. Women have become the main means through which men can remember their true selves, and the loss of deep relationships between men and women is an example of the split in modern living that is partly result and cause. Women should not carry the burden of responsibility for these injuries, but they do. Men feel a sense of loss of dignity if they are asked to play a feeling or caregiver role or are asked to feel their own emotions, as though doing so was somehow beneath them or not part of their world. This puts the expression of emotions into the female arena. And yet there is very little evidence that these disparities are based on biology or genetics.[14,15] It is not unlike the concept of race; less than 1% of the human genome is dedicated to those characteristics that we call racial, and they are all superficial characteristics. The fact of race is becoming more and more unclear and difficult to define.[16] The same should be true for gender roles that are mainly based on the same cultural hierarchy of power. We do not know how many wars would not be fought if men were engaged in the rearing of their own children.

In the end, no one is completely parenting the children, and the wisdom traditions of truthful living are being lost due to lack of time for listening and the development of a self that would provide an example. Children are forced back on themselves to develop their own beliefs about themselves and their world, beliefs often derived from media influences. Parenting is being driven by fiduciary needs and the effort to survive; and, therefore, parenting is often driven by fear.[17] The parenting that does occur is mostly by women. The love that occurs in the home is often only from women. Love has become a four-letter female word and not a human word. This is such a terrible loss to men.

Adults, and especially men, are not parenting themselves through self-care and inner work. No example for this kind of active inner life and self-development, for mindful living, is given to children. And women and men are out of touch with not only themselves but with one another. Men and women often no longer understand each other or have the time to develop an ongoing and deepening relationship. Slipping into roles helps resolve this lack of understanding but is only a temporary solution.[18] When women are providing more resources in a home and family, the stressors on the male component in the home sometimes become unbearable. Men have lost their sense of wholeness that would enable them to be comfortable with this. Women enable this. There must be a living creative dynamic relationship between husband and wife, mother and father, that is organic in nature and can flex with every nuance and change in a family. Male and female relationships are often not alive in this way and cannot cope with the stresses of life due to this lack of dynamism.

This gives an unhealthy example to children, who learn to a large extent who they are and how they should behave in their families. Mothers and fathers are often out of touch with their children and do not know about their children's lives because they frequently do not share in those lives. Everyone is running, literally and figuratively. The name of the game is continually about performance and "making it." There is a pervasive sense of loneliness for everyone involved.[19] Women carry the main burden of these conflicts and losses. Their frustration, grief, and depression are palpable realities.

Women who live these lives, even when those lives are generally happy, are often the last to bed in their households and the first to get up. They are the last to bed because late night is the one time many women have to themselves, to feel where they are in it all and who they truly are — very basic needs of self-care. They are up early in order to get everything done for everyone to get off and on their way. These sleep cycles contribute to hormonal imbalances, lowered immunity, chronic exhaustion and depression, improper eating habits and obesity, and premature aging.[20] Modern women steer by the torch of chaos and doubt.

When other issues like ethnicity, sexual orientation, poverty, single-motherhood, and illness are added to this mix, it becomes even more complex. The rates of advanced breast cancer and prostate cancer among blacks in the US are significantly higher than for whites.[21] These rates do not indicate only a difference in access to health care and early screening or in genetics. No one knows for sure why this discrepancy exists. Although the US was built on the backs of African-American peoples and they have contributed immensely to the culture of this country, there is a continued disparity that remains a source of tension and pervasive angst. The deep wounds that have been endured by nonwhite peoples are as palpable as a tumor. Imagine being a black American and a member of the only group of people here in the US that do not know where they came from or what their heritage is. Imagine being a nonheterosexual individual who grew up having to live a secret life, who grew up not being able to discover or be their true self, who grew up in self-hatred and rejection. The point is that many people, just by being who they are, suffer insults that are in their own etheric and emotional body and in the etheric body of the culture contributing to the latent stresses that cause disease. From this perspective, it is interesting to note that breast cancer and prostate cancer rates are both so high. This deep geology of the modern cancer epidemic is the basis for the way of life that has created the epidemic. It is this geological evidence that Chinese medicine is so good at discovering, mining, and explaining.

Chinese medicine has for centuries had an elegant, logical, and clinically useful explanation of how these etheric body or energetic injuries translate from the emotions to the physical. *Liver Qi, heart Qi*, and *lung Qi* oppression all are etiological components of static conditions that contribute to cancer, especially breast cancer. Usually these injuries come from one form or another of inner conflict and even self-hatred, and translate to inner oppression. These injuries are vicious circles. They can be blatant or very subtle and even unconscious. The unconscious programming that we all endure contributes to the tracks that are worn in our minds and bodies over a lifetime. Many of these tracks are cultural; and these tracks are the lifetime evolutionary data for diseases caused or contributed to by these deep wounds as they march across our lives. In Chinese medicine, what happens in the etheric body is what drives life, health, and disease, because *Qi* is the place where spirit and matter meet, and *Qi* is the precursor and driver of all physiological processes.[22] Whereas conventional medicine looks at the measurable biological components of the diseases we call cancer, for example the DNA mutation, Chinese medicine looks at the precursors of those physical realities. It looks at what caused the physical injury, the DNA mutation, in the first place.

In modern psychotherapeutic theory, these explanations can be further deepened to show the connection between an ongoing emotional reality and who we become and the state of our physical manifestation. The theory of shamebinds[23,24] is one such analysis that has poignant meaning in the context of gender and how that might contribute to the etheric body injuries that Chinese medicine identifies. In this chapter, the shame binds are interpreted specifically in terms of girls and women. But they are not specific to the female gender. This section could also be applied to boys and men in the context of prostate cancer and the issues brought up in the next chapter.

Self-hatred is a major track of injury that comes from shame. Whenever a feeling — anger, joy, fear — is met with a response from a significant other that induces shame, an affect shame may result. An affect shame bind serves to control the later expression of the feeling involved. Innate affects include: interest–excitement; enjoyment–joy; surprise–startle; distress–anguish; fear–terror; anger–rage; shame–humiliation; bad-smells–disgust.[25] Any of these feelings, or feelings that are derivatives of them, may become shamebound. Shame binds are the equivalent of *knotted Qi* or unresolved emotions, which Chinese medicine so elegantly explains. In a sense, and within a very different cultural reality, the childhood programming and injuries that result from judgment are very well explained in Chinese medicine and form the basis for how emotions can cause physiologic pathology.[26]

Since *liver Qi stasis* is connected with five of seven possible diagnostic patterns for breast cancer[27] and is considered a strong component of breast cancer etiology in Chinese medicine, it is valuable to delve more deeply into how this pathology may come about in women and how it can be compounded by judgments based on race or ethnicity, marriage status, or sexual orientation, all important issues when one is looking at breast cancer statistics. It is important to remember that these shame binds are present for everyone, male and female, and contribute in varying ways, as social and personal programming, to internal injuries that can manifest as disease. They can contribute to mental habits and interpretations that drive our internal and also our external world. It is important to realize that the tracks of emotional injury that women as a group suffer have an effect in men and what they perceive as their feminine side, and these injuries can contribute to disease in anyone, male or female. However, since we are speaking here of women specifically, the context is oriented toward women.

In any case, no one should ever be made to feel responsible in terms of personal guilt for these interpretations that can be made. Shame is already a major element of living for all of us. In fact, it is a primary cultural motivating tool.[28] These interpretations are spoken of here in an effort to understand the internal terrain of women, which can help us understand how to treat for the prevention of breast cancer by freeing the *Qi* transformation mechanism.[29]

It is also important to realize that the underlying beliefs and philosophies that live in our consciousness that are responsible for injury to the female psyche and body are also responsible for the injury to the Earth's body. The two are inseparable because women and the natural world both exemplify the receptive side of life. And the intent of this writing is to provide a ground on which this truth can stand and become clear. Chinese medicine states that *liver Qi stasis*, a manifestation of depression and constraint, is dominant in the patterns responsible for creating the internal ecological environment for breast cancer. These same patterns also contribute to the underlying mechanisms of our way of life which ends in environmental destruction and the exposures, like endocrine disruptors, that lead to breast cancers.[30]

Drive–Shame Binds[31–34]

When hunger or sex is connected with shame, these two drives may become shamebound. Since food and nurturance and mother are inextricably linked, food comes to symbolize nurturance, security, safety, and love. When the relationship needs are not met, a greater dependence on food is likely to develop. For the compulsive eater, addiction to food is a constant reminder of the individual's neediness that actually transcends the food itself. The hunger fuels deep feelings of shame bound to the relationship needs, as well as shame about eating.

Young girls and women are seen as objects of sex. This objectification of females is so embedded in our society that, unless it is horribly manifested, we are not even aware of it. We are habituated to it. The roles of men and women are to a large extent based on these early trainings and programmings. Knowing one's self as a complete being within this context is almost impossible; children take on the characteristics that are expected of them, whether these be mental, emotional, or physical expressions. These characteristics, for girls, are most linked to mother and often to food and one's gender role and role as a sexual human being. Anorexia nervosa and bulimia nervosa are manifestations of the shame that girls feel about their true selves or loss of their true selves, physical and emotional. For some girls and young women, anorexia becomes a way to deny femaleness because many anorexics no longer have a menstrual cycle, remain childlike in body type, and are nonrelational, and this is actually the purpose of their anorexia. If we observe the classic body of modern models, it is straight and thin, with many female characteristics eliminated by a lack of flesh and muscle; secondary sex characteristics like breasts are almost nonexistent, and underarm hair is shaved away, along with leg hair. This is the standard by which girls measure themselves. To achieve this goal, many girls and young women must suppress their true female bodies, their true sexuality and selves. These ideals are a form of misogyny that is internalized by many girls and women.[35]

At the other end of this cycle is obesity. Obesity is considered an important risk factor in breast cancer causation.[36] Fat cells are storage units for estrogen and this is one way that hyperestrogenicity occurs. Estrogen is a proliferative factor in breast cancer causation, and estrogens are endogenous hormones. Xenoestrogenic influences that are fat-soluble are now entering the human body in astonishing amounts through pharmaceutical drugs, water, and the food stream.[37] These xenoestrogenic chemicals often have a very long half-life and, since they are fat-soluble and lipophilic, are stored in fat cells for many years. Many of them increase the number of estrogen receptors in body tissue, like the breast, and thereby become carcinogenic. Some are xenoestrogenic *in utero* and, in smaller amounts than thought necessary or possible, they can affect embryonic development with negative results much later in life.[38,39]

Obesity is often an expression of familial food habits, an effort to nurture one's self in a way that is unhealthful, and may even be a latent manifestation of an obsessive–compulsive disorder. It may also be an unconscious revolt on the part of some girls against the "twiggy" figure and all that it means — the flip side of the coin. And it may provide protection, in the form of body armor, against relationship. Whether it is anorexia, bulimia, or obesity, all of these expressions can be manifestations of self-hatred. A lack of acceptance of self and an inability to properly nurture one's self are emblematic in Chinese medicine of *spleen* injury. They are expressions of boundary issues that indicate impacts on the *spleen/pancreas*, the primary organ unit that is responsible for holding things in place and forming boundaries. The spleen is the functional unit that when properly nourished teaches us how to nurture ourselves. The very center, the Mother, has been injured when these manifestations occur in girls and young women.

Self-love is a human right. It must come before any other expression of love for those outside of the self. Women are asked to love and care for everyone but themselves. The training for this mind-boggling task begins at birth. The reversal of this training is what the current revolution is about. Feminism is not about hating men. It is about loving women and the receptive within oneself, whether one is male or female. It includes love and respect for the sacred feminine, the receptive, the Earth, the connection between nature and mind and mind and heart; and it is about birth and regeneration. It is about creating a world in which men and women and children and the world we call nature are all equals.

Interpersonal Need Shame Binds[40]

Shame can be internalized when a person's attempt to have an interpersonal need met is thwarted or unacknowledged. Following are interpersonal needs:

- The need for a relationship in which an individual feels loved and cherished as a person is the most fundamental need. Shame results when a child fails to experience such a relationship.
- The need for touching and holding is a biologically based need and allows an individual to feel safe, comfortable, and protected. Shame results when the type and quality of touch is withholding or abusive.
- The need for identification and the desire to be like the parent allows the parent to transmit and the child to receive a "personal culture," a place to belong. Shame results not only from the inconsistencies in what the parent says and does but also from any secrecy or withdrawal on the part of the parent.

- The need for differentiation is one whereby the individual feels that he/she has a separate identity. Separation is seen as a vital aspect of human development. Shame results from parental over-protectiveness and overpossessiveness. When parents resist physical, emotional, and cognitive autonomy on the part of the child, the child may experience a deep sense of shame for being different.
- The need to nurture is defined as one in which the child wants to be allowed to give nurturance rather than just receiving it. Shame results when attempts to nurture a significant adult are rejected, ridiculed, or ignored.
- The need for affirmation is the need to be valued and to feel worthy. This affirming process is initially developed through significant others but eventually the individual must learn how to self-affirm. Shame results from nonacceptance. The child who has never felt truly accepted by his/her parents will have a difficult time affirming and accepting the self.
- The need for power is the need to have some measure of personal control over one's life, rather than to remain in or return to the helpless state of the small child. Shame results when children are given too few choices, or are given too many choices beyond their maturity level.

Boy and girl children are loved differently. Let's face it, — even in our own culture, when a sign goes up that says "It's a boy," the meaning is inherently different than if that sign says "It's a girl." Expectations for the newborn are inherently different. Somehow the joy is significantly changed based on the gender of the newborn. Women have traditionally hoped to fulfill their husband's hope that a male heir will be born. Wives still change their surnames in most cases to that of their husband. So, being loved as a person usually comes *after* being loved as a girl or a boy. When girls learn this for the first time, if they have the opportunity to remain untainted by cultural habituation, it is a profoundly stunning blow. Otherwise, the inherent shame of being born not a person but a girl is unconscious to a large extent. Perhaps this is a coping mechanism on the part of girls as they adjust to being second. One way to experience this is to live in another culture where one is in the minority based on color or some other physical and unchangeable reality that distinguishes one from everyone else. We call this "culture shock" but it may be more than cultural and can be "color" shock or some other form of shock caused by differences. Paying close attention to how we respond or react when other cultures are expressing themselves, without editing, within the context of their own culture, can give us clues as to the depth of this early programming. Being able to live without editing one's self is freedom. Girls edit themselves in order to be acceptable. And these constraints injure the *Qi* flows of the *heart, liver, spleen, lung, chong,* and *ren* channels. These *Qi* flows are all implicated when injured in breast cancer etiology. This is not to say that boys do not also edit themselves; and this editing will be covered in the next chapter.

Domestic abuse is about reclaiming power on the part of usually male persons who have been programmed from day one to believe that they are the dominant person in a relationship. Men who dominate women are injured by an unanswered need for love, relationship, comforting, and by racism and class issues as these are expressed in the workplace and community. Male abusers are usually men who hate their own vulnerability[41,42] and as a result both love and hate women. Through abusive nurturing, domestic abusers use the need for interpersonal bonds against women who have been equally injured by self-hatred. The two parties are injured in similar ways but the status of women in our culture allows them to be injured in such a way as to allow the door to inappropriate touch and abuse to open. The shame inherent in this situation is a burden that is equal within each party but the woman carries the shame for both more poignantly through the abuse and a programmed need to love. Usually, men become ashamed only when they are caught or called out on the underlying reasons for their behavior. And then their shame is not only about the abuse but, more poignantly, about the need for love and being cherished that went unattended usually as a child. The shame is about the need itself. The vulnerability that drives abusive behavior is the issue, and it in turn is driven by the need for power — the primary goal of abuse and rape. This kind of power shields abusers from their own pain. The abuse and injury to another is itself a projection of one's own pain and vulnerability. Vulnerability has come to be synonymous with powerlessness.[43] Women are trained to be vulnerable and to love and shield those who are vulnerable. Men are trained to be "unwoman." Men who are vulnerable are put down, pansies, and equated with women. This is misogyny. It harms not only women but also men and all of our children. And it harms Mother Nature, the Earth, and all of its fauna and flora that are intimately connected in the web of life. Misogyny is a hatred of vulnerability and, therefore, connection. This hatred of vulnerability and connection allows many men and some women to split[44] from their own actions, whether those actions take the form of rape and abuse in the home or the form of destroying and contaminating the Earth through abusive collective actions.

Women are trained culturally to be vulnerable in these ways. They are trained not to have boundaries, to be there for everyone. This training leaves women open to being used and abused; and it begins in the home and from one's own mother and father. In a sense, because this is a generational issue handed down for centuries, it is women who must break the cycle. Women must stop training men and boys to treat them in these ways based on their own behaviors. Women must stand against this behavior and learn to love themselves, partly through developing and having boundaries, through separating themselves from others. When we think of the ultimate nature of cancer, it is one in which all boundaries have been lifted and cells that are injured, usually by external forces, are running amuck without constraint. These cells are like teenage mutant ninjas who were born healthy but have been injured by the abuse of the environment, whether that environment be the internal human body or the external wounded body of nature in which we live. They are one and the same. We often make cancer the enemy; but the true enemy is the influence that damages normal behaviors and connections that underlie cancer. Cancer is the result, not the culprit.

Girl children have few role models outside of their culture and their mothers to teach them new ways of being. When women hate some part of themselves and express this by not allowing themselves to live full lives, by allowing men and boys to expect them to care for everything but themselves, they teach their girl children how to do the same. And they teach their boy children to have these expectations and to treat women as children and slaves, albeit often slaves who are loved. This personal culture handed down for centuries is one that the some native American peoples call injuries coming from the "bloodline." These bloodline psychic injuries take on individual family traits and require continual healing by reviewing one's individual life and that of one's ancestors, so that threads of injury can be detected and worked with and healed. There is no shame in this review and healing. It is the only way in which true and permanent healing can take place that protects our daughters and sons from being part of this immensely vicious circle. It is part of the crisis of femininity.

The need for an identity, separate from mother and wife, is something that many women come to later in life, when their children have left home. Marriage relationships often shatter or go through a stressful re-evaluation during this time. Women reach "the end of their rope," a rope tied around them in very early life, like an umbilical to slavery, to the concept that their lives were predetermined and had something to do with child-rearing and, therefore, marriage. For those women who did not choose this path, an equally stressful and lonely living ensues, as a reaction to the very same problem. This autonomy came to women who chose the path less traveled not through good parenting but through the school of hard work and self-doubt. The self-confidence that is expected of male children and men has to be learned by girls and women, who often must support themselves alone. Finding an identity beyond childbearing and parenting is often a shame-filled path no matter what a woman does. All women, mothers or not, truly do steer by the torch of chaos and doubt.

Self-affirmation is often learned through nonacceptance and pure determination. Girls who are not accepted for who they are as persons by their parents and families and society feel shame coupled with a schizophrenic need to find oneself. These splits in an individual are complex and confusing to girls and women. One is asked to be acceptable and do acceptable things and, at the same time, find one's self and excel. This is often logistically a contradictory message. Of course, boys and men experience this issue, too, but not to the extent that girls and women do. We end up with Britney Spears–like young women exhibiting lewd and lascivious dance moves in scanty clothing while simultaneously trying to be a mother and spouse and making billions of dollars. It is insanity for a child, girl, young woman, woman.

The power that can come from manifesting one's true self is lost in these complicated and contradictory moldings of a self. The choices hold no life; they are not dynamic, because they are not true. They are caricatures of fantasies based on programming inherited from generation to generation and from culture to culture. As the world gets smaller, these caricatures become simultaneously larger and smaller. Women and children are the largest group of people sold into slavery and the sex trade. This trade goes on across the world. Women and children are the largest group of people killed, injured, and maimed in war. At the same time, it is women who are saving the world. For example, almost all microinvesting is coming from women and going to women who are saving themselves, their families, and their cultures. Women, in general, are working on millions of fronts to save their families and to save their homes and lands. In many ways, women and the receptive *Yin* side of life are the last frontier, seeking freedom in the world revolution to become one.

Purpose Shame Binds

A sense of purpose is central to the lives and actions of human beings. Their purpose, what they imagine for themselves and anticipate in the future, pulls them forward in different, often-changing directions. Purpose is experienced through imagined scenes like daydreams, fantasies, and heroic dreams. Scenes imagined with deep, enduring affect motivate the self to enact them. The imagined scenes that are played over and over again shape the contours of a person's life and provide a frame in which to become.

Scenes of purpose become fused with shame when children are ridiculed for the various daydreams, fantasies, or imagined vocations that are voiced to adults. When children are ridiculed for imagining creatures or monsters, imagination itself can become shamed. When imaginative play is continually disparaged or demeaned, scenes imagined in the future become associated with shame. When the affect of interest or excitement is shamebound, curiosity, risk-taking, and exploratory behaviors are stifled. When there are purpose shame binds, the motivation for learning, creativity, and the acquisition of skills is damaged.[45] Girls learn early on that their options are limited based on purpose shame binds. No one knows the cumulative loss to all of humanity.

For some women the purpose of having and raising children can be a primary calling. For some women the primary calling is never found. And for other women a calling is not paramount to their lives, because of poverty, early experiences that extinguished the spark that drives the need for a calling, or the burden of so many children that leaves no space for developing the base from which a calling could be discovered. In other words, the loss of hope becomes more comfortable than maintaining hope in a hopeless situation. For those women who never have children, usually the hope that comes in parenting children is not extinguished or lost but circumstances have maneuvered to eliminate the possibility of having children. Whatever category one falls into, the idea of being a hero as a woman and fulfilling a heroic dream or vision is not often manifested. Partly this is because loving is not seen as a heroic life calling. However, perhaps loving should be our only life calling. The fulfillment of a heroic vision is often linked primarily to a material success or victory and not to living a life that consistently expresses and manifests love.

Beyond the dream of becoming a mother, other dreams and visions for a particular future are often ridiculed or driven out of a girl. It is only recently that girls have been supported and rewarded for life dreams that do not include child-rearing. Even in the 1960s, the only women who were playing professional classical music in orchestras were piccolo and harp players. Any female CEOs who existed at that time were newly appointed in the cosmetic or fashion industry, or were the women who had founded those companies. Almost all doctors were men, and medical research in various diseases and women's health issues, including designing the contraceptive pill and the tampon, was all done by and conceived of by men. Now that there are women astronauts and doctors and researchers, the role of child-rearing still falls primarily on women. And so the curiosity and resulting exploration of these possible life paths is still somehow complicated by the issue of mothering and parenting, which is primarily placed on women and not men. It is a form of hierarchical denigration of women, of children, and of the tasks of mothering and nurturance that persists in our world. And it lends itself to denigration of all life that is part of the receptive.

Results

The sociological constraints and philosophical questions that arise from the meaning of gender, and therefore family, are complex. Reproductive decisions are in this realm and impact mainly women. *Liver Qi constraint* is a common outcome for women living these complex realities. When *liver Qi stasis* is present over time, *heart Qi stasis* will manifest via the *five phases*. *Lung Qi stasis* arises from constraint as well. Grief and a lifetime lived within the context of the suffocation of the manifestation of one's true self can cause injury to the *Lung Qi*. *Liver* and *heart Qi stasis* alongside *lung Qi stasis* cause a form of clumping in the chest, which then leads to *internal heat* and *blood and phlegm stasis*, a precursor condition for cancer, especially breast cancer. In fact, the temperature of breast tissue of women diagnosed with breast cancer is significantly higher than that of women without breast cancer. Inflammation caused by stasis is considered a primary underlying condition in the pathology of all cancers. These internal conditions act like magnets for *latent pathogenic factors* like hormonal influences coming from external xenoestrogenic impacts.

Even when these realities happen only within the etheric body and only in the channel, a template is set for other external injuries to have a greater impact. *Spleen deficiency* is a frequent underlying condition in *liver Qi stasis*, especially in women. The *liver channel* runs through the axilla; the *heart and lung channels* also run through the axilla; the stomach and *spleen channels* run through the breast; the *lung channel* begins in the upper outer quadrant of the breast. All of these realities can lead to stasis in the chest and to *liver* and *kidney Yin* deficiency, and thus to abnormal hormonal levels. Based only upon emotional insults, the scene is set for breast cancer. Although conventional science does not attribute emotional injuries to breast cancer causation, in Chinese medicine the concepts of *Qi* and of channel pathology, which do not exist in conventional medicine, provide a means of explaining injuries that are very much considered precursors and promoting factors, setting the ecological stage for imbalances typically thought of as necessary for breast cancer. If we consider that these very same emotional realities, as stated in Chapter 1, are what allow for the ongoing denigration of the Earth, then these underlying constraints placed on women are all part of a field of magnetism. *Latent pathogenic factors*, like endocrine disruptors and other chemicals that are carcinogenic and ubiquitous in our contaminated world, are expressions of thoughtlessness, greed, hatred for the receptive in life, disrespect for the Mother Earth, nature, woman, and immorality. Therefore, treatment of these conditions on the individual and also cultural level is immensely important in prevention. It is important to remember that the female body is more sensitive to chemical exposures than the male body, and it is partly because of all of the factors mentioned above that this is true.

Chinese Medicine

Depression

Breast cancer is considered a multifactorial disease. However, in the context of Chinese medicine the very real concepts of stasis caused by constrained emotions mentioned above have an organic translation in the internal environment of the human body. *Liver Qi stasis, Yin deficiency, spleen deficiency*, and *dampness* all are magnets for latent pathogenic factors to enter deeper terrains in the correct circumstances. If xenoestrogenic influences are considered latent pathogens — that is, the exposure enters the body and sits silently for a period of time before becoming symptomatic — then a possible environment for their storage and impact is present in women who are chronically run-down, sleep-deprived, living on poor diets high in certain fats, and unhappy. One manifestation of this unhappiness and exhaustion is depression, and certainly the pharmaceutical companies that produce antidepressants are cashing in on this dilemma in the industrialized world, especially among women.

Depression, anxiety, and insomnia present a unified front in the unhappiness of women. They often come as a unit, and the following is an attempt to analyze the clinical manifestations and treatment of these three distinct diagnoses from the perspective of Chinese medicine.

Depression is a symptom that is descriptive of a state of mind or being. However, it is also a condition/diagnosis in Chinese and conventional medicine. In Chinese medicine, depression leads to *Qi* stagnation, which is traditionally divided into two main patterns[46]:

- *Plum pit Qi*
- *Organ agitation.*

The etiology for *plum pit Qi* is that the symptom of depression and unresolved anger or frustration injures the *liver*. Obsessive thinking over the emotional content of this depression or frustration injures the *spleen*. *Liver* injury manifests as *liver Qi stasis* that transforms into *fire*. *Spleen stasis* generates *dampness*. And *dampness* and *fire* combine to form *phlegm*. The *phlegm* lodges in the throat and leads to something caught that will not go away by swallowing or coughing. This becomes *plum pit Qi* and is a kind of classical "scream therapy" conundrum. In fact, singing can be a therapeutic tool for the *plum pit Qi* type of depression. Exercise that moves *Qi* and *blood* and provides a means by which the emotional constraints of normal living can be discharged may be another way to manage *plum pit Qi*. Of course, eliminating the constraint is primary.

Organ agitation has a different etiology that is more pertinent to most women. Long-term depression leads to reduced appetite from *spleen stasis* and a *stomach–spleen disharmony*. The reduced nourishment then leads to the *Qi* and blood losing their source of nourishment. This ends in either *spleen Qi deficiency* or *kidney Qi deficiency*. The pattern of *organ agitation* was first mentioned in *Prescriptions from the Golden Chamber*.[47] The text states that women tend toward crying easily and becoming melancholy. The main organ affected is the *heart*, which controls the tears, and this leads to *heart Yin deficiency*. *Gan mai da zao tang* is the main formula for this presentation.

The *Nei Jing* says that the *heart* desires moderation or slowing down, and eating sweet foods will slow it down. This rule from the *Nei Jing* is often applied to women who are premenstrual and have a sweet craving. The *heart* is hurried and oppressed and jittery during premenses, because the *heart* is the ruler of the blood. If the *liver Qi* is static the *heart* will also become constrained. When there is *liver Qi constraint* it can be especially constrained during that part of the menstrual cycle when the *Qi* should be moving the most and the smoothest — the follicular or *Yang* phase. When women are depressed and simultaneously agitated during the premenstrual time, the desire for sweets is the body's attempt to slow down and address the underlying *spleen deficiency* which may be contributing to the *liver* and *heart Qi stasis*. *Organ agitation* is treated by smoothing the *Qi* and tonifying the deficiency of the *spleen*.

Many systems of medicine utilize treatment to confirm a diagnosis. Chinese medicine is no different. If a patient is treated for depression that is caused by *organ agitation*, and the typical *liver Qi stasis* points are used for releasing an *excess* condition, the patient often will start crying during treatment. Some practitioners take this as a healthy release. In many cases, however, it is a sign that mistreatment has occurred. P 6 and Lv 3 are points used to disperse *excess*. P 6 is a point used to disperse *"men,"* or a chest stifling sensation. The name of this point is *Neiguan* — "Inner gate." The gate is the opening between the *middle* and the *upper Jiao*. The solar plexus is the site of constraint along with the chest, with the *heart* and *lungs* residing in it. Opening this gate is a profound action. Lv 3 is a point that spreads the *liver Qi* with the additional effect of opening the gate between the *middle* and the *upper Jiao*. *Organ agitation* is a condition of deficiency and not *excess*. It is a condition of *heart Qi deficiency* with underlying *spleen Qi deficiency*. Tears are the charge of the *heart*, and when a patient who is *Qi-deficient* is treated with dispersing points, the *heart* will discharge tears and further *Qi* will be lost. This is not therapeutic. Differentiating organ agitation due to *heart Qi deficiency* and *liver Qi stasis* that is due to excess is very important in terms of choosing the correct treatment principles for each. And crying as a release and crying as a symptom of *heart Qi deficiency* needs to be differentiated.

Gb 2 and Bl 20 are two points that are able to wash, clean, and clear away sufferings from under the *heart*. Bl 20 tonifies the *spleen*. Gb 2 can be used instead of the lower body points like Lv 2 and Lv 3, which spread the *liver Qi* too strongly and end up dispersing it in deficiency; Gb 2 will regulate and harmonize the *Qi* instead. Women suffer from this condition of agitation due to *deficiency* because women's *spleen* and *heart Qi* is more pressed. Women bleed monthly, form new life inside their bodies, nurture life outside their bodies, work hard, and are trained to care; these are all *spleen/middle Jiao/mother/heart/kidney* activities. These realities make women more susceptible to *organ agitation*. It is also these realities, as translated onto the physical and material plane, that make women more susceptible to injury from chemical exposures like endocrine disruptors.

Depression has many indications[48]:

- Some patients tend toward melancholy;
- *Others toward* anger;
- *Others toward* fear;
- *Others toward* apprehension and doubt;
- Still others toward insomnia.

This variation requires an in-depth history and explanation of symptoms. How do people feel depressed? Symptoms of depression correlate with different organs:

- A tendency to cry correlates with *heart Qi deficiency*;
- A tendency to anger correlates with *liver Qi stasis*;
- A tendency to feel fear correlates with *kidney Qi deficiency*;

- A tendency to *"men"* correlates with *phlegm* or *liver/heart Qi stasis;*
- A tendency to apprehension correlates with *phlegm* or *gallbladder/heart Qi stasis;*
- A tendency to quietness means *Yang Qi deficiency;*
- A tendency to insomnia means *phlegm* or *heart blood deficiency* or *liver fire* blazing;
- A tendency to melancholy means *heart Qi deficiency* or *kidney Yang deficiency.*

These combine according to the relationships expressed in the *five-phase* theory.

The normal condition of the *Qi* in the body is moderated and circulating throughout. Emotions that are not coped with or remain unresolved will disrupt the regular movement of the *Qi* and blood. The organ that is weakest acts like a magnet for this disruption of *Qi* and blood flow. The condition of depression will develop in that organ. All organs have some relationship to the *heart*, since the *heart* rules the blood. If the blood becomes weak, then this can affect the *spirit* since the *heart* stores the spirit (*shen*). Depression is a form of *knotted Qi* and relates not only to the *liver* but also to many other organs. Knowing more accurately how a particular depression manifests itself gives information that is very valuable in treatment and in advice for living. When something is understood, change can take place. Chinese medicine is wonderful at providing a nonjudgmental language that helps patients understand their own actions and behavior and the importance of changing them.

When a patient complains of depression, there are three basic considerations:

- Is it *excess* or deficiency?
- What is the constitution of the patient?
- Are there accompanying problems?

An excess type of depression is less prevalent, involves the *heart* and *liver*, and is usually about more recent problems. It is a form of

Qi stasis that manifests with a floating or surging pulse that is also wiry and forceful. The main symptoms are irritability and anger. For instance, this manifestation is exemplified by the patient who comes in fuming about the person who just cut them off in traffic. You can feel the *fire* and see the steam spouting out of their ears.

A deficiency type of depression is more prevalent and happens more commonly in women. It is usually about less recent problems that may have been going on in one form or another for a long time, even years. It is not so much about *Qi* stasis but about organ *deficiency*. The pulse is deep and fine and forceless. The patient is not fuming and yelling but is quiet and melancholy, even somewhat disoriented; the emotional material relevant to their state is old and forgotten or constant and ongoing but in a subliminal way. The psychic losses women suffer from childhood on into adulthood are obvious fodder for this type of depression. If women had better access to their anger, they might manifest the *excess* type of depression. And this would place their depression in the *Qi* realm rather than in the organ *deficiency* realm. Perhaps we could say that this is one of the manifestations of women being different endocrinologically. Perhaps simultaneously women are different endocrinologically because they live different lives than men and this in part is also what makes them express disease differently. It is not possible to say since we are mixing medical systems theories, but it seems probable and is part of an immensely complex interaction of mind, body, learning, programming, and *Qi* dynamics.

A *Yang-deficient* constitution can easily lead to knotting of *Qi* and organ agitation. A *damp phlegm* constitution can easily lead to the development of *phlegm* and *plum pit Qi*. Those with deficiency conditions may develop excess conditions like *Phlegm*, *Dampness*, or *blood stasis*. A referral to a psychotherapeutic model practitioner is necessary. This allows a patient to work from the inside out, and that is exactly how these conditions should be healed. Acupuncture is an excellent modality for treating the *Qi* aspect of this type of depression. Herbal medicine is used to treat the underlying deficiencies.

It is important not to disperse in *deficiency* depression types. Advise your patient not to eat many cold or raw foods, as these foods exacerbate the problem of *Qi stasis* by depleting the *middle Jiao*. In a *deficiency* condition the long and slow course combined with psychotherapy is the path of recovery. A combination of needles and moxibustion is applied to *back shu* points in one treatment for *deficiency* depressions.

Emotional Constraint

Emotional constraint is another diagnostic category that is often given the diagnosis of depression or *liver Qi stasis*. *Constraint* has a very broad meaning in Chinese medicine and includes any form of stagnation. Historically, it has been thought to affect all of the organs. In the Yuan Dynasty there were six types of *constraint*:

- *Qi constraint,*
- *Damp constraint,*
- *Heat constraint,*
- *Lung constraint,*
- Blood *constraint,*
- Food *constraint.*

Emotional constraint can cause any one of these *constraint* syndromes, depending on which organ or level of disease attracts injury.

Emotional constraint, as a pattern within the context of depression, is often accompanied by changes in perception regarding pain. And so patients with constraint often end up seeing practitioners who use the modality of acupuncture. Differentiating pain syndromes is important not only relative to type and place and quality of pain but according to an understanding of the cause. A condition or disease can cause pain but emotional or psychological issues can also play a major role in the cause and perception of pain.

People with chronic pain will often develop *constraint*, and in conventional medicine this would be considered a form of depression treated with antidepressants. The question becomes whether a patient has pain because of a psychological predisposition or whether being in pain for long periods of time has caused psychological problems.

Men and women suffer chronic pain and therefore *constraint*. Men must continue working or engaging in other activities that exacerbate their pain condition. Women must continue working and taking care of their families no matter what — often even when ill. Either way, understanding the origin of the pain is important and treating any underlying emotional issues that change perceptions about the pain is also required.

If a patient has pain and this causes a depressive emotional state, the condition should be easier to treat than one caused purely by an emotional problem as the root cause. Many patients with *constraint* will often interpret relaxation as a more intense throbbing and discomfort and less as a release or relief. Patients who are unable to relax cannot do so because the content of their emotional *constraint* will become more palpable if they relax. All sensations are interpreted as uncomfortable. In the acupuncture setting, a patient with *constraint* will become more uncomfortable during treatment. In addition, a patient with *constraint* will not improve with correct acupuncture treatment for a pain syndrome. Women can suffer from emotional *constraint* as a result of PTSD, depression, or anxiety. Almost always, these conditions result from injuries that were due to self-hatred in one form or another. These are hugely important conditions to treat as part of treating the pain. Emotional pain caught in the cellular memory is akin to the *shen* aspect in relation to the *San Jiao* and it is, therefore, ubiquitous in an afflicted individual. Touching this pain can be complex and requires an interweaving of several therapeutic modalities.

Emotional constraint is a pathology of the *liver* and *gallbladder*, and is related to a lack of the spreading function of the *liver*. *Constraint*, therefore, is the only accurate diagnosis for the symptom of depression when caused purely by excess *liver Qi* stagnation. Most patients who report depression as a symptom are treated as though they had excess *liver Qi stasis* or *constraint*. In other words, depression equals excess *liver Qi stasis*. This is incorrect. With *liver constraint*, *heart* problems will result as a mechanism of *shen cycle* flows and *spleen* problems will result as a mechanism of *Ko cycle* flows. The vast majority of patients who report depression are deficient and treating for *excess liver Qi stasis* is incorrect treatment that exacerbates their underlying deficiencies.

When the *spleen* function is adversely affected by the *liver*, as in a transverse rebellion, the transformation and transportation activities of the *spleen* are affected, and *dampness* and *phlegm* result. This is a *Qi* problem. When the *heart Qi* is affected by the *liver Qi*, the resulting *liver/heart Qi* stasis is a manifestation of the mother–son relationship. The *heart* loses its nourishment and this leads to a blood-level problem.

In early-stage *constraint* the *Qi*-level problem can result in *dampness* and *phlegm*. Over time, however, the *heat* from *constraint* and dampness and *phlegm* will damage the *Qi* and then a blood-level problem will evolve. When severe, this can cause chronic diseases that are characterized as consumptive diseases in Chinese medicine (not to be confused with consumption or tuberculosis). These processes evolve from many things including overwork, chronic *blood stasis* (from many causes), and chronic emotional constraint. Excess constraint is seen more frequently in men and is caused by immense frustration, intense anger, physical and emotional abuse as a child, and many of the shame binds which men are programmed to manifest differently. The patient is constantly wound up and ready to explode, there is chronic irritability with blowups sometimes so severe that the person cannot hold a job. Many young men, especially black young men, suffer from this kind of constraint. It is probable that they are suffering from a kind of culturally institutionalized PTSD. Until we understand this and address the problem of racism and of poverty in our world, our prisons will continually be full of these young men.

In *liver constraint* there is distension and even pain in the chest and flanks that is generalized and not fixed. The tongue body is thin and the coating may be greasy. The pulse is wiry and forceful. The focus is on smoothing the *liver Qi*. However, all of the medicine in the world will cure the patient only if the root of these injuries is found and released and resolved. These kinds of injuries that happen so early in childhood preclude a safe and understandable way to view them, release them, and escape them when they happen. Going back to the origin of the behavior is the only way to stop the suffering, and a highly skilled therapist is required. However, acupuncture is an especially supportive therapy that can kick-start and lift the spirit of the patient to untangle these knots of emotional injury lodged in the cellular memory of the body.

Deficiency constraint is more pertinent to women than men, because women are generally not allowed access to their anger and rage. The presentation of the patient is more disoriented and confused, quiet and inward. These patients are upset as opposed to angry, wondering what they did to elicit such behavior from another. The empowering response would be anger but the patient feels personal fault, melancholy, and sadness and expresses this with crying and sighing. The patient does not swell with anger and outrage; she ducks and hunches her shoulders like a victim. The tongue body is pale with a thin coating because the *spleen* is too weak to raise a coating and the blood and *Qi* are not well nourished. The pulse is thin and thready, and if it is wiry it is forceless. Whereas smoothing the *liver Qi* is important in the excess presentation, here the treatment is to tonify the *spleen* in order to nourish the *liver blood*. Nourishing the *liver blood* helps to move the *Qi*. This condition is so common among women that it is sometimes difficult to find someone who does not experience it. And yet the conditions of constraint and the varying patterns of depression equally snarl the machinery of life. It is important to free the *liver Qi* that is static, for whatever reason, and to benefit the *spleen* in order to clear the terrain of the *liver* channel and the *middle Jiao*, for it is here that many promoting factors for breast cancers have their beginnings. Women who are under this type of stress on a daily basis have high cortisol levels. And high cortisol levels have been found to be linked to breast cancer and metastatic breast cancer.[49]

It is important to remember that women do not cause their own breast cancer by being injured in these ways. These injuries are systemic to our world and way of life. Blame causes shame and shame binds the truth in a web of complicity. Promoting factors are those things that create an ecology that allows carcinogenic factors and hits to take hold and proliferate. It is important to remember that this terrain acts as a magnet for *latent pathogenic factors* and is not, in and of itself, the cause of cancer. However, treating and clearing the terrain and repairing the ecology of the *liver*, *liver* channel, and *middle Jiao* will disallow the intensification of external hits from carcinogens, many of which are xenoestrogenic endocrine disruptors. It is also immensely important that women do not get caught in a web of self-destructive guilt about these realities. A woman must not be allowed to believe that she herself caused these injuries. However, helping women to free themselves from these injuries allows the *Qi* dynamic to be free, and this freedom of *Qi* movement allows the organ systems, especially those most related to breast cancer, to remain as healthy as possible, even in the presence of carcinogenic hits.

Anxiety

Anxiety states include many different disorders: panic disorder, obsessive–compulsive disorder (OCD), and posttraumatic stress disorder (PTSD) to name a few.[50] In Chinese medicine these disorders have traditionally been characterized as spiritual disorders. Spiritual disorders have to do with disruption of the spirit housed in the void of the *heart*, the only place in the human body where there is a void in which to find the quiet necessary to house the *shen*, or the spirit.[51]

The character for the *heart* in Chinese medicine is the only one for an organ in which the flesh radical is missing. This implies a special place reserved for the *heart* as an anatomical organ, and one in which there is something more than just the physical function of pumping the blood. The void of the *heart* is connected to the great void, the *Tao*, and this connection allows the spirit to be present and to impart spiritual influences and power to the blood. Blood, as a body fluid, is different from all other fluids because it is infused with the power of the *spirit* of the *heart* and the *Tao*. This *jun* aspect of the *heart* is the stillness aspect which houses the spirit and the *Tao*. The *zhu* aspect of the *heart* is the moving and pumping aspect of the *heart* that drives all of the anatomical units of which conventional medicine speaks. However, even in the *zhu* aspect, the *heart* is given special authority or function or expectation. The character for *zhu* is a lamp stand with a rising flame: a *human* being who spreads the light. These are the Chinese medicine expressions of the Great Chain of Being.

The mind and the *heart* have a strong connection. The mind is a relatively outer level of being that relates to the sensory orifices and data collection. The mind is in relation to material existence. The *shen* aspect of the self is in relation to the *Tao* and is capable of introspection. It arises out of the *kidney Jing* which is the primordial connection to the *Tao* and is housed in the void of the *heart*. The functions of the mind and *heart* — external and internal life — must be aligned with the *Tao*. And it is only then that the truth can be accurately perceived. The mind is meant to serve our lives rather than rule them. It rules the life only when there is a split between the *Yin* and the *Yang*, the outer and the inner, the mind and the *heart*. Many Eastern spiritual paths and meditation forms seek to maintain the *Tao* in the *heart* in an effort to foster the connectedness of mind and *heart* and enable peace.[52]

When harmony prevails, the mind initiates action via the will of the *kidney* based on the truth we find in the *heart*. The *heart* can acknowledge only truth. This is part of what makes it a void and a safe place for the spirit to reside. The *heart–kidney* axis is one of spiritual stability and power. The *shen* and the *jing* have a deep relationship exemplified by the *shen* and *ko* cycles.

The blood carries *Qi* and *shen* to the whole body. The quality of the *Qi* and *shen* that permeate the blood will impact the quality of all the other organ systems. In embryology the *heart* is the first solid organ (*zang*) created and it has a major influence on the building and creation of the other *zang* organs because of its nourishing capacities as well as its energetic influences through the *shen*. So *shen* is partly rooted in prenatal *Qi* and inhabits every aspect of the body. It is anchored by essence, blood, and *Yin*. The quality of the *shen* can be compromised if any of these vital substances is deficient. The shen through its connection to the *Tao* is necessary for life to begin and evolve.

Injuries to the *shen*, the spirit, are what cause psychiatric disorders. All of the shame binds cause injury to the spirit and to the function of the whole human being, since the spirit is the primary animating force for life. The female aspect of life has for several thousands of years been placed in a compromised position because female human beings are not allowed to live fully from the Tao, the sacred residing in their *hearts*. Females are allowed to manifest and express a lesser being as interpreted by the mind. This damage to the sacred feminine in modern life is very much a part of what our current crisis in the family, in world cultures, and in the natural world is about. It is a global *shen* disturbance caused by hatred of that which is the receptive. Elie Weisel said that "the opposite of love is indifference," and the use of the word "hatred" here is not too strong, no matter if there is hatred or indifference. The two are the same. And this affects all of us, male and female. As a result, there is no quiet place left for the sacred to reside and chronic anxiety and other forms of *shen* disturbance are endemic. These energetic-level disturbances cause material diseases, and the modern epidemic of cancer is emblematic of disturbances that allow the rape of the Earth, of women, of children, of our health, and of the very concept of vulnerability in the name of greed and abuse. Greed, abuse, and indifference are forms of hatred.

Depression and anxiety go hand in hand symptomatically in conventional medicine. But in Chinese medicine they may be separate manifestations: depression is a *Qi* problem and anxiety is a *shen* problem. Anxiety is caused by the irregular movement of *Qi* that agitates the *shen*. It may arise out of *deficiency*, *excess*, or *stasis*. Whatever the cause, anxiety can be exacerbated by tiredness and general stress. Anxiety is usually described as running at a high idle with the sympathetic nervous system inappropriately on alert. Common presentations are mental strain, insomnia, exhaustion, panic attacks, increased *heart* and respiratory rates, palpitations, tremors, muscle tension, and so on.[53] Unknown causes of anxiety may be imaginary or real but not necessarily conscious. PTSD, phobias, sexual abuse, paranoia, and withdrawal from pharmaceutical drugs can all cause anxiety and even hallucinations. Anxiety is common in everyday life and for reasons that can be expected, such as exams and public speaking. When anxiety becomes chronic or out of proportion to a given stimulus, it may be the result of pathology. And pathology may result. To some extent, just living in the modern world may produce anxiety.

People who are chronically depressed often experience anxiety and vice versa. And people who are chronically anxious and depressed experience insomnia. All of these *Qi* and *shen* disorders are linked.

Fire and phlegm fire are excesses that disturb and agitate the *heart shen*, causing it to be more irregularly active and intense. *Fire* often evolves from *heart fire* combined with either *liver* or *stomach fire*. In the case of the *liver*, the *fire* results from emotional stresses, smoking, drug abuse, alcohol abuse, a high-fat and greasy diet, lack of exercise, and a generally hectic and stressed "type A" lifestyle. *Phlegm fire* results from *spleen deficiency* and *stasis* that gives rise to *phlegm* and then combines with *heart fire*.

Deficient heart Qi, heart blood, and heart Yin are all deficiencies that evolve from lack of sleep, overwork, stress, illness, and malnutrition. These deficiencies do not allow the *heart shen* to be adequately anchored by blood, *Yin*, *Qi*, or essence. Deficient *heart Qi* is often combined with *kidney deficiency* and/or *spleen deficiency*. Deficient *heart Yin* is often combined with deficient *kidney Yin*. These *deficiencies* are ones to which women are especially prone. The combined lives that many women are forced to live in the modern world, where they "burn the candle at both ends" can result in these deficiencies that contribute to anxiety. When we consider the character for *zhu*, the lamp stand or human exuding light to the world, this metaphor becomes even more poignant.

Stagnation gives rise to irregularity of movement that disturbs the free circulation of *Qi* and *shen*. This can result in the accumulation of *phlegm*. *Heart Qi stasis* is commonly combined with *liver Qi stasis* via the *shen* cycle, or with *liver Yang* rising, or with *heart phlegm*. This is where depression and anxiety may become linked in the Chinese medicine analysis of anxiety. When the *Qi* problem of depression becomes linked to the *shen* problem of anxiety through *liver Qi stasis* or *phlegm*, an interactive relationship evolves where both are occurring partly as a result of each other.

Some people are more prone to anxiety than others. Anxiety manifests differently in different people, depending upon which *zang* organs are involved and what type of agitation is occurring — *excess, deficient*, or static.

There are clinical presentations involving anxiety that can provide clues to diagnosis:

- Anxiety and the *heart*
- ○ Emotions — agitation, panic, hysteria;
- ○ Physical — insomnia, palpitations, hypertension, cardiac pain, pallor.
- Anxiety and the *kidneys* = *heart* anxiety rooted in *kidney* fear
- ○ Emotions — apprehension, fear, easy startlement;
- ○ Physical — trembling, urinary frequency, loose stools.
- Anxiety and the *liver* = combination of fear, anger, anxiety
- ○ Emotions — fear, anger, anxiety, *gallbladder* uncertainty, indecision, hypersensitivity;
- ○ Physical — headaches, stiffness, tremors, muscle and joint pain, insomnia.
- Anxiety and the *spleen* = anxiety that interferes with one's ability to think clearly
- ○ Emotions — worry, anticipation of problems real or imaginary, insecurity, fear;
- ○ Physical — digestive problems, insomnia, fatigue, nausea.
- Anxiety and the *lungs* = a condition resulting from fear of loss, imagined or real, and manifesting as grieving before an event that warrants it actually occurs
- ○ Emotions — fear of loss;
- ○ Physical — Asthma, difficulty in breathing.

The symptoms of psychological diseases occur in a continuum of relativity. Following is a schematic to try and demonstrate this continuum in regard to anxiety.

Relative *Yin* --- **Relative *Yang***

Type:	Anxiety and deficiency	Anxiety and stasis	Anxiety and excess
Treatment:	Calm and tonify	Calm and move	Calm and disperse

The source of anxiety lies in a *shen* disturbance and, therefore, treatments are primarily for *heart deficiencies, stasis,* and *excesses.*

Following are TCM acupuncture strategies (energetic treatment works well for energetic-level conditions) for treatment of the main patterns of anxiety.

(1) *Heart fire*

- Emotions — agitation, feelings of desperation, restlessness, impulsiveness, difficulty in concentrating;
- Physical — nervous talking, palpitations, a red face, heat rising from the whole body;
- Tongue — red or dark-red, with a yellow dry coating;
- Pulse — full and rapid.

Points:

- Du 20 — reduce; vents *heat* and clears the mind;
- CV 15 or 14, or Bl 43 — reduce; calms the mind, clears *heat,* and adjusts the *Qi* of the upper *Jiao*;
- Ht 8 or Ht 9 — reduce; clears *heart fire*;
- Ht 3 — reduce; regulates the *heart* and calms the spirit;
- P 3 — even; regulates the *heart*;
- Lv 2 — reduce; clears *heart fire*; add for *liver fire* signs;
- St 44 — clears *stomach fire*; add for *stomach fire*;
- P 6 — even; transforms *heart phlegm* and calms the spirit;
- Ht 5 — reduce or even; clears *heart fire* and calms the spirit;
- P 3 and Ht 3 — even; regulates the *heart* and calms the spirit; add for *heart phlegm.*

(2) *Heart Qi stasis*

- Emotions — anxiety, depression, irritability;
- Physical — sensations of epigastric and chest fullness ("men"), palpitations, chest constriction;
- Tongue — normal or slightly dark;
- Pulse — wiry and full.

Points:

- CV 17 — regulates the *upper Jiao* (use only in excess conditions);
- P 6 and Sp 4 — moves the *Qi*, regulates the *heart*, and calms the spirit;
- Lv 3 and Lv 14 — moves *liver* blood; for *liver Qi stasis*;
- Lv 3 and Gb 34 — subdues *liver Yang*; for *liver Yang* rising;
- Ht 5 — clears *heart phlegm* and calms the spirit; for *heart phlegm*.

(3) *Deficient heart* Qi

- Emotions — exaggerated emotional response, anxiety;
- Physical — palpitations, condition worse with fatigue, cold hands and feet;
- Tongue — pale;
- Pulse — empty.

Points:

- CV 4 — tonifies the *Source Qi*;
- CV 17 — regulates the *upper Jiao* (use only with short retention so as not to disperse *Qi*);
- Ht 7 — tonifies the *heart* and calms the spirit;
- St 36 — tonifies *Qi* and blood.
- K 3 — tonifies *kidney Qi* and *Yin* with BL 15, 20, 23;
- K 27 — tonifies the *kidneys* and lifts the *Qi* to the chest;
- Sp 3 — tonifies *spleen Qi*;
- Gb 40 — regulates the *liver/gallbladder*.

(4) *Deficient heart blood*

- Emotions — anxiety, poor memory, easy startlement, sadness, confusion, depression, inability to concentrate;
- Physical — palpitations, insomnia, fatigue, dizziness, a pale face;
- Tongue — pale and dry;
- Pulse — thin and possibly choppy.

Points:

- CV 4 — nourishes blood and calms the spirit;
- CV 14 — regulates the *heart* and calms the spirit.

Some common anxiolytics from botanical medicines:

- Ashwaganda — *Withania somnifera;*
- Kava kava — *Piper mythysticum;*
- Lemongrass — *Cymbopogon citratus;*
- Panax ginseng — Chinese ginseng; not to be used when the patient is hypertensive;
- Ginkgo biloba — GBE extract;
- St. John's wort — *Hypericum perforatum;* not to be used alongside MOAs;
- Siberian ginseng — *Eleutherococcus senticosus.*

Insomnia

The *Wei Qi* circulates externally 12 times during the daytime and internally 12 times during the night.[54] This circulation pattern allows the organs, especially the *liver,* to be replenished and to detoxify during the night while *Yin* and blood are nourished. *Wei Qi* circulatory patterns are disrupted when people do not sleep well or enough. When people do not sleep well conditions can arise that are precursors to chronic disease. These include *Qi deficiency* that leads to immune deficiency, *Yin deficiency* that is a magnet for *latent pathogenic factors* and also is a cause of hormonal imbalances, *liver* and *kidney deficiency* that can lead to *stasis of Qi* and blood, and *spleen deficiency* that can lead to damp accumulations and obesity and diabetes.

In conventional medical terms, sleep is divided into two types: nonrapid eye movement (NREM) sleep and rapid eye movement (REM) sleep. NREM sleep occurs during the initial phase of sleep and is characterized by slow EEG waves, lowered respiratory and heart rates, and lowered muscle tone. REM sleep occupies the remainder of the sleep time. The rate and depth of respiration are increased during REM sleep but muscle tone is depressed even further than in

NREM sleep. REM sleep always follows NREM sleep and ends each sleep cycle. Norepinephrine pathways in the brainstem are implicated in REM sleep. Serotoninergic (melatonin) pathways are implicated in NREM sleep. Most dreaming occurs during REM. Most nightmares and sleepwalking occur during NREM stages 3 and 4. People who do not dream often have B vitamin deficiencies. Interruption of REM sleep produces hyperactivity and emotionally labile behavior.[55]

Delta sleep is a deeper level of REM sleep and is the only time when growth hormone is released from the pituitary.[56] Most primary tissue rehabilitation happens during this time. And it is the main time when the liver (Western medicine) detoxifies itself. Lack of delta sleep can lead to chronic illnesses due to a buildup of oxidative stress and the lack of rehabilitation of normal tissue and function.

In conventional treatment for insomnia, there are five different diagnoses possible that are indicative of the cause. Initial insomnia is one category of insomnia in which a patient cannot fall asleep. It would probably coincide with a *spleen* and *heart Qi deficiency* type of insomnia in Chinese medicine. The early morning waking type of insomnia is just that and probably coincides with a *Yin-deficient* type of insomnia. The inverted sleep pattern type of insomnia occurs especially in the elderly or those on sedation who have lost the circadian rhythm of a night *Yin* quiet cycle; they sleep during the day and not at night. Primary insomnia is longstanding and has an apparent relationship to a somatic or psychic event like PTSD, and probably coincides with several different Chinese medicine categories but especially that of *heart* and *gallbladder deficiency heat* with *phlegm*. Lastly, there is secondary insomnia, which is secondary to another problem, most commonly pain, anxiety, and depression.

Women are especially prone to insomnia, because of a propensity for spleen deficiencies that snowball into deficiency *liver Qi stasis*, *phlegm/damp*, *heart Qi deficiency* and *stasis*, and *blood deficiency*. Women are also more likely to be diagnosed with depression and anxiety, and depression and anxiety are also indicative of the previous list of issues.

The patterns of insomnia in conventional medicine are treated with benzodiazepines like Halcion, Valium, Ativan, and Restoril. These drugs have a negative effect on memory and sometimes on behavior. Antihistamines are also used, because of their side effect of drowsiness. Tryptophan and valerian help with serotonin synthesis in a more natural way, without the side effect of possible addiction or dependency. For some people who cannot sleep because they suffer from what has come to be called restless leg syndrome, folic acid deficiency has been found to be a possible cause. And people who are hypoglycemic also wake in the night if their blood sugar falls too low. Night eating while asleep may indicate hypoglycemia. Melatonin treats serotonin-related insomnia.

It is important to ascertain the actual symptoms that accompany what a patient is calling insomnia. Some people report that they have insomnia but actually sleep the right number of hours per night. Their problem is that they awake feeling tired. The issue may be the quality of their sleep. Normally, most adults require 8 h of sleep per night. This changes based on the constitution of the patient and their lifestyle. A monk who is meditating 12 h per day may not need to sleep 8 h. A coal miner may need to sleep more hours per day. Insomnia may also relate to the routine of the patient at nighttime. Some people watch television in bed and then cannot go to sleep. Stimulating activity late at night is generally not conducive to the quiet needed to switch off and into a *Yin* activity like sleep. A night routine will help patients develop patterns that enable them to have a better chance of sleeping well.

Patterns

There are four main kinds of insomnia, called the "four toos."[57] These are too much thinking, too much work, too much food, and too much anger. In the "too much thinking" realm there are several signs and symptoms that are indicative of this type of insomnia:

- The day continues in the mind while the person is trying to go to sleep;
- Often, there will be a lifestyle change prior to the development of the insomnia, and this is due to anxiety over the change;
- There may be a constitutional factor;
- The person chews over their thoughts but never digests them;

- There is a hard time getting to sleep;
- There is a tendency to wake easily;
- There is also a tendency to awake feeling groggy and unclear.

There are several patterns that fall into the general realm of *thinking too much.*

(1) *Deficient spleen* Qi *and heart blood*

- Symptoms — palpitations, poor memory, a face that is pale or lacks luster, easy sweating, fatigue, a tendency to loose stools;
- Signs — a pale tongue with a thin coating; a thin and weak pulse.

The *spleen* is injured from thinking too much and is unable to nourish the *heart,* creating *heart blood deficiency* symptoms. The *heart blood deficiency* develops from thinking too much, and/or from blood loss due to trauma, childbirth, or menorrhagia. Damage to the *heart* and *spleen* leads to *blood deficiency,* causing the spirit to float. This results in frequent dreams, wakefulness, forgetfulness, and palpitations. The blood does not nourish the *upper Jiao,* leading to a pale face and tongue body. The *spleen* loses function, leading to poor appetite and symptoms of *Qi* and *blood deficiency.*

The treatment principles are to tonify the *Qi* and to nourish the blood with a focus on the *spleen* and *heart.* The common formula used to treat this presentation is *Gui Pi Tang.*[58] Commonly used points are Bl 15, 20, 37, and 39 (the last two for excessive dreaming). Include Ht 7 and Sp 6.

(2) *Heart and gallbladder deficiency heat with phlegm*

- Symptoms — the person is terrified of sleeping alone, wakes easily, is not just thinking but is literally afraid but may have no idea why they are afraid, and may think that they are going crazy; there may be generalized anxiety, a tendency to dizziness, or a tendency to acid regurgitation or even vomiting, often following abuse or a scary experience;
- Signs — a pale and swollen tongue; a thin and weak pulse.

This is a type of *Hun* disturbance.[59] The *gallbladder* pertains to one's resolution and courage and the ability to make decisions. Problems with it are often inconsistent. *Phlegm* in the *stomach* can lead to *heat* in the *gallbladder*. *Phlegm heat* causes constraint that interferes with the rising of the *clear Yang*, manifesting as dizziness. The *turbid Yin* rises, causing digestive symptoms ranging from belching to distension and bloating in the epigastric area, and to nausea or positional eructation. *Phlegm heat* disturbs the chest and *heart*, and causes irritability, insomnia, palpitations, and anxiety. GERD and esophagitis can be underlying problems that cause this disorder. A hiatal hernia can also cause positional eructation. When these last conditions contribute to this type of insomnia, it is called "high pillow disorder." Otherwise, it is a *hun* disorder.

The treatment principles are to transform *phlegm* and to adjust the *gallbladder*. Points used can be Bl 19 and 43. Bl 47 is the *hun* point, and Gb 34, 40, and 41 all deal with head problems, including mental problems, related to the *gallbladder*. The herbal formula commonly used is *Wen Dan Tang*.[60]

In the *working too much* realm of insomnia, there is commonly only one pattern. *Yin deficiency* with glowing *fire* is further divided into two subsets of the main diagnosis: *heart Yin deficiency*, and *heart* and *kidney Yin deficiency*.

The general symptoms include: irritability, difficulty in falling asleep due to mental restlessness, a tendency to toss and turn due to physical restlessness; the person wakes easily and is a light sleeper. All of these symptoms indicate that the *Yang* cannot enter the *Yin*.

(1) *Heart Yin deficiency*

- Add the following symptoms to the above — palpitations, forgetful, "*fan*," dry mouth, dry throat;
- Signs — a red tongue; thin and rapid a pulse.

The treatment principle is to nourish the *Yin* of the *heart*. The primary formula for treating this presentation is *Tian Wang Bu Xin Tang*.[61] In the case of blood and *Yin deficiencies*, the main means of treatment is usually herbal medicine. However, common points for treating this condition would be those that nourish the *Yin* and calm the spirit.

(2) *Heart and kidney disharmony*

- Add the following symptoms to the set under "working too much" — low back pain, five-center *heat*, tinnitus.

Kidney Yin deficiency leads to *heart fire* uprising and dry mouth, restlessness, forgetfulness, backache, and palpitations. People with *heart* and *kidney Yin deficiency* insomnia will have not only *kidney* signs and symptoms but more severe signs and symptoms. They may not be able to sleep at all. They may spend the entire night tossing and turning. The lack of sleep starts a vicious circle in which the more one does not sleep the more one cannot sleep. "Burning the candle at both ends" is a common saying; it may contribute to this pattern. People who are constitutionally *Yin-deficient* are more susceptible to this pattern. *Liver fire* can become a subset of *kidney Yin deficiency* and *heart fire.*

The treatment principles are to enrich the *Yin* and to cause the *fire* to descend. In the case of *liver fire*, soothing the *liver* may be an additional aspect of treatment. Common points are: Ht 7 or P 7, Ht 8, K 3 and K 6, and Bl 23. For *heart* and *kidney Yin deficiency*, use the formula *Zhu Sha An Shen Wan*[62] or an acceptable replacement. For *liver fire* as a subset of *kidney* and *heart fire* due to *Yin deficiency*, use *Suan Zao Ren Tang.*[63]

In the *too much food* realm of insomnia, there is one pattern.

(1) *Food stasis insomnia*

- Symptoms — there is not usually a problem in falling asleep or waking, the person may sleep 7–8h per night, they wake and still feel tired, they do not sleep enough and sleep is not restful, they feel easily hassled, there may be stomach problems and epigastric distension, there may be foul smelling belches, there may or may not be *phlegm*: (a) they may spit up *phlegm* and have a frog in the throat; (b) they may have a *"men"* sensation; (c) there may be disorientation and dizziness; and there is often a history of overeating, depression, or improper foods; Signs — a tongue with a greasy and thick coating; a slippery and wiry pulse.

Food stasis is a problem with dietary habits. It can be a short-term and once-in-a-while event or can occur chronically as a result of long-term improper eating habits. Too much greasy food, raw foods, and high-fat and highly refined foods that cause obesity and athero-sclerosis contribute to food stasis syndrome. This syndrome implies *dampness* and *phlegm* obstruction.

The treatment principles are to transform *phlegm* and to harmonize the *stomach*. Common points are CV 12, St 40, St 36, St 45 (which is a special point for this type of insomnia), P 6 (*yintang* for dizziness), and Li 4 (for dizziness due to a *yangming excess* condition). The most common formula used is *Bao He Wan*.[64]

In *too much anger* insomnia, the primary pattern is, of course, *liver fire*.

(1) *Liver fire insomnia*

- Symptoms — the person cannot get to sleep, they have frequent headaches, there is dizziness, irritability, a bad temper, *liver* and *gallbladder* channel problems, there may be hypochondrium distension or pain, tinnitus, vision or eye problems, a bitter taste in the mouth;
- signs — a tongue with a yellow thin coating and red and edges; a rapid wiry forceful tongue.

Liver fire happens as a result of unresolved emotional material causing pent-up frustrations and anger. It can also occur because of *damp–heat*. In many of these types there are overlaps. No one person is a pure manifestation. In this particular type, the person will not come for treatment of insomnia but some other *liver*-related problem that is accompanied by insomnia. With all of these insomnia patterns, the important thing is to find the primary pattern and focus on treating that. If other patterns become more clear as a result of treatment, then emphasis can be switched as the pattern or patterns are revealed.

Treatment in the *liver* fire type of insomnia includes points like Lv 2, Gb 44 (which lowers the *Qi*), Gb 20 (which treats *liver/gallbladder* problems with the head), Ht 7, and Ht 4; last two nourish the spirit points.

There are some less commonly seen types of insomnia:

Consumptive insomnia is due to *Qi* and *blood deficiency*. Because the heart controls the pulse, when it is undernourished it loses vital force and function, resulting in manifestations like anxiety and palpitations. The *heart blood* provides the foundation for the activities of the spirit. When it is deficient, the spirit has no place to reside because the void of the *heart* is unquiet or nonexistent. This causes irritability and insomnia. Others symptoms may include emaciation and shortness of breath. Blood and fluids are intimately related and deficiency of one can lead to deficiency of the other. Low fluids lead to constipation of the dry type, dry mouth and throat, no tongue coating, a pale tongue, and a forceless pulse. This is not the same pattern as *Gui Pi Tang* with a *spleen* and *heart deficiency* caused by *blood deficiency*. The history of severe chronic or acute illness is the key to diagnosis. The treatment is Zhi Gan Cao Tang.[65]

Qi-level heat lingering in the superficial yangming is another less commonly seen cause of insomnia. Heat constrained in the *Qi-level* leads to fever. *Heat* constrained in the chest causes insomnia. Tossing and turning while asleep, and tossing and turning to get to sleep are symptoms of this presentation. There is a yellow tongue coating and a high and fast pulse. This pattern is due to the aftermath of an excess disease of external origin. We do not see it often here in the developed world but it is not uncommon where epidemic diseases occur. The treatment is *Zhi Zi Dou Chi Tang*,[66] which clears *heat* and nourishes the fluids.

Clinical experience shows that the use of ion pumping cords from the Japanese acupuncturist Yoshio Manaka[67] is a valuable form of intervention for insomnia.

- In *heart/*spleen *deficiency*, use P 6 and Sp 4;
- In the *Yin deficiency* type, use K 6 and Lu 7;

- In the food stasis type, use P 6 and Sp 4;
- In the *liver/gallbladder* type, use SJ 5 and Gb 41.

If your diagnosis is correct and you are using ion-pumping cords, the patient should fall asleep on the table. Usually the red clip is placed on the more important channel.

Breathing shallowly can contribute to stress and constraint. Breathing exercises and *Qi* gong are very useful for adjusting the breathing mechanism and therefore the *Qi* mechanism, and help tremendously to "soothe the savage beast." Sleep is an important rehabilitative part of life. It helps the body to regulate hormones, improve immune function, restore organ function, detoxify and depurate the products of oxidative stress, and clear stress hormones,[68] and it allows the spirit to nourish itself and recenter the soul.

Conclusions

All of these emotional and spiritual disorders snarl the machinery of life. It is immensely important to treat them, because they set the stage for liver patterns that are so intimately involved in breast cancer etiology (internal), and for *latent pathogens* to enter and have a larger effect on the human body (external). They are also part of the cultural milieu that allows humans to contaminate their own nests and the nests of others, to damage the Earth without constraint, and to not look at the long-term effects of these actions. They allow a split to occur between actions and intent — one that can be lethal. These issues begin in the etheric and emotional bodies of people. And their healing begins in the etheric and emotional bodies of humans.

The underlying patterns of *liver Qi stasis, spleen deficiency, dampness,* and *Yin deficiency* all act as magnets for *latent pathogenic factors,* as stated first in the *Shang Han Za Bin Lun* and later (more completely) in *Wen Bing Xue.* A *Yin-deficient* constitution leads to empty heat, which attracts inwardly unresolved pathogens. *Spleen deficiency* leads to a propensity for *damp* accumulations; and *damp-ness* can attract or transform external pathogens to *wind–dampness* which can lead to *damp–heat* in the interior. *Qi stasis* also generates heat and stasis, leading to a vicious circle that includes injury to the *middle Jiao* and the *liver–spleen* axis. The result is the attraction of latent pathogenic factors through the levels, as stated in the theory of the four levels from warm disease theory.[69] All of the following external influences are examples of *latent pathogenic factors* or entities that can become *latent pathogenic factors*. They are enabled by the constitution formed in a lifestyle that many modern women live. This acquired constitution results in *liver Qi stasis, spleen deficiency, dampness*, internal *damp–heat*, and *Yin deficiency* — all magnets for the new and multitudinous chemical and hormonal factors we are exposed to in modern life. These patterns of dysfunction are the primary patterns considered by Chinese medicine to be foundational for breast cancer.

External Influences

Known Links to Breast Cancer Causation

The influence of multiple external exposures in modern life may help to explain why the incidence of breast cancer has risen so dramatically in the last 60 years, from 1 in 40 women in the 1940s to 1 in 8 women in 2005. It was in the last 60 years that "better living through chemistry" and better living through technology became a reality in the Western world. Since that time the rates of almost all cancers have been on the rise. There are only two cancers whose rates have dropped in the US — lung and cervical. These have dropped, as said previously, because of public health efforts to encourage people not to smoke and because of early screening that detects precancerous cervical conditions, allowing early treatment.

The idea of prevention has become a semantic slippery slope when it comes to cancer. The longer latency period for many cancers, the multifactorial etiology, and a lack of concentrated research data in many cancers as to direct causes are all apparently insurmountable problems on identifying and interacting with these causes to prevent a *cancer*. In breast cancer almost 99% of attention is given to research on treatment but very little is given to research on prevention. The rates of incidence for breast cancer have risen steadily since the advent of the chemical industry and industrial agriculture. Less than 4% of breast cancers are due to genetic predisposition. Half of all breast cancers occur in women with no known risk of breast cancer. And the complexity of determining causes in hormonally sensitive tumors implies that the timing, duration, and pattern of exposure to substances that impact reproductive development are as important as the dose of the substance. This is a new and burgeoning area of research and requires long-term studies that are geographical, epidemiological, and age-related, carried out through time following the same people in the same place and making linkages to environmental activities.[70]

We now know that an endocrine-disrupting impact during a critical window of development can cause permanent damage to organs and interactive processes within the body. DES, used to prevent miscarriage in women who were prone, is one example, but today there are many more. Prenatal development is an exquisitely sensitive process regulated by an intricate system of hormonal signals. Many chemicals and hormonally mimicking substances have been added to the armamentarium of modern industries and agriculture. Today there are more than 100,000 new chemicals on the Earth, manufactured primarily in the US and for which the human body and other animal bodies have no defense.[71,72] Studies by the US Centers for Disease Control and Prevention show that women have higher levels of many of these chemicals in their bodies than do men.[73]

Some chemicals have had a now-proven impact on breast cancer rates. DDT and its breakdown product DDE, atrazine, and some other agricultural chemicals are now implicated. Perhaps we could say that the human breast has become the canary in the coalmine providing a vast amount of information about how these chemicals impact human health. The precautionary principle that demands proof of safety *before* a chemical is used does not exist in the US Women's bodies, as well as other animal bodies and the Earth itself, are the laboratory studies, without any controls, for finding information, after the fact, about how these chemicals work in the macrocosm and microcosm of life.

One example of how the long-term effects of environmental exposures impact the rates of breast cancer is a case control study of 3200 women aged 35–79 in western New York state that showed that exposure to high levels of PAHs (polycyclic aromatic hydrocarbons, resulting from combustion engine exhaust) at birth was associated with an increased risk of postmenopausal breast cancer.[74] These results could only be obtained through monitoring over the long term, and this study was conducted from 1959 to 1997. Clustering patterns of premenopausal breast cancer in western New York were more closely related to place of residence at birth and at menarche than at any other period of life.

It is not clear how we would speak of these exposures in Chinese medicine. Certainly, the clinical concept of latent pathogenic factors again comes to mind. Exposures that disrupt the endocrine system come through the environment and so they are external pathogens. They remain latent in the body, usually in fat cells because they are often lipophilic, and for long periods of time before manifesting symptoms. Some of them look so much like normal body hormones that they are misinterpreted and fill receptor sites for hormones when, in fact, they are not hormones. Whereas human estrogen breaks down within 24 h, xenoestrogens persist and can remain stored in the body for years, some of them up to 48 years.[75,76] The more one is exposed to xenoestrogens, the more xenoestrogens are stored. Some of them actually exert influences up to 1000 times greater than normal endogenous estrogens, leading to much higher estrogenic influences in a woman's lifetime.[77]

According to the theory of conventional medicine, promoting factors can create an environment in which a cancer is more likely to occur. Promoting factors fall into the realm of what we call *spleen deficiency, Yin deficiency, dampness,* and *liver Qi stasis,* all of which are acquired constitutional patterns that, according to *Wen Bing Xue,* invite *latent pathogens* inward. These acquired constitutional conditions are certainly promoting factors from the conventional point of view, and they are internal. *Spleen deficiency* refers to the many conventional medical manifestations of hypercholesterolemia, early diabetes, hyperinsulinemia, and atherosclerosis along with other similar conditions that are terrains in which *cancers* occur and take hold more readily.[78] *Yin deficiency* refers to abnormal hormonal levels resulting from *liver* and *kidney Yin deficiency*. *Dampness* refers to *spleen* and *kidney deficiency* accumulations due to injuries in water and food metabolism. And *liver Qi stasis* refers to the manifestations we talked about earlier in this chapter.

Determining at what level a *latent pathogenic factor* is lodged is more complex. Traditionally, the four levels that come out of *Wen Bing Xue* seem not to include a level that works well for these kinds of chemical exposures. Many endocrine disruptors are lipophilic and are stored in fat tissue. One thought is that the *San Jiao* may be the place where the latent pathogen sits and smolders and then begins to move — attracted to the least strong organ or group of organs. The *spleen, liver, chong* and *ren* in Chinese medicine are highly stressed channel and organ functional units in women, especially during the prenatal period, during menarche, and during pregnancy. In postmenopausal women, *Yin deficiency* and *kidney deficiency* are added to the picture. These are theoretical questions for Chinese medicine practitioners to discuss and evaluate as we try to find out what we can contribute to the modern issue of chemical toxicants in the internal and external environment and to the epidemic of cancers. The reader is referred back to Chapter 1 and the discussion of the *San Jiao*.

In terms of the nature of an exposure, we must rely on our ability to analyze conventional science's analysis. Following is a long list of scientific data from Western science evaluations of certain exposures and their relationships to breast cancer. Some of these are hormonal disruptors and some may fall into the realm of *toxins*. Most of them do not have immediate effects that are symptomatically discernible. The complexity of these exposures and their impacts make them especially problematic in terms of discernment and treatment. Understanding the next step beyond eliminating exposures to these chemicals will take time and effort. Many are already ubiquitous and are found in the human body.

General

Breast cancer may result from altered development in breast tissue itself rather than only from a genetic mutation. The tissue organization field theory (TOFT) proposes that carcinogens alter the interaction between cells in the stroma and those in the epithelium of the breast, disrupting normal development and predisposing the organism to cancer.[79] This is a new analysis of how various types of chemicals work to cause cancer.

The younger the organism is, the more vulnerable the developing cells are to environmental exposures. The critical windows are prenatal, prepubertal, adolescent, and through a woman's first full-term pregnancy. Fetal toxicology is also a burgeoning area of research. And the idea that women's bodies may be different from men's and more sensitive to environmental exposures is now being proven.[80]

There is no research that definitively states that synthetic chemicals or radiation is responsible for the fact that the breast cancer risk in the US has tripled in the last 40 years. However, taken together, all the different types of research provide compelling evidence that exposure to certain chemicals contributes to an increase in the risk of breast cancer. The Standing Committee of European Doctors has stated: "It has now been scientifically demonstrated that there is indeed a link between chemical products and the appearance of diseases such as cancers, infertility, degenerative diseases of the central nervous system, MS, and allergies."[81]

There are three types of research that have contributed knowledge about breast cancer: ecological research, environmental research, and epidemiological research. What is required is integration of the information derived from all of these types of research in order to gain real working information valuable for preventing breast cancer.

Known Links to Breast Cancer

Ionizing Radiation

Ionizing radiation is the most-studied carcinogen and mutagen. It includes gamma radiation used in weapons testing, nuclear medical procedures (such as bone, thyroid, and lung scans), and X-rays, CT scans, fluoroscopy, and radionuclide research.

Ionizing radiation may enhance the ability of hormones or other chemicals to cause cancer.[82,83] Since genomic instability is the hallmark of cancer cells, it is thought that ionizing radiation is involved in car-cinogenesis.[84,85] There is no such thing as a safe dose.[86–88] And radiation damage to genes is cumulative over a lifetime.[89]

Radiation exposures of 1 rad to the breast are equivalent to the breast irradiation received during 3300 h of flying.[90] Therefore, the typical mammogram of 0.2 rads is equal to the radiation dose received by the breast during 660 h of flying. Increased radiation exposure may have contributed to the 90% increase in breast cancer incidence in the US between 1950 and 2001.[91] X-rays can be reduced to ALARA "as low as reasonably achievable" standards and still produce high quality images. In 1976, women were exposed to 2 rads during mammography. In 2005, they were exposed to 0.2 rads.[92]

CT scans were introduced in the 1970s. They contribute about 10% to diagnosis by radiologic procedures, but about 65% of all radiation exposures.[93] The type of cancer resulting from diagnostic or treatment radiation procedures depends on the area exposed and the age at exposure. Infant X-rays and fluoroscopy expose the whole body. Women over the age of 55 derive less benefit from radiation therapy to prevent recurrence in terms of a lowered rate of local recurrence.[94] SEER data showed a 16-fold increase in the risk of angiosarcoma of the breast and chest wall following radiation to a primary breast cancer.[95] MRI and ultrasound should at least be considered as possible alternatives to diagnostic and treatment options.

Chemicals

Estrogens (estradiol, estriol, and estrone) and progesterone are the main hormonal influences on breast tissue. In the 1950s, estrogen replacement therapy (ERT) was used to treat the symptoms of menopause, which were considered to be a result of estrogen "deficiency." Studies showed that ERT caused a marked increase in uterine cancer and so progestin was added to ERT, forming hormone replacement therapy (HRT). It was thought that opposing estrogen with a form of progesterone would reduce and resolve this problem. In 2002, the National Toxicology Program of the US added HRT and steroidal estrogens, found in many oral contraceptive pills, to the list of known human carcinogens.[96] The International Agency for Research on Cancer (IARC) listed HRT and steroidal estrogens as carcinogenic in 1987, 15 years earlier. The information that drove these decisions confirmed evidence from the 1930s about the use of estrogens or progesterone in treatment.[97] The entire history of hormonal therapies and contraceptive therapies for women also confirms the tremendously stressful issues that women face in our world. The feminist revolution from the 1960s and 1970s, during which women were reclaiming their bodies and the right to determine more freely how their bodies would be used, has ended up being a far more complicated issue than anyone ever imagined. Now we are beginning to realize the heavy price paid by women for having reproductive responsibility placed entirely on their own bodies rather than shared by the two genders.

The longer the exposure to estrogens, the greater the risk of breast cancer. This means that girls who menstruate before the age of 12 have longer exposure (see the section on early puberty); women who enter menopause after the age of 55, or have children late or not at all, have longer exposure; and women who use HRT after menopause have longer exposure. Natural estrogens supplemented by HRT or the oral contraceptive pill increase the risk of breast cancer.[98] If both are used in a woman's lifetime, the risk of breast cancer is increased even more.[99,100]

In 2003 Sweden halted a study of HRT in women with a history of breast cancer after finding a three-times-greater rate of recurrence for women in the study.[101] In the same year, the Million Women Study in the United Kingdom reported that *all* menopausal HRT increased the rate of breast cancer and the greatest risk was among users of estrogen/progestin in combination. This study established that women who used estrogen/progestin HRT for 10 years were 4 times more likely to develop breast cancer than those who used ERT.[102] The Women's Health Initiative found that, among 16,000 women age,[50–79] half of whom were on Prempro and half on a placebo, there was a 49% increase in risk in the Prempro group. The study was stopped after 5 years.[103]

These studies indicated that both endogenous and exogenous hormones and substances that acted like hormones increase the risk of hormonally related cancers and breast cancer. When it came to oral contraceptives, numerous studies showed an increased risk of breast cancer.[104–106] The risks were greatest among current and recent users, those using OCPs for over 5 years, premenopausal women, those with a family history of breast cancer, and women with the BR CA1 and 2 mutations.[107,108]

High body fat levels in postmenopausal women also may increase risk, because fat is a reservoir for any synthetic lipophilic (fat-seeking and fat-soluble) chemicals like organochlorines that can mimic effects of natural estrogens. Since breast tissue is primarily fatty tissue, it can become a repository for these contaminants. In post-menopausal women a correlation has been found between high body fat, free circulating estrogens, and higher risk of breast cancer.[109,110] However, if we look at epidemiological studies worldwide, the breast cancer rates are not higher in cultures where women are traditionally fatter as they age. One example is Italy, where women tend toward overweight or even obesity. Italy does not have a higher breast cancer rate possibly because almost all food from small family farms is grown without chemical inputs.

Xenoestrogens

Xenoestrogens are found in plastics containing p-nonyl-phenol, and pesticides, fuels, detergents, cosmetics, and some prescription drugs. They are endocrine disruptors.[111] A high risk of breast cancer has been found in postmenopausal women with the highest levels of total effective xenoestrogen burden (TEXB-alpha). The pesticides aldrin and lindane are associated with the highest risk.[112–114]

A number of metals also have estrogenic effects on breast cancer cells, including copper, cobalt, nickel, lead, mercury, tin, and chromium. Methyl mercury alters growth-related signaling in MCF-7 breast cancer cells.[115] These statistics are significant, in that these metals are commonly found in industrial and urban areas. And mercury in the Puget Sound area, which currently has the highest rate of breast cancer in the US, blows in via ocean-driven weather systems from China, where coal is burned in the production of electricity for energy to run its burgeoning economy. Mercury is a by-product of coal burning,[116] and much of it ends up in the rain and snow falling on Puget Sound and into the mountain reservoirs that provide the public water supply.

In Cape Cod, on the other side of the US, women were found to have a 20% higher risk of breast cancer than the rest of Massachusetts. The Silent Spring Institute studied this issue and found synthetic estrogens (xenoestrogens) in septic tank contents, groundwater, and some private wells.[117,118]

Indoor air and household dust samples were found to contain 52 compounds in the air samples and 66 compounds in the samples taken from Cape Cod homes. These compounds included phthalates, parabens, alkylphenols, flame retardants, PAHs, bisphenol-A, and banned and currently used pesticides. The Silent Spring Institute found the highest risk of breast cancer in women on Cape Cod who had lived there for 25–29 years. Industrial agricultural and residential land use contamination exposures were suggested as reasons for the higher risk.[119]

Chronic exposures to widespread and persistent xenoestrogens may help explain the increase in breast cancer in industrialized countries. DES (mentioned earlier) was used from 1941 to 1971 for the prevention of miscarriage in pregnant women. Daughters of women who took DES were diagnosed, usually in their 20's, with higher rates of an extremely rare form of vaginal cancer than were their peers whose mothers did not take DES. Some of the women who took it in the 1950s were diagnosed with breast cancer, and their breast cancer may have been linked to the use of DES.[120] DES was also used in the cattle feedlot industry to speed up weight gain for many years after its use in humans had been banned. Unfortunately, DES is a xenoestrogenic and lipophilic chemical that is absorbed by the fat cells of any animal; thus, it has entered humans via the food stream.[121]

Bisphenol-A (BPA) is one of the most pervasive chemicals in modern life. Two billion pounds are produced in the US each year. BPA is the building block of polycarbonate plastic used in epoxy resins, polyester, and styrene manufacture. It is found in the lining of metal food cans and some plastic food containers (including some baby bottles), microwave ovenware, and eating utensils. BPA is an unstable polymer and is lipophilic, leaching into foods when heated.[122] It is found in umbilical cord blood at birth and in placental tissue.[123] The CDC has found BPA in 95% of over 300 urine samples tested.[124]

Intrauterine exposure to BPA has been linked to drastic changes in the development of the reproductive and mammary glands. Fetuses and embryos whose growth is regulated by the endocrine system are most vulnerable and there may be lasting effects from exposure to synthetic estrogens or other chemicals that disrupt endocrine function like BPA.[125] In 2005 Tufts University scientists found that exposing mice to extremely low levels of BPA altered development of the mammary gland in female offspring at puberty. These changes included an increased sensitivity to estrogens, a decreased level of apoptosis (cell death), and an increased number and size of the terminal end buds. If found in humans, these changes would increase the risk of breast cancer; and based on urine samples, studies are underway to evaluate the levels in humans. Exposure to BPA of mice in the study was 2000 times lower than the level which the EPA has designated as safe.[126]

BPA acts through the same response pathways as natural endogenous estrogen.[127] Two recent studies showed that low-dose BPA increases breast cell proliferation *in vitro* via the membrane estrogen receptor.[128]

Disagreements with the above research literature have come almost exclusively from the plastics industry's own scientists. As of December 2004, 115 studies on the health effects of BPA had been published. Among them 94 out of 104 government-funded studies conducted in Japan, Europe, and the US found adverse health effects from low BPA levels. None of the 11 studies funded by the industry reported adverse health effects at low-level exposure. The vast number of studies on BPA done since 2004 have shown that it is hazardous. However, the FDA has yet to completely reject the use of BPA in plastics and in the food industry.[129]

Polyvinyl chloride

Polyvinyl chloride (PVC) is used to produce food packaging, medical products, appliances, cars, toys, credit cards, rainwear, and piping. Vinyl chloride is a by-product of manufacture and can be released into air and water. It is found in air, near hazardous waste sites and landfills, and in tobacco smoke. Animal studies show that long-term exposure to vinyl chloride at low levels increases breast cancer risk.[130] Vinyl chloride is also linked to an increased rate of mortality from breast and liver cancers.[131,132]

Pesticides

From 1950 to 1970, aldrin and dieldrin were used for the growing of corn and cotton crops. Both were banned in 1975 except for use in termite control, and in 1987 they were banned altogether. Therefore, the human body burden regarding these two pesticides comes from past exposures or from lingering environmental residues.

The Copenhagen Center for Prospective Studies, in collaboration with the CDC, examined a rare bank of blood samples taken from women prior to development of breast cancer.[133] In the late 1970s and early 1980s, 7500 Danish women age 30–75 had blood samples taken. Researchers detected organochlorine compounds in most of the 240 women of this group who were eventually diagnosed with breast cancer prior to the study's publication in 2000. Researchers found dieldrin in 78% of the women who were later diagnosed with breast cancer. The women who had the highest levels of dieldrin long before cancer developed had more than double the risk of breast cancer compared to women with the lowest levels. This study also showed that exposure to dieldrin correlated with aggressiveness of the breast cancer. The higher the levels of dieldrin, the higher the rate of mortality from breast cancer.[134]

Investigation continues into the potential links with other chemicals and pesticides and breast cancer risk on Long Island, another hot spot. An increased risk was found in women living within one mile of hazardous waste sites containing organochlorine pesticides when compared to women living farther away. A second study showed that the highest tertile of total PCB concentration in surgical specimens of adipose tissue from women with nonmetastatic breast cancer was associated with a higher risk of recurrence. However, the higher risk of recurrence was not associated with pesticide levels.[135]

A case control study of 128 Latina agricultural workers in California newly diagnosed with breast cancer showed a higher risk from chlordane, malathion, and 2,4-D. The rates were higher in young women and in those with early-onset breast cancer than in unexposed women.[136]

A large prospective study by the National Cancer Institute looked at 30,000 women in Iowa and North Carolina who were farm wives. It found an increased risk in women using 2,4-D, 5-TP, dieldrin, and captan. Risk was also modestly elevated in women whose homes were closest to areas of pesticide application.[137]

Cosmetics and Personal Products

Nearly 90% of the ingredients used in cosmetics and personal products have not been tested for human health effects. The industry is largely unregulated. Some ubiquitous ingredients have been shown to be estrogenic *in vitro*[138,139] and *in vivo*:[140]

Parabens are a group of compounds used as antimicrobial preservatives in food, pharmaceuticals, cosmetics, and underarm deodorants. They are absorbed through skin contact and from the gastrointestinal tract and through the blood. They are found in measurable amounts in human breast tumors.

Placental extracts from human, equine, and porcine sources and other estrogenic chemicals are also found in cosmetics, hair products, and products marketed especially to women of color. They may be linked to precocious puberty or early menarche, both of which increase the risk of breast cancer.[141,142]

Phytoestrogens may counteract the effects of synthetic xenoestrogens. Adding soy to the diet has lowered estradiol levels in the body.[143,144] Some studies show that plant-estrogen-like compounds may reduce the risk of breast cancer. At the same time, genistein (found in soy) and daidzen — both phytoestrogens — have been found to cause oxidative damage to DNA and this is thought to play a role in tumor initiation.[145] Genistein may interfere with the antitumor activity of tamoxifen. This is important to consider when treating to prevent a recurrence in women already diagnosed and treated for breast cancer. It is linked to questions that many women have regarding the use of tamoxifen, for women who are not good candidates for tamoxifen, and women who wish to prevent recurrence with integrated care. Then this question becomes: What is the best approach, — natural medicine or pharmaceutical antiestrogenic treatment, — and can they be combined and how?

Solvents

Organic solvents have become ubiquitous and are now especially problematic with the manufacture of computer components. Benzene, toluene, and trichloroethylene have all been shown to induce mammary tumors in laboratory animals.[146] Many of these solvents are also used in the cosmetic industry.[147]

A Taiwanese study from 2003 showed a high risk of breast cancer among electronics workers exposed to chlorinated organic solvents.[148] Also, a government study at Scottish semiconductor plants showed a 30% increase in breast cancer among their female workers.[149] In Denmark, women between the ages of 25 and 55 employed in solvent-using industries had double the risk of breast cancer.[150] The increases were found in workers in the fabricated metal, lumber, furniture, printing, chemical, textile, and clothing industries.

A 1995 US study found an increased breast cancer risk with occupational exposures to styrene[151] and with several organic solvents, including formaldehyde and carbon tetrachloride. These findings were validated by studies in Finland, Sweden, and Italy.

A Duke University and National Institutes of Environmental Health Sciences (NIEHS) collaborative study showed that the solvent ethylene glycol methyl ether (EGME) and its metabolites act as hormone sensitizers *in vitro* and *in vivo*. It found increased cellular sensitivity to the effects of exposure to estrogens and progestins. EGME is used in the semiconductor industry and is a component in varnishes, paints, dyes, and fuel additives. Researchers at Duke and the NIEHS found that the increased hormonal activity was as much as eightfold.

They cautioned women exposed to EGME while taking HRT, oral contraceptives, or tamoxifen. They made similar findings for valproic acid, an anticonvulsant medicine used in treatment for bipolar disorder and migraines.[152,153]

Aromatic Amines

These chemicals are found in plastics and in chemical industries. They appear in environmental pollution like diesel exhaust, combustion of wood chips and rubber, tobacco smoke, and in grilled meats and fish.

There are three types. One type — o-toluidine — causes mammary tumors in rats.[154] Heterocyclic amines are found with PAHs when meats and fats are cooked at high temperature.[155] This is why eating a lot of grilled or barbequed meats can cause cancer. The most critical time of exposure to these chemicals in the female body is from menarche to the first full-term pregnancy, including adolescence. It is very important to avoid exposure to aromatic amines during this window of time.[156]

1,3-Butadiene

The internal combustion engine, petroleum refineries, the processing of synthetic rubber products, and some fungicides cause this air pollutant, which is a carcinogen when inhaled.[157] Women are more vulnerable to the carcinogenic effects, and younger women are even more vulnerable.[158]

All of the above have definitively been linked to breast cancer causation. Some of them have been known for over 70 years without evidence-based changes being made to manufacturing processes or to medical decision-making processes and treatment. This is a disconnect between the knowing of science and the meaning of wisdom based on the void of the heart. It is a split. If we are to use linear thinking to understand the world we have made, then we should make sure that it comes full circle and the knowledge is used for good, not harm.

Probable Links to Breast Cancer Causation

DDT/DDE and PCBs

The organochlorine pesticide DDT and its breakdown product DDE and polycarbonated biphenols (PCBs) are two chemicals and types of chemicals that disrupt hormonal function. DDT and PCBs have been banned in the US for three decades now but are still found in the fat tissue of humans and other animals, as well as breast milk.[159] DDT was banned in 1972 as an extremely dangerous persistent pesticide used to control insects on farms and in swamps. It has a very long half-life, and in 1995 it was found in measurable amounts in 82% of all the homes studied.[160] It is still manufactured and used for malaria control in 17 countries.[161]

A US study examined blood drawn from children and adolescents at the time of active DDT use. Increased breast cancer risk paralleled increasing concentrations of serum DDT, and risk was significantly higher in women exposed before the age of 15 than in women exposed after.[162]

Some studies did not find links between DDT/DDE and PCB exposures and breast cancer. But levels were measured only at the time of diagnosis for the cancer. Researchers did not consider effects of chemical mixtures and did not assess key metabolites. They looked only at blood levels — not at the levels of fat tissue, which accumulates at higher levels and for longer periods of time.

PCBs are classified into three types, depending on their effects on cells. There are more than 200 PCB congeners, with as many mechanisms of effect. All of these chemicals alter normal metabolism by disrupting either hormones or enzymes. A 1999 study was the first to show that certain types of PCBs promote the proliferation of breast cancer cells in culture by stimulating the production of key proteins or structures in cancerous tissue.[163]

Numerous studies have shown that PCBs are carcinogenic. They were banned in 1976 but remain in daily use in as many as two-thirds of all insulation fluids, plastics, adhesives, paper, inks, paints, dyes, and other products manufactured before 1976. One-third of PCBs have been discarded but the other two-thirds gradually make their way to landfills and waste dumps as things containing PCBs are discarded.

The Nurse's Health Study revisited the issue of PCBs and breast cancer risk, and revised their conclusions regarding the link between PCBs and DDE and breast cancer. It used studies of PCBs and DDE in blood, and concluded that there was an unlikely link between these chemicals and breast cancer rates. In 2002 new evidence regarding individual differences in susceptibility due to genetic differences prompted researchers to call for more studies.[164] In 2003 a New York study implicated PCBs in breast cancer recurrence among women with nonmetastatic breast cancer. Women with one PCB congener in their adipose tissue were three times as likely to have recurrent breast cancer as women with lower levels.[165]

PAHs

PAHs are found in soot and fumes from diesel combustion and other fuels. They create a distinctive type of damage in genetic material where the compounds directly bind with the basic building blocks of DNA, forming DNA adducts. Women with the highest PAH body burdens had a 50% higher risk of breast cancer.[166] Early life exposure to PAHs is associated with an increased risk of premenopausal breast cancer.[167] Some PAHs may have estrogenic effects in addition to causing DNA damage.[168] Tobacco smoke also contains PAHs and that may explain a potential link between higher risks in active and passive smoking.[169]

A large California study showed that teachers who started smoking during adolescence or at least five years prior to their first full-term pregnancy had an increased risk of breast cancer.[170] Smoking acts as an antiestrogenic and damages the ovaries. This may lower breast cancer risk but simultaneously the carcinogens in cigarette smoke increase a smoker's breast cancer risk. Passive smokers, on the other hand, do not get a large-enough dose of smoke to depress estrogen levels. The Air Resource Board of California's FPA found that the ETS is consistent with a causal association and breast cancer and appears to be stronger for premenopausal women.[171]

Dioxin

Dioxin is an incineration product of PVC, PCBs, and other chlorin-ated compounds, and also comes from industrial processes that use chlorine, and from the combustion of gasoline and diesel. It is found in the body fat of every human, including newborns. Dioxins are known carcinogens and hormone mimickers. TCDD was classified in 2000 by the EPA as a known carcinogen.[172]

Exposure to dioxin comes through consumption of animal prod-ucts: meat, poultry, dairy, and human breast milk.[173] It enters the food chain when vehicle exhaust or soot from incinerated chlorinated compounds falls on field crops which are then fed to animals. A study of women exposed to a chemical plant explosion in 1976 in Seveso, Italy showed a 10-fold increase in the risk of breast cancer. The women involved in this industrial accident continue to be followed.[174]

Ethylene Oxide

This is a fumigant used to sterilize surgical equipment. It is also found in some cosmetics. It is a known mammary carcinogen. A large number of women (7576) working in commercial sterilization facilities were found to have an increased incidence of breast cancer.[175]

Possible Links to Breast Cancer

Chemicals that have been found to be possible links to breast cancer causation include heptachlor, triazines, some sunscreen ingredients, phthalates, and some food additives.

Heptachlor

Heptachlor is an insecticide used in the 1980s for termite control. The EPA restricted the use of this chemical to fire ant control in 1988. Agricultural use of heptachlor continued until 1993, because growers were allowed to use up pre-existing stocks. Heptachlor still contaminates soil and humans. HE is a breakdown product of heptachlor and is fat-soluble, accumulating in fat and breast tissue. It is found even in adolescents age 12–19 and in umbilical cord blood from newborns.[176]

Heptachlor does not act like estrogen but affects the way the liver processes estrogen, allowing circulating estrogen levels to rise, thereby increasing breast cancer risk. It has also been shown to disrupt cell-to-cell communication in human breast cells in tissue culture. This disrupts cell growth regulation, and may increase breast cancer risk.[177]

Heptachlor was used a pesticide on Hawaiian pineapple fields since the late 1950s. The chopped-up leaves of the harvest were made into a kind of silage for dairy cows on Oahu. From 1981 to 1984, heptachlor levels in Oahu milk and dairy products exceeded the FDA-allowed level of 0.3 ppm 10-fold. Followup studies found that heptachlor levels in the breast milk of women on Oahu averaged 200 ppm and were as high as 400 ppm in some women. Breast cancer in Hawaii has among the highest rates in the world. From 1975 to 1985, the incidence of breast cancer increased by 35% among all racial groups in Hawaii.[178] Heptachlor still contaminates the soil and crops in some parts of that state.

Triazine Herbicides

Atrazine, simazine, and cyanizine are atrazine herbicides that are the most-heavily-used herbicidal chemicals in agriculture in the US. All three have been shown to cause mammary cancer in animals.[180] Simazine is used extensively in Florida, California, and the Midwest, and it contaminates the surface groundwater. In 1994 the EPA banned it as an algicide in swimming pools, hot tubs, and whirl-pools.[179] Rats are found to have elevated prolactin levels when fed simazine.

More than 80 million pounds of atrazine are used annually in the US to control weeds in corn and soybeans in the Midwest. Atrazine is banned in the European Union and in Israel, where the breast cancer rate dropped after it was no longer used.[181] It was once classified as a carcinogen in the US but industry pressure on the EPA forced a controversial risk assessment process resulting in the reregulation of atrazine as a permissible chemical. Elevated levels are found in the spring and summer in drinking water and groundwater in the Midwest. The Environmental Working Group found atrazine in the public drinking water supplies of 28 of 29 Midwestern cities tested.

Atrazine is a known endocrine disruptor that disrupts pituitary and ovarian function. Exposure to atrazine during gestation delays the development of rat mammary glands in puberty, widening the window of sensitivity to breast carcinogens.[182]

Sunscreens

Some sunscreens contain chemicals that are estrogenic and lipophilic. They have been found to be accumulating in humans and in wildlife.[183] One of these chemicals, 4-MBC, has recently been found to accelerate cell proliferation in estrogen-dependent breast cancer cells (MCF-7).[184] Earlier Swiss researchers who tested six commonly used UV sunscreens found that five of them showed estrogenic activity in breast cancer cells and three showed estrogenic activity in laboratory animals.[185]

Phthalates

These are endocrine-disrupting chemicals that are used to render plastics soft and flexible. They are found in soft plastic chew toys for infants. They are also in nail polish, perfume, skin moisturizers, flavorings, solvents, and plastics in cars and in homes. Phthalates are now found in indoor air and dust and in humans. Levels are highest in children age 6–11 and in women.

Some phthalates have hormone-disrupting effects. Three types increase cell proliferation in MCF-7 breast cancer cells (BBP, DBP, DEHP). They inhibited the antitumor action of tamoxifen in MCF-7 breast cancer cells.[186] Estrogen, testosterone, and other hormones have a relationship to cancer and many studies have indicated that hormonal factors are central to breast cancer risk. Since many phthalates disrupt hormonal processes, they may increase the risk of breast cancer.[187]

Food Additives

The US and Canadian beef, veal, and lamb industries have used *synthetic hormones* since the 1950s to hasten the fattening of animals and, therefore, weight gain, which is important to profits since animals for slaughter are sold by weight. Animal fat can retain pesticides and other environmental toxicants consumed by an animal. Many of these chemicals are lipophilic and become more concentrated as they move from plants to animals and then to humans, since we are at the top of the food chain in the developed world.

These hormones used to fatten animals may elevate the risk of breast cancer.[188] The European Union has banned imports of US and Canadian beef since 1999 because of these concerns. The European Union has made the precautionary principle their policy regarding all kinds of chemicals.[189] A process is now in place that requires manufacturers to evaluate the effects of their products before they are able to sell them.

Despite opposition from physicians, scientists, and consumer advocacy groups, the FDA in 1993 approved Monsanto's genetically engineered hormone product *rBGH* (recombinant bovine growth hormone) for injection into dairy cows to increase milk production. rBGH has subsequently been renamed *rBST* (recombinant bovine somatotrophin). The controversy surrounding this product and its use arises from its potential carcinogenic effects.

Drinking any milk raises body levels of IGF-1, a naturally occurring hormone in cows and humans. Increased levels of IGF-1 have been shown to be associated with increased risk of breast cancer. Premenopausal women with the highest levels of IGF-1 were found to be seven times more likely to develop breast cancer than women with the lowest levels.[190] In postmenopausal women there was no increased risk. Three studies that came out in 2005 from the UK, Sweden, and the US also showed an association between circulating IGF-1 levels and risk of breast cancer in premenopausal women. All three studies confirmed the earlier studies.[191,192]

Injecting a cow with rBST stimulates the production of IGF-1, which increases cell division and decreases cell death (apoptosis). Both of these changes increase cancer risk.[193] Drinking milk from injected cows increases IGF-1. Animal evidence indicates that digestion does not break down IGF-1 because casein, the principal protein in cow's milk, protects IGF-1 from the action of digestive enzymes.[194]

Zeranol

Zeranol (Ralgro) is a nonsteroidal growth promoter with estrogenic activity. Researchers at Ohio State University found that abnormal cell growth was significant at zeranol levels 30 times lower than the FDA has approved as safe.[195] A more recent study showed that zeranol is comparable to natural estrogen and the synthetic DES in its ability to transform MCF-10A human breast epithelial cells. Results demonstrated that zeranol can create neoplastic changes in breast cells *in vitro*.[196]

A Harvard study of dietary fat intake in 90,000 women suggests cause for concern regarding hormone use in the meat industry. Premenopausal red meat consumption may increase the risk of breast cancer later in life. The risk was found to be one-third higher among women with the highest animal fat intake, derived mainly from red meat and milk.[197]

A Danish study concluded: "The very high potency of zeranol suggests that zeranol intake from beef products could have greater impacts on consumers than the amounts of the known or suspected endocrine disruptors that have been found in food."[198]

Electromagnetic Fields

Electromagnetic fields (EMFs) are a type of nonionizing radiation and low-frequency radiation without the energy to break off electrons from their orbits around atoms to ionize, or charge, the atoms. The mechanisms of EMFs are not fully understood. Microwaves, radio waves, radar, and power frequency radiation associated with electricity are all examples of EMFs. The International Agency for Research on Cancer has classified EMFs as possible carcinogens. In 1998 the NIEHS EMF Working Group recommended that low-frequency EMFs (like power lines) be classified as possible human carcinogens.[199]

Conclusions

The interplay between timing of exposures, multiple exposures, low-dose exposures, chronic exposures, and cumulative exposures of all of the above impacts on human health needs to be studied. And less invasive screening for breast cancer and all other cancers, and more effective screening for breast cancer, need to be developed.

Environmental health teaching programs need to be established at the state and federal levels. We need to practice healthy purchasing by adopting precautionary purchasing laws at the local, state, and federal levels for businesses, government, consumers, and hospitals. Only products should be purchased that are free from chemicals linked to cancer. Workers should be protected from hazardous exposures. We need to educate the public regarding health effects from radiation and how to reduce exposure to ionizing and nonionizing radiation.

Corporations should be held accountable for hazardous practices. Incentives should be offered at the local, state, and federal levels for clean green practices. We need to strengthen right-to-know legislation and public participation in decisions regarding toxic exposures. And we need to enforce the existing environmental protection laws.

Greater transparency in funding of scientific and medical training, research and publications should be required. And a comprehensive chemicals policy based on the precautionary principle needs to be created.

REACH (Registration/Evaluation/Authorization of Chemicals) is a new policy put into effect by the European Union in 2006 which requires all of the above protections. In May 2004 hundreds of members of the European parliament, scientists, physicians, ethicists, and citizens from Europe, Canada, and the US signed the International Declaration on Chemical Pollution Health Dangers, known as the Paris Appeal. This statement would ban all products that are certainly or probably carcinogenic, mutagenic, or contain reproductive toxicants for humans. It would apply the precautionary principle to all chemicals that are persistent and bioaccumulative.

The Falling Age of Puberty in Girls

Early puberty — especially early menarche — is a known risk factor for breast cancer.[200] Although there are no studies that go back even 50 years, there does exist a body of historical evidence from Europe and the US that shows that the age of onset of puberty has declined over the last 150 years, from age 17 in 1830 in Europe to age 13 in 1960. Among European girls, the average age of menarche (the first menstrual period) ranged from 12.3 years in Greece to 13.3 years in Finland in 2003. In the US in 1900, the average age of menarche was 14.2 years. By 1970, the mean age of menarche was 12.8 years.[201] In 1922, a prospective longitudinal study was launched that followed 3650 public school first graders in three Massachusetts cities for 19 years.[202] In 1937, the average age of menarche was 13.5, which, at the time, was the youngest average age recorded anywhere.[203]

The National Health and Nutrition Examination Survey (NHANES) showed that by 1970 the mean age of menarche in US girls stood at 12.8 years.[204] Using the original NHANES and more recent renditions of the studies, women were grouped according to age cohorts. Those born prior to 1920 were in the oldest group, while those born in 1980–84 were in the youngest cohort. The mean age of menarche declined by 10 months from the pre-1920 cohort to the 1980–84 cohort for whites, by 12 months for Mexican Americans, and by almost 15 months for blacks. In the older cohort, black women, in their 80s now, had a higher average menarchal age than whites — the reverse of contemporary patterns.[205]

Nutritional changes and infection control, both of which drive the onset or delay of menarche in mammals, are not able to explain all worldwide trends during the first half of the 20th century. For example, in Japan the age of menarche declined during a period of rapid industrialization after 1900 that ushered in increased poverty, higher rates of infant mortality, and tuberculosis outbreaks. Several studies have shown declines in menarchal age as a result of rapid industrialization. At present, the fastest rates of decline are occurring among countries that are newly industrialized, such as South

Korea, where girls are now reaching menarche more than four years earlier than they did in 1920.

In the US nutrition alone cannot explain the racial differences in age at menarche or the differences in ongoing rates of decline. US white girls have shown far more gradual decreases over the past few decades than black or Mexican girls.[206] Far more specific studies need to be done that reveal patterns of change within specific populations and even within specific individuals.

Menarche is a late event in the march to sexual maturity. This makes it an unreliable marker for the onset of puberty. Thelarche (the growing of breast buds) and pubarche (the growing of pubic hair) are puberty's manifesting events. Increasingly, unique factors contribute to the timing of thelarche and menarche, whereas, in the past, the two had more factors in common. The decoupling of puberty's onset from menarche suggests that environmental signals may be influencing thelarche and menarche in different ways. This implies that trends in menarche may reveal little about the temporal changes in puberty.[207]

These concerns have prompted new studies of pubertal time trends that revisit the limited and deficient historical data available. Tanner and Marshall in England developed the Sexual Maturity Rating Scale for girls in the 1960s.[208] Their comprehensive findings have become a standard for what is considered normal puberty. Tanner and Marshall reported that the mean onset of breast development was 11.1 years. By the 1990s, many US pediatricians were seeing that girls were experiencing puberty considerably earlier than the Tanner–Marshall norm. Using the methods of Tanner and Marshall, a large study of more than 17,000 girls and pediatricians in 65 office practices was initiated by Marcia Herman-Giddens, a child abuse specialist.[209] What was found was that the mean age of thelarche was 10 years in white girls (more than a year younger than what Tanner and Marshall had found 30 years earlier) and 8.9 years in black girls. Pubarche was also considerably earlier, although the mean age of menarche had not changed much from the 12.8 years reported by NHANES from the 1970s. Under the old guidelines, 14 percent of US girls would be considered precocious. In 1999, the cutoff age for precocious puberty, as defined by the onset of breast development, was pushed back from 8 to 7 for white girls and from 7 to 6 for black girls. Europe did not adopt this revision. And the original study by Herman-Giddens was critiqued as flawed.

The criticisms were twofold: inspection was based on inspection rather than palpation and some chubby girls may have been misidentified; the cutoff age for the study was 13, and so latebloomers were excluded, thus skewing the data. However, the major findings were upheld in another study that analyzed data collected as part of a nationally representative sample — NHANES. The NHANES data also suffered from its own deficiencies, because it did not include girls under the age of 8 and thereby eliminated some early bloomers. Statistical corrections were used to compensate for the various omissions in the data sets.

The conclusions of these varied studies suggest that US girls are maturing earlier, with significant racial differences.[210] The average age of pubertal onset (as marked by thelarche and pubarche) in US girls appears to have fallen faster in the last half-century than menarchal age.[211] Pubertal onset and menarche are not as tightly coupled with each other as they were in the past. Factors associated with the onset of puberty and with the onset of menarche may be similar but, increasingly over the past 50 years, there are unique factors associated with the development of each.

What Is Happening?

When neurons in the hypothalamus begin translating signals into chemical signals in the form of gonadotropin-releasing hormone, (GnRH) the hypothalamus–pituitary–gonad (HEG) axis stirs to life and puberty begins. What is it that moves the hypothalamus to begin this process? The intrinsic and extrinsic factors that modulate this work are an incomplete body of work. Endocrinologists are not certain whether the HPG axis is actively arrested during childhood (between infancy and puberty) or it is lying dormant, waiting to be awakened. Some researchers have suggested a kind of thermostat — a "gonadostat" — mechanism that gradually changes its sensitivity over time.[212] Is this hormonal? Monkeys castrated at birth still experience the reactivation of the HPG axis even in the absence of any gonadal hormones. The CNS itself seems to provide much of the drive for puberty.

Leptin is a protein hormone produced by body fat that likely plays a role. But it may be a more reliable predictor of caloric availability necessary for the onset of puberty and, therefore, pregnancy and lactation. Kisspeptin is produced by neurons in the two areas of the forebrain. It binds to receptors on GnRH neurons in the hypothalamus and this stimulates GnRH release. Kisspeptin levels increase dramatically at puberty. The regulation of kisspeptin-making neurons in the forebrain is accomplished by estradiol from the ovaries and testosterone from the testes. Estradiol stimulates these two areas of the forebrain in opposite ways, speeding up or slowing down signals to the hypothalamus. Kisspeptin neurons may be the gonadostat. But the complexity of this system is not completely known and is also not static. Leptin seems to affect kisspeptin production, and kisspeptin neurons have receptors for leptin; kisspeptin production, goes down in times of undernutrition.[213,215]

Melatonin also appears to influence pubertal timing. It is secreted by the pineal gland and is regulated by light–dark cycles. It is secreted during darkness, in response to signals received by the pineal gland from the retina of the eye. Melatonin levels display circadian (diurnal) patterns and also seasonal patterns. Melatonin functions as a clock and a calendar. The hypothalamus displays many receptor sites for melatonin. Melatonin levels remain very high throughout childhood and drop precipitously during puberty and remain low throughout adulthood. The pineal gland itself is one of the first structures in the body to calcify.

Melatonin may be an inhibitory signal for pubertal development. Some researchers believe that elevated melatonin levels in childhood maintain the dormancy of the HPG axis.[215] This model posits that the decline in levels of melatonin is the activating signal that releases the HPG axis. Melatonin seems to modulate kisspeptin signaling to drive pubertal development.

Another neurotransmitter critical to pubertal timing is gamma-aminobutyric acid (GABA), which actively suppresses GnRH neurons prior to puberty. Many researchers believe that it is the primary signal responsible for the childhood hiatus of the HPG axis.[216]

All of the above available information comes together to some extent when we look at causes of early puberty. The evolutionary history of mammals indicates that sexual maturation among females is governed by a complex of internal and external signals that either permit or inhibit sexual maturation. Genetics alone cannot explain racial and ethnic differences. Menarche is one year earlier in US black girls than in South African black girls from well-off families. And, on average, girls in Kenya reach menarche four years later than US black girls.[217]

Low Birth Weight and Premature Birth

Premature birth and low birth weight are well-established risk factors for precocious puberty in girls, especially precocious pubarche.[218] Both of these factors dramatically increase the chances that a girl will develop pubic hair before the age of seven. Compensatory catchup growth may be a predisposing factor for pubarche. We know that obesity or overweight, or excessive weight gain during childhood is a predisposing factor for pubarche. However, of the girls of normal weight who exhibited precocious puberty, two-thirds had a history of prematurity or low birth weight. Therefore, with or without subsequent rapid weight gain, being born as a very small baby is a predisposing factor for early pubarche.

Hyperinsulinism may underpin all of these associations. With rapid weight gain, insulin sensitivity decreases. Blood insulin levels rise to compensate. Insulin regulates not only glucose uptake but also the secretion of androgens from the adrenal gland. The adrenal cortex has receptors for insulin and insulin growth factors.[219] Increased blood levels of insulin from rapid weight gain may boost androgen production from the adrenals. These hormones trigger the growth of pubic hair. Hyperinsulinism may also play a role in altering the timing of sexual maturation in girls who are not overweight or obese.

Hyperinsulinism brought on by restricted prenatal growth is part of a sequence of events described by David Barker, a British epidemiologist, as part of his hypothesis about the fetal origin of adult diseases.[220] His idea is that fetal response to prenatal stress may divert resources to the developing brain at the expense of other tissues. This results in a low-birth-weight baby but enduring changes in function that predispose the individual to adult-onset diseases. The risks of diabetes, obesity, hypertension, and heart disease are all increased with low birth weight. Many of these conditions are promoting factors for cancer. Barker calls this "fetal programming."

This idea has been expanded to consider the effects of prenatal chemical exposure on gene expression and imprinting and thereby growth and development. For example, exposure to high levels of ambient air pollution in early pregnancy has been linked to low birth weight, as have prenatal exposures to tobacco smoke, wood preservatives, alcohol, and drinking water contaminants.[221]

The incidence of low birth weight is rising in low-risk, nonsmoking mothers in the US, as is that of prematurity. These incidences may be contributing to the rise in early pubarche among US girls, for which low birth weight and prematurity are predisposing factors. In the US, low birth weights have risen by 16% and premature births by 18% since 1990. Since 1981, premature births have jumped by 30%. The racial disparities are significant: 17.8% of US black babies arrive prematurely, while only 11.5% of US white babies do.[222]

Prematurity has many causes, including exposure to chemicals that shorten gestation time. These include industrial chemicals, pesticides, and air pollutants.[223] Maternal consumption of mercury-contaminated fish has been demonstrated to shorten human gestation and contribute to prematurity. A phthalate plasticizer used to soften vinyl, namely DEHP, has been linked to preterm birth.

Obesity and Weight Gain

The obesity rates in children have tripled in the last 30 years.[224] The trend of increasing body mass parallels the trend of early puberty. A higher percentage of black girls are now obese or overweight. As a group, black girls also reach puberty sooner than white girls.[225] A recent national study of pre-school-age children from urban, low-income families found that 35% were overweight by the age of three. Hispanic children were the fattest. And, as a group, Mexican-American girls are currently exhibiting the most rapid ongoing decline in age at menarche.[226]

No studies link body mass, obesity or sedentariness with early puberty but there are reasons to believe that these factors are linked. In the case of pubarche, weight gain rather than BMI appears to trigger early onset. Obesity has been associated with earlier menarche and thelarche. Pubertal 6–9 year-old girls have higher BMI scores than prepubertal girls of the same age.[227]

The onset of puberty itself possibly triggers increased body fatness. Several studies have shown that fatter children tend to experience menarche sooner than thinner children. High BMI during childhood also predicted earlier menarche in Australian girls who were followed from prenatal life at 18 weeks to adolescence at age 14. This study showed that the lower-than-expected birth weights coupled with rapid weight gain in childhood showed the strongest association with young age at menarche. A University of Michigan study followed 354 girls from their third birthdays through sixth grade. It found that higher body fatness at age 3 was associated with earlier thelarche. The faster that body fatness increased between ages 3 and 6, the greater the chances that breast budding would begin by age 9. In this study, nearly half of the girls in the cohort had entered puberty by age 9.[228]

Many studies have shown that early maturing girls are more likely to become obese in adulthood.[229] Girls who eat more animal protein in early childhood have earlier menarche than those who eat less.[230] The girls who enter puberty with breast development first and pubic hair development second tend to be fatter than girls who enter puberty through the pubic hair pathway. Body fat itself is estrogenic. Fat tissue manufactures the enzyme aromatase, which converts androgens to estrogens. Fat cells secrete leptin. Leptin not only regulates food intake but also serves as a permissive agent for HPG activation and therefore breast development. Obesity represents a dysfunctional energetic state and results in leptin resistance and elevated circulating leptin levels.

Hyperinsulinism

There are compelling reasons to believe that the increased fatness of US girls is not the whole story behind the falling age of puberty. The BMI profiles for US and Danish girls are about the same but Danish girls reach puberty a year later. Fatter girls do reach puberty sooner but obesity cannot explain the differences between the timings of puberty in US and Danish girls. Furthermore, although early maturing white US girls are heavier at the time of puberty, this is not the case for black girls. Leptin levels are higher in blacks, and black girls still have an earlier onset of puberty. They also have decreased insulin sensitivity even after adjusting for body fat. These racial disparities suggest another hypothesis for early puberty: the falling age of puberty is not a direct consequence of increasing fatness per se, but a result of increasing hyperinsulinism among US children.[231]

Calorie-dense diets and sedentary lifestyles contribute to the development of hyperinsulinism and insulin resistance.[232] This can lead to type 2 diabetes. Emerging evidence suggests that exposure to chemical pollutants can also contribute to hyperinsulinism. Chlorinated pesticides and PCBs have been associated with insulin resistance in nondiabetic adults, as have phthalates.[233] Studies have also found connections between exposure to dioxin-like compounds and risk of diabetes. These fat-soluble chemicals bind to genes in the liver that are involved in the regulation of glucose uptake.[234] NHANES data revealed a strong dose–response relationship between blood levels of dioxin-like compounds and diabetes in adults. The prevalence of diabetes was 3–5 times higher in individuals with higher concentrations of contaminants. Obesity was a risk factor for diabetes only for individuals with a blood concentration of pollutants above a certain level. In people with very low levels of pollutants, there was no association between obesity and diabetes. This suggests that obesity may confer the risk of diabetes by serving as a vehicle for fat-soluble chemicals.[235]

Obesity does have roots in dietary choices that are individual and cultural. But there may be some environmental links as well. "Environmental obesogens" refers to chemical contaminants that act to disrupt homeostatic control over energy balance or stimulate the growth of fat cells. Organotins are a family of chemical compounds made of tin and carbon that are used as antifungal agents, wood preservatives, and heat stabilizers in the manufacture of vinyl plastics. Mice exposed to the pesticide dieldrin doubled body weight; hexachlorobenzene had the same effect. Endocrine disruptors that are antiandrogens may direct more nutrition to a fattier body composition.[236] Prenatal exposure to the plastic compound bisphenol-A speeds growth in juvenile female mice such that they are heavier at puberty than untreated females. New evidence shows that prenatal exposure to bisphenol-A can cause low birth weight followed by rapid, overcompensating growth leading to obesity. The modulation of lipid metabolism is now recognized as yet another route by which endocrine-disrupting chemicals can exert their effects.

The above are all examples of how connections between internal disease issues like obesity and diabetes and external pathogens like chemical exposures set up an interplay that is very similar to the Chinese medicine concept of latent pathogenic factors.

Formula Feeding

Formula-fed infants have higher body fat than breastfed babies and this difference persists into adolescence. Breastfed babies tend to self-regulate their energy intake and are less likely to overeat. Formula feeding in infancy also alters lipid metabolism in ways that have lifelong consequences. Individuals who are formula-fed have higher blood cholesterol levels in adulthood.[237] A recent national study found that prolonged bottle-feeding was an important predictor of childhood obesity.[238] The breastfeeding rates among US white and black mothers are different. In 2004, 71.5% of US white infants were ever breastfed. However, only 50.1% of US black infants were ever breastfed. These differences existed within all of the socioeconomic groups studied.

It is unknown if formula feeding is a risk factor for early puberty. Questions have been raised about soy-based infant formulas. And one-quarter of US infants are fed a soy-based formula at some point during their first year. Soy contains high levels of genistein and daid-zen, both of which are phytoestrogens or substances with structural similarities to estrogen. The human data on the risks and benefits of soy consumption for adults and infants are conflicting. Infants fed soy formulas do absorb and excrete phytoestrogens and exhibit altera-tions in cholesterol synthesis. No differences in pubertal maturation rates were found in women in Iowa who had been fed soy formula as infants when compared with those fed cow milk formula.

Mother's milk provides fewer calories than either soy or cow's milk formulas. But it may contribute growth factors that modulate the programming of the HPG and HPA axes during infant puberty, as well as the neural circuitry that both controls and responds to their hormo-nal messages. Breast milk contains melatonin — a puberty inhibitor.

Physical Inactivity

US girls eat more than they used to and exercise less. Black and Hispanic girls from low-income homes have lower indices for physical activity. By the age of 16 or 17, half of black girls and almost one-third of white girls engage in no habitual physical activity at all.[239] Recess and physical education classes both significantly increase moderate-to-vigorous activity patterns in children but these two traditional elements of school are a lesser part of the curricula than in the past. Today only one in five adolescents participate in PE in their schools. Illinois is the only state that requires PE from kin-dergarten through high school. There is no federal law that requires PE to be provided in schools.

Exercise is protective against early puberty. Leanness and physical activity are difficult to separate but girls who are anorexic, or who are gymnasts, runners, or ballet dancers, all have delayed puberty.[240] Elite swimmers and ice skaters also have delayed puberty and these girls tend to be of normal weight. Competition has its own set of stresses, physical and psychological, and it is difficult to isolate the relative contribution of each to pubertal timing.

Exercise delays thelarche but not pubarche, so the puberty-delaying effects of exercise seem to be limited to its effect on the HPG axis.

Strenuous training can inhibit the GnRH pulse generator, maybe by raising melatonin levels. But the role of energy expenditure in pubertal onset is not clear. It may modify the set point of the GnRH system in ways that delay pubertal development.[241] Endorphins may also modulate hormonal impulses. Leanness and exercise appear to work together to delay puberty.[242] There is enough evidence to recommend individual and social changes to the built environment and to educational curricula that will encourage physical activity in girls.

Family Dysfunction and Child Sexual Abuse

Girls in stressful home environments and those who have suffered child sexual abuse reach menarche sooner. Studies in this area are primarily confined to anthropological and psychological research that utilizes menarche as the marker for pubertal maturation, and although the data is consistent there exists very little data about the impact of stress and child abuse on the actual onset of puberty.

However, these studies are still impressive in their consistency across geographical and cultural boundaries.. European and US data corroborate each other. These data have been corroborated in French-speaking Canada and New Zealand as well. War conditions in Bosnia caused delays in menarchal ages among girls who were exposed to extreme psychological stress accompanied by physical injury and poverty.

Father absence, but not mother absence, is consistently associated with early menarche, and the longer the absence the earlier the first menstruation. More time spent by fathers in childcare, more father–daughter affection, and more paternal involvement in the family all appear to be protective against early puberty.[243]

Divorce and single-parent households notwithstanding, it is not clear that father absence is more common now than in previous times. From time immemorial, countless fathers have been absent because of the demands of war, hunting, fishing, farming, shipping, slave labor, wage labor, homesteading, or mining. It seems unlikely that father absence alone could be responsible for driving down the average age of pubertal onset in US girls. But it does seem plausible

that father absence may be contributing to the ongoing racial disparities in pubertal timing between white and black girls.

Cortisol is released as part of a stress response. It may modulate
hormones in ways that encourage early puberty. Early childhood
experiences are known to shape the basal rhythms of the HPA axis
and set its reactivity. Maltreated children have altered HPA axes and
respond to stress differently.[244]

Some researchers propose an evolutionary explanation in which
females growing up in adverse family environments with uncertain
futures may have reliably increased their reproductive success by
accelerating physical maturation and reproduction. Their idea is that
father presence may have inhibited puberty in daughters as part of an
ancestral mechanism for incest avoidance. Stepfather presence was
correlated with early puberty in one study but not in another. A recent
study reported that half- and stepbrothers accelerated menarche,
while the presence of sisters, especially older sisters, was associated
with delayed menarche.

Television Viewing and Media Use

A dramatic increase has been documented in erotic marketing messages aimed at preteen girls. Early–maturing girls seek out sexual
media imagery significantly more than late-maturing girls. Exposure
to sexy media material is also known to accelerate sexual initiation
among white adolescents.[245] In contrast to the wealth of studies that
have documented the impact of media violence on boys, scant
research has investigated the effects of sexualized media on girls. US
children watch an average of 3 h of television per day. Daily screen
time is far higher when video games and other types of media are
included. These numbers are high even for children under the age of
two. Children who are nonwhite and from low-income families
watch even more television each week than white children and those
from higher-income families.

Television and video viewing is associated with overweight and
obesity among preschoolers and school-aged children. US girls who
watched more than 2 h of TV per day had a significantly higher BMI

and were 13 times more likely to be overweight by age 11 than girls who watched less TV.[246]

An Italian study found that children aged 6–13 who were denied access to TV, computers, and videos for one week experienced a 30% increase in melatonin levels.[247]

Environmental Exposures

The HPG and HPA axes are vulnerable to endocrine disruption. Chemicals in the environment may contribute to early puberty by shortening gestation time, lowering birth weight, and increasing the risks of obesity and insulin disregulation. They may also alter the timing of sexual maturation through direct impact on the HPG axis. Low doses of estradiol can induce breast development, while high doses can inhibit it. Intermittent exposures may have different effects than continuous exposures. The neuroendocrine instrument that controls pubertal timing is, by its very nature and complexity, innately vulnerable to perturbation by endocrine-disrupting chemicals.[248]

Studies have demonstrated that children during the quiescent period have an exquisite sensitivity to sex hormones. Estradiol concentration in prepubertal girls is 100 times lower than previously thought. However, estrogen receptors are expressed in target tissues throughout childhood. Prepubertal girls are highly sensitive to sex hormone exposures, which may influence the timing of pubertal maturation.[249] Even in infancy, girls respond differently than boys to estrogen exposures, indicating that fetal programming has already begun to organize the endocrine system. Girls are sensitive to estrogenic environmental chemicals which contribute a higher portion of sex hormone levels in a prepubertal child than previously thought.[250]

Accidental exposures of mothers who were pregnant at the time of exposure who bore girls had elevated levels of PBBs. The girl children who were exposed to PBBs during pregnancy and nursing began menstruating a year earlier than other girls. The exposure was also associated with earlier pubarche.[251]

Three other studies from Italy in the 1970s found 3–7-year-old boys and girls who all attended the same school in Milan had developed breasts. Elevated blood levels of serum estradiol were documented. Poultry contamination was suspected but never confirmed. Some of the girls went on to exhibit early menarche.

Dioxin exposure is known to interfere with an enzyme necessary for the production of GABA in the brain. Dioxin exposures have been documented and are ongoing and ubiquitous. Testosterone creams for enhancing strength, libido, or athletic performance are commonly used by fathers. Premature pubarche in both male and female children has been linked to exposure to these creams. The route of exposure was passive dermal transfer from the father's skin. The level of exposure was quite low indicating the sensitivity of children to these exposures that are hormonal in effect.[252]

Estrogen and placenta-containing products are used by the African-American community and may help to explain the predominance of early sexual development among US black girls.

Pesticides, packaging, and building materials all contain hormonally active agents. These agents subject all of us, including children, to low-level background exposures. Children's lower body weight and sensitivity to hormonal agents make them at higher risk for injury from these substances. Bisphenol A is one of them and has been spoken of earlier. The discovery of bisphenol A in the urine of young girls is troubling. Prenatal PCB levels were related to increased height and weight at the time of puberty. Thelarche and pubarche did show acceleration at the highest levels of exposure to the metabolized pesticide DDT. Prenatal exposure to DDT metabolites lowered the age of menarche by one year.[253]

The European Union has forbidden the use of exogenous hormones as promoters of animal growth since 1989. But estradiol and other synthetic hormones are still used as growth promoters in the US beef industry. This is why the EU does not allow US beef to be imported to Europe. As more and more information becomes available about the exquisite sensitivity of children's hormonal systems, federal risk assessments about safe threshold levels for these estrogens in meat should be restudied.

In the dairy industry, rBGH has been used since 1993. It is not approved for use in Canada or the EU. The lower overall consumption of dairy over the last three decades makes this less of a problem. And the issue of early thelarche began prior to 1993. However, various growth factors in bovine milk probably cross the gut wall and interact with human receptor sites. Cows treated with rBGH (rBST) have highr levels of IGF-1 in their milk. Bovine IGF-1 does enter the milk and probably does cross the gut wall. If this escapes the digestion and enters the bloodstream, it can elevate IGF-1 levels in humans. IGF-1 appears to be a part of the mechanism for estradiol signaling and is required for the priming actions of estradiol on the HPG axis. There is emerging evidence that IGF-1 all by itself plays a role in regulating pubertal onset. The continued discovery of new mechanisms for sex hormone regulation gives reason for precautions against exposure to excess levels of animal hormones and growth hormones.[254]

Early puberty is a phenomenon that may best be understood as an ecological disorder. This disorder does not result from a single toxicant, or set of toxicants. It is a sequence of multiple and interpenetrating environmental stressors that exist within a causal web and can thus be defined as an "ecological manifestation of multiple changes in the dynamic system in which people are conceived, develop, live and grow old." There is much more that needs to be known. But obesity, television, sedentariness, family dysfunction, preterm birth, formula feeding, and chemical exposures are higher in poorer communities and communities of color, where poverty, racism, unemployment, and toxic substance exposures are high and access to nourishing food and safe places to exercise is low. In particular, black children are disproportionately exposed to physical environmental stressors and it is also this group that reaches puberty earliest among US girls.

Conclusions

Cancer, to a large extent, is an epidemic disease of the developed world. But, as the Western lifestyle and *modus operandi* spreads through globalization, the rates of many cancers are rising across the entire world. It is a public health crisis that is emblematic of the terrible predicament in which we find ourselves. The modern world has been greatly influenced by, and is perhaps an expression of, the Industrial Revolution and the philosophy of domination. This philosophy ended in bringing forth modern science by a small group of people during the Age of Enlightenment, coupled with the culmination of the Industrial Revolution. This coupling has created a crisis. Nowhere does this crisis become more observable than in the quest for understanding of how to stop the epidemic of breast cancer. This crisis is now everywhere and impacts almost every type of cancer and many other diseases as well. Although the science that was born out of the Age of Enlightenment, and its resulting way of life, may have grossly contributed to the breast cancer epidemic, we are still looking to modern science to find a cure.

The cure is in prevention. Prevention comes from changing the way in which we live, and understanding the roots of why we live as we do now. Global climate change, the cancer epidemic, poverty, racism, and sexism are all expressions of the same problem. The internal reality that drives these problems in life is a split between the mind and the heart that allows us to live an untruthful life, an immoral life, and a life that hurts others, ourselves, and our planet. This split is between male and female, mind and heart, the constructed world and the natural world, the receptive and the linear mind. It is artificial and arbitrary; it is a construct of a cultural mind that has lost its connection to the heart, and a culture that is based on domination and fear. The changes that are required to reverse the damage done by this split are immense. These changes may not completely eradicate breast cancer or any other cancer, but it may reduce the incidence of these cancers to the very low levels at which they occurred prior to the 20th century. Prevention is very much a phenomenon of the following:

- Research into causes — interior and exterior;
- Research into how the female body works;
- Clinical medicine, including Chinese medicine, which teaches all people — men and women and children — about the causes of cancer and ways to avoid cancer;

- Community activism that addresses the particular problems that contribute to cancer in any given neighborhood;
- Political activism to teach decision-makers and others in positions of oversight about the issues creating the problem of cancer — both internal and external;
- The establishment of agricultural and environmental policies that support all life;
- Universal healthcare;
- Use of the precautionary principle regarding the utilization of any new chemicals in food, industry, agriculture, medicine, personal products, etc.;
- The eradication of racism;
- The eradication of poverty;
- Defining the Commons and how they are to be preserved.

References

1. Baldwin C, (ed). *Our Turn, Our Time: Women Truly Coming of Age.* Beyond Words; Atria. Final chapter — "Council of Grandmothers," by Kit Wilson.
2. The Iroquois Confederacy. *Sojourn Mag,* Winter, 1998. www.light-party.com/spirituality/iroquois.html
3. Cancer facts and figures. American Cancer Society. www.cancer.org/research/cancerfactsfigures.index
4. Heller A. The great dichotomy: breast cancer versus prostate cancer. www.voices.yahoo.com/the-great-dichotomuy-breast-cancer-versus-prostate-cancer-106207
5. Fu H. (1899) *Yi Jing (Book of Changes).* Transl. by James Legge. Hexagram Number 2 — Kun the receptive.
6. Steinem G. (1995) *Moving Beyond Words.* Touchstone.
7. *Women Working, 1800–1930.* Harvard University Library. Open Collections Program.
8. Ludden J. (2012) Working mom's challenges: paid leave, child care. *NPR.* Sep. 15.
9. Caregiver salary. www.indeed.com/salary/caregiver.htmal

10. Planned parenthood. Birth control pills. www.plannedparenthood. org/health-topics/birthcontrol/birth-control-pill-422
11. *Contraception: An International Reproductive Health Journal.* Nov. 2012; Vol. 86(5).
12. Bureau of Labor Statistics. *Occupational Outlook Handbook.* Kindergarten and elementary school teachers. Similar occupations.
13. Glaser S. What should teachers be paid? *The New York Times.* www.6thfloor.blogs.nytimes.com/20903/08/what-should-teachers-be-paid
14. Simov R, Nath C. (2004) Gender and emotion in the United States: Do men and women differ in self-reports of feelings and expressive behavior? *AJS* **109(5)**: 1137–1176.
15. Else-Quest NM *et al.* Gender differences in self-conscious emotional experience: a meta-analysis. *Psychol Bull.* Advance online publication. doi:10.1037/a0027430.
16. Minorities, race, and genomics. Human Genome Project Information. www.ornl.gov/sci/techresources/human-genome/c/si/minorities. shtml
17. Masheder M. (2009) *Recapturing Childhood: Positive Parenting in the Modern World.* Merlin.
18. Ickes W. (1993).Traditional gender roles: Do they make and then break our relationships? *J Soc Issues* **49(3)**: 71–85.
19. Modern way of life leading to loneliness. Mental Health Foundation. May 2, 2010. The Lonely Society. www.mentalhealth.org.uk/publications/the-lonely-society
20. Gomez-Gonzalez B *et al.* (2012) Role of sleep in the regulation of the immune system and the pituitary hormones. *Ann NY Acad Sci* **1261**: 97–106.
21. Cancer health disparities. www.cancer.gov/cancertopics/factsheet/ disparities
22. Rochat E. (2006) *A Study of Qi in Classical Texts.* Monkey.
23. Bradshaw J. (1988) *Healing the Shame That Binds You.* Health Communications, Inc.
24. Kaufman G. (2004) *The Psychology of Shame: Theory and Treatment of Shame-Based Syndromes.* Springer Series. Springer.
25. *Ibid.*

26. Wang YH, Kang YC. (2010) *Treatment of Depressive Disorders with Chinese Medicine.* People's Medical Publishing House.

27. Lahans T. (2007) *Integrating Conventional and Chinese Medicine in Cancer Care.* Churchill Livingstone.

28. Wong Y, Tsai J. Cultural models of shame and guilt. psych.stanford.edu/-tsailab/pdf/ywo7sce.pdf

29. Larre C, Rochat E. (1996) *Seven Emotions.* Monkey.

30. Rochat E. (2009) Wu Xing, *the Five Elements in Classical Texts.* Monkey.

31. Hassan I. (2007) Compass of shame: a study of affect and normal consciousness and its use in the treatment of shame reactions and post-traumatic stress. ISSTD Conf.

33. Nathanson D. (1992) *Shame and Pride: Affect, Sex, and the Birth of the Self.* Norton, New York.

34. Kluft R. (2008) The use of Tomkin's innate affect theory and Nathanson's compass of shame in facilitating the understanding and treatment of DID and DDNOS. ISSTD Webinars Series.

35. Holland J. (2006) *Misogyny: The World's Oldest Prejudice.* Carroll and Gaaf.

36. Obesity and cancer risk. National Cancer Institute. www.cancer.gov/cancertopics/factsheet/risk/obesity

37. Spangler C. Xenoestrogens and breast cancer: nowehere to run. www.fwhc.org/health/xeno.htm

38. news.wsu.edu/pages/publications.asp?action-release&publicationsid=31639

39. Institute of Medicine. (2012) Breat cancer and the environment. A life course approach. National Academies Press.

40. *Op. cit.,* No. 1. Chaps. 31–34.

41. Understanding men who batter. Minnesota Coalition for Battered Women. www.mcbw.org

42. Clare A. (2000) *On Men: Masculinity in Crisis.* Chatto and Windus, London.

43. *Ibid.*

44. Burland JA. (1994) Splitting as a consequence of severe abuse in childhood. *Psychiatr Clin North Am* **17(4):** 731–742.

45. Erikson E. (1993) *Childhood and Society. www.* Norton and Company.

46. Ma SC. Lecture notes.

47. *Jin Gui Yao Lue* (*Essentials from the Golden Cabinet*). Transl. by Nigel Wiseman, Sabine Wilms, Fang Ye. Paradigm.

48. Wang YH. (2010) *Treatment of Depressive Disorders with Chinese Medicine.* People's Medical Publishing House.

49. Richter R. Stress hormone may contribute to breast cancer deaths. Stanford University. www.news.stanford.edu/news/2000/june28/breast-628.htmal

50. Garmany G. (1956) Anxiety states. *Br Med J* **1(4973)**: 943–946.

51. Larre C, Rochat E. (1996) *The Heart.* Monkey.

52. Hardy G. Great minds of the Eastern intellectual tradition. The Great Courses. www.thegreatcourses.com/tgc/course_detail.aspx?cid=4621

53. Anxiety disorders. National Institute of Mental Health. www.nimh.nih.gov/health/topics/anxiety-disorders/index.shtml

54. *Ling Shu.* Chap. 76.

55. Stages of sleep: REM and non-REM sleep. www.webmd.com/sleep-disorders

56. Iver KS, McCann SM. (1987) Delta sleep-inducing peptide (DSIP) stimulates growth hormone (GH) release in the rat by hypothalamic and pituitary actions. *Peptides* **8(1)**: 45–48.

57. *Op. cit.,* No. 46.

58. Bensky D, Barolet R. (1990) *Formulas and Strategies,* 1st ed. Eastland, p. 255.

59. *Op. cit.,* No. 48.

60. *Op. cit.,* No. 58, p. 435.

61. *Ibid.,* p. 378.

62. *Ibid.,* p. 384.

63. *Ibid.,* p. 379.

64. *Ibid.,* p. 457.

65. *Ibid.,* p. 257.

66. *Ibid.,* p. 73.

67. Manaka Y. (1995) *Chasing the Dragon's Tail.* Paradigm. Including Lecture Notes from Yoshio Manaka presentations.

68. Slee and disease risk. Healthy Sleep. www.healthysleep.med.harvard.edu/healthy/matters/consequences/sleep-and-disease-risk

69. Ma SC. Lecture notes on latent pathogenic factors.

70. Calabrese EJ. (2003) Toxicology rethinks its central belief: hormesis demands a reappraisal of the way risks are assessed. *Nature* **421**: 691–692.
71. Carpenter DO *et al.* (1998) Human health and chemical mixtures: an overview. *Environ Health Perspect* **106(S6)**: 1263–1270.
72. Bennett M. (2002) The identification of mammary carcinogens in rodent bioassays. *Environ Mol Mutagen* **39(2–3)**: 150–157.
73. Centers for Disease Control and Prevention. (2003). Second National Report on Human Exposure to Environmental Chemicals. DHHS. NCEH Pub. No. 02-0716. Jan. 7; pp; 1–257.
74. Bonner MR *et al.* (2005) Breast cancer risk and exposure in early life to polycyclic aromatic hydrocarbons using totally suspended particulates as a proxy measure. *Canc Epidemiol Biomarkers Prev* **14**: 53–60.
75. Hsu PY *et al.* (2009) Xenoestrogen-induced epigenetic repression of micro-rna-9-3 in breast epithelial cells. *Canc Res* **69(14)**: 5936–5945.
76. Furic A *et al.* (2012) Environmental exposure to xenoestrogens and estrogen-related cancers: reproductive system, breast, lung, kidney, pancreas, brain. *Environ Health* **11(suppl 1)**: 58.
77. Endocrine disruptors and human health: Is there a problem? *Toxicology*, 2008.
78. Risk factors. National Cancer Institute. www.cancer.gov/cancertopics/nytk/cancer/page3
79. Soto AM, Sonnen-Schein C. (2011) The tissue organization field theory of cancers: a testable replacement for the somatic mutation theory. *Bioassays* **33(5)**: 332–340.
80. Linking early environmental exposure to adult diseases. National Institute of Environmental Health Sciences. www.niehs.nih.gov/health/materials/linking_early_environmental_exposures
81. Reducing cancer through environmental policy change. Health and Environment Alliance. Committee of European Doctors on Environmental Health. www.env.health.org/IMC/pdf//20110315_heal_briefing_on_environmental_cancer
82. Calaf GM. (2000) Establishment of a radiation- and estrogen-induced breast cancer model. *Carcinogenesis* **21**: 769–776.

83. Segaloff A *et al*. (1971) The synergism between radiation and estrogen in the production of mammary cancer in the rat. *Canc Res* **31**: 166–168.
84. Gofman JW, O'Connor E. (1985) *X-rays: Health Effects of Common Exams*. Sierra Club Books p. 375.
85. Little JB. (2003) Genomic instability and radiation. *J Radiol Prot* **23**:173–181.
86. US Environmental Protection Agency: Federal Radiation Protection Guidance for Exposure of the General Public (1994). Notice, Federal Register. Dec. 23, 1994.
87. Brenner DJ *et al*. (2003) Cancer risks attributable to low doses of ionizing radiation. *Proc Natl Acad Sci* **100(24)**: 13761–13766.
88. National Radiological Protection Board (Britain). (1995) Risk of radiation-induced cancer at low rates for radiation protection purposes. *Documents of the NRPB* **6(1)**: 25.
89. Boice JD. (2001) Radiation and breast carcinogenesis. medical and pediatric oncology. *Oncology* **36**: 508–513.
90. Gofman JN. (2000) Are x-ray procedures equivalent in extra radiation dose to taking an airplane trip? www.ratical.org/radiation/CNR/RMP/plane+xrays.html
91. Summary of changes in cancer incidence and mortality, 1950–2001. SEER Cancer Statistics Review. 1975–2001. National Cancer Institute.
92. Bailor JR III. (1976) Mammography: a contrary view. *Ann Intern Med* **84**: 77–84.
93. National Cacner Institute. (2002) Radiation risks and pediatric computed tomography (CT): a guide for health care providers. www.cancer.gov
94. Veronisi G *et al*. (1993) Radiotherapy after breast-preserving surgery in women with localized cancer of the breast. *NEJM* **328**: 1587–1591.
95. Huang J, MacKillop W. (2001) Increased risk of soft tissue sarcoma after radiotherapy in women with breast carcinoma. *Cancer* **92**: 532–536.
96. National Toxicology Program. (2002) Tenth Report on Carcinogens. NIEHS. NIH.
97. Krieger N *et al*. (2005) Hormone replacement therapy, cancer, controversies, and women's health: historical, epidemiological, biological, clinical, and advocacy perspectives. *J Epidemiol Community Health* **59**: 740–748.

98. Collaborative Group on Hormonal Factors in Breast Cancer. (1996) Collaborative Reanalysis of individual data on 53,297 women with breast cancer and 100,239 women without breast cancer from 54 epidemiological studies. *Lancet* **347**: 1713–1727.

99. International Agency for Researh on Cancer. (1999) IARC Monographs on the Carcinogenic Risks to Humans, Vol. 72. *Hormonal Contraception and Post-menopausal Hormonal Therapy.* Lyon.

100. Brinton LA *et al.* (1998) Breast cancer risk among women under 55 years of age by joint effects of usage of oral contraceptives and hormone replacement therapy. *Menopause* **5(3)**: 145–151.

101. Holmberg L, Anderson H. (2004) HABITS (Hormonal replacement therapy after breast cancer — is it safe?) Trial stopped. *Lancet* **363**: 453.

102. Million Women Study Collaborators. (2003) Breast cancer and hormone replacement therapy in the Million Women Study. *Lancet* **362**: 419–427.

103. Writing Group for the Women's Health Initiative Investigators. (2002) Risks and benefits of estrogen plus progestin in healthy postmenopausal women. *JAMA* **288(3)**: 321–333.

104. Kumle M *et al.* (2002) Use of oral contraceptives and breast cancer risk: the Norwegian–Swedish Women's Lifestyle and Health Cohort Study. *Canc Epidemiol, Biomarkers Prev* **11**: 1375–1381.

105. Althuis MD. *et al.* (2003) Breast cancers among very young premenopausal women (United States). *Canc Causes Contr* **14**: 151–160.

106. Newcomer, LM *et al.* (2003) Oral contraceptive use and risk of breast cancer by histologic type. *Int J Canc* **106**: 961–964.

107. Grabick DM *et al.* (2000) Risk of breast cancer with oral contraceptive use in women with a family history of breast cancer. *JAMA* **284**: 1791–1798.

108. Narod SA *et al.* (2002) Oral contraceptives and the risk of breast cancer in BRCA1 and BRCA2 mutation carriers. *J Natl Canc Inst* **94**: 1773–1779.

109. Holmes MD. (1999) Association of dietary fat intake and fatty acids with risk of breast cancer. *JAMA* **281(10)**: 914–920.

110. Endogenous Hormones Breast Cancer Collaborative Group. (2003) Body mass index, serum sex hormones, and breast cancer risk in postmenopausal women. *J Natl Canc Inst* **95**: 12–18, 26.

111. *Hormonally Active Agents in the Environment.* National Academy Press. 1999.

112. Soto M *et al.* (1994) The pesticides endosulfan, toxaphene, and dieldrin have estrogenic effects on human estrogen-sensitive cells. *Environ Health Perspect* **102(1994)**: 380–383.

113. Zava DT *et al.* (1997) Estrogenic activity of natural and synthetic estrogens in human breast cancer cells in culture. *Environ Health Perspect* **105(Suppl 3)**: 637–645.

114. www.ourstolenfuture.org/newscience/human/cancer/2001

115. Martin MD *et al.* (2005) Estrogen-like activity of metals in MCF-7 breast cancer cells. *Environ Toxicol* **20**: 32–44.

116. Basic Information. Mercury and coal burning. www.epa.gov/hg/about.htm

117. Brody JG *et al.* (1998) Endocrine disruptors and breast cancer. *Forum Appl Res Publ Policy* **13(3)**: 24–31.

118. Rudel RA *et al.* (1998) Identification of alkylphenols and other estrogenic phenolic compounds in wastewater, septage, and groundwater on Cape Cod, MA. *Environ Sci Technol* **32(7)**: 861–869.

119. Rudel RA *et al.* (2003) Phthalates, alkylphenols, pesticides, polybrominated diphenylethers, and other endocrine disrupting compounds in indoor air and dust. *Environ Sci and Technol* **37**: 4543–4553.

120. Celton T *et al.* (1993) Breast cancer in mothers prescribed diethystilbesterol in pregnancy. Further follow-up. *JAMA* **269**: 2096–2100.

121. American beef: Why is it banned in Europe? Cancer Prevention Coalition. www.preventcancer.com/consumers/general/hormones_meat.htm

122. Broton JA *et al.* (1995) Xenoestrogens released from lacquer coatings in food cans. *Environ Health Perspect* **103**: 608–612.

123. Schonfelder G *et al.* (2002) Parent bisphenol A accumulation in the human maternal–fetal–placental unit. *Environ Health Perspect* **110**: A703–A707.

124. Calafat AM *et al.* (2005) Urinary concentrations of bisphenol A and 4-nonylphenol in a human reference population. *Environ Health Perspect* **113**: 391–395.

125. Markey CM *et al.* (2001) *In utero* exposure to bisphenol A alters the development and tissue organization of the mouse mammary gland. *Biol Reprod* **65**: 1215–1223.

126. Munoz de Toro M *et al.* (2005) Perinatal exposure to bisphenol A alters peripubertal mammary gland development in mice. *Endocrinol Online* doi:10.1210/ea.2005-0340.

127. Rivas A *et al.* (2002). Estrogenic effect of a series of bisphenol A analogues on gene and protein expression in MCF-7 breast cancer cells. *J Steroid Biochem Mol Biol* **82**: 45–53.

128. Watson CS *et al.* (2005) Signaling from the membrane via membrane estrogen receptor-alpha: estrogens, xenoestrogens, and phytoestrogens. *Steroids* **70**: 364–374.

129. Bisphenol A (BPA): use in food contact application. FDA. www.fda.gov/newsevents/publichealthfocus/ucm064437.htm

130. US Centers for Disease Control and Prevention. (1997) Public Health Statement for Vinyl Chloride, CAS #75-01-4, Agency for Toxic Substances and Disease Registry.

131. Chiazze L, Ference LD. (1981) Mortality among PVC fabricating employees. *Environ Health Perspect* **41**: 137–143.

132. Infante PF, Pesak J. (1994) A historical perspective of some occupationally related diseases of women. *J Occup Med* **36**: 826–831.

133. Hoyer AP *et al.* (1998) Organochlorine exposure and risk of breast cancer. *Lancet* **352(9143)**: 1816–1820.

134. Hoer AP *et al.* (2000) Organochlorine exposure and breast cancer survival. *J Clin Epidemiol* **53**: 323–330.

135. Muscat JE *et al.* (2003) Adipose concentration of organochlorine compounds and breast cancer recurrence in Long Island, NY. *Canc Epidemiol, Biomarkers Prev* **12**: 1474–1478.

136. Mills PK, Yang R. (2005) Breast cancer risk in Hispanic agricultural workers in California. *Int J Occup Environ Health* **11**: 123–131.

137. Engel CS *et al.* (2005) Pesticide use and breast cancer risk among farmers wives in the Agricultural Health Study. *Am J Epidemiol* **162**: 121–135.

138. Byford JR *et al.* (2002) Estrogenic activity of parabens in MCF-7 human breast cancer cells. *J Steroid Biochem Mol Biol* **80**: 49–60.

139. Dabre PD *et al.* (2003) Estrogenic activity of benzyl-paraben. *J Appl Toxicol* **23**: 43–51.

140. Dabre PD *et al.* (2004) Concentrations of parabens in human breast tumors. *J Appl Toxicol* **24**: 5–13.

141. Li ST et al. (2002) Hormone-containing hair product use in prepubertal children. *Arch Pediatr Adolesc Med* **156**: 85–86.

143. Jaga K, Duvvi H. (2001) Risk reduction for DDT toxicity and carcinogenesis through dietary modification. *J Reprod Soc Health* **121(2)**: 107–113.

144. Murata M et al. (2004) Genistein and daidzein induce cell proliferation and their metabolites cause oxidative DNA damage in relation to isoflavon-induced cancer of estrogen-sensitive organs. *Biochemistry* **43**: 2569–2577.

146. Labreche EP. (1997) Exposure to organic solvents and breast cancer in women: a hypothesis. *Am J Ind Med* **32(1)**: 1–14.

147. Envirosense. Cleaning agents and cosmetic manufacturers. US EPA. www.es.epa.gov/techinfo/facts/cleaning.htmal

148. Chang YM et al. (2003) A proportionate cancer morbidity ratio study of workers exposed to chlorinated organic solvents in Taiwan. *Ind Health* **41**: 77–87.

149. Health and Safety Executive. (2001) Cancer among current and former workers at National Semiconductor (UK) Ltd, Greenock: results of an investigation by the Health and Safety Executive.

150. Hansen J. (1999) Breast cancer risk among relatively young women employed in solvent-using industries. *Am J Ind Med* **36**: 43–47.

151. Tenth Report on Carcinogens. (2002) Styrene was added to the national toxicology program list of chemicals "reasonably anticipated to be a human carcinogen."

152. Walrath J et al. (1985) Causes of death among female chemists. *Am J Publ Health* **15**: 883–885.

153. Jansen MS et al. (2004) Short-chain fatty acids enhance nuclear receptor activity through mitogen-activated protein kinase activation and histone deactylase inhibition. *Proc Natl Acad Sci* **101**: 7199–7204.

154. National Toxicology Program. (2003) Chemical associated with site-specific tumor induction in mammary gland. www.ntp-server.niehs. nih.gov/htdocs.sites/MAMM_html

155. Layton DW et al. (1995) Cancer risk of heterocyclic amines in cooked foods: an alaysis and implications for research. *Carcinogenesis* **16**: 39–52.

156. DeBruin LS (2002) Perspectives on the chemical etiology of breast cancer. *Environ Health Perspect* **110**: 1990–128.

157. National Toxicology Program. (2005) Eleventh Report on Carcinogens. www.ntp-server.niehs.nih.gov

158. Melnick RL *et al.* (1999) Multiple organ carcinogenicity in inhaled chloroprene (2-chloro-1,3-butadiene) in F344/N rats and B6C3F1 mice and comparison of dose–response with 1.3-butadiene in mice. *Carcinogenesis* **20**: 867–878.

159. Zheng T *et al.* (1999) DDE and DDT in breast adipose tissue and risk of female breast cancer. *Am J Epidemiol* **150**: 453–458.

160. Simcoe NJ *et al.* (1995) Pesticides in household dust and soil: exposure pathways for children of agricultural families. *Environ Health Perspect* **103**: 1126–1154.

161. Roll Back Malaria Partnership. (2001) Final DDT agreement endorses RBM objectives. *Roll Back Malaria News 3.* Feb. World Health Organization. www.rbm.who.int

162. Cohn B *et al.* (2002) Timing of DDT exposure and breast cancer before age 50. *Proc Int Soc for Environmental Epidemiology* (abstract): *Epidemiology* **13**: 5197.

163. Robinson PE *et al.* (1990) Trends of PCB, hexachlorobenzene, and benzene hexachloride levels in adipose tissue of the US population. *Environ Res* **53**: 175–192.

164. Laden F *et al.* (2001) 1,1-dichloro2,2-bisethylene and polychlorinated biphenyls and breast cancer: combined analysis iof five US studies. *J Natl Canc Inst* **93**: 768–776.

165. Muscat JE *et al.* (2003) Adipose concentrations of organochlorine compounds and breast cancer recurrence in Long Island, NY. *Canc Epidemiol Biomarkers Prev* **12**: 1474–1478.

166. Rundle A *et al.* (2000) The relation between genetic damage from polycyclic aromatic hydrocarbons in breast tissue and breast cancer. *Carcinogenesis* **21(7)**: 1281–1284.

167. Han D *et al.* (2004) Geographic clustering of residence in early life and subsequent risk of breast cancer (United States). *Canc Causes Contr* **15**: 921–929.

168. Villeneuve DL *et al.* (2002) Relative potencies of individual polycyclic aromatic hydrocarbons to induce dioxin-like and estrogenic responses in three cell lines. *Environ Toxicol* **17**: 128–137.

169. Hanaoka T *et al.* (2005) Japan Public Health Center–based Prospective Study on Cancer and Cardiovascular Disease Group. Active and passive

smoking on breast cancer risk in middle-aged Japanes women. *Int J Canc* **114**: 317–322.

170. Reynolds P *et al.* (2003) Active smoking, household passive smoking, and breast cancer: evidence from the California Teacher's Study. *J Natl Canc Inst* **96**: 29–57.

171. California Environmental Protection Agency, Air Resources Board. (2005) Proposed identification of environmental tobacco smoke as a toxic air contaminant. www.arb.ca.gov/toxics/ets/finalreport/finalreport.htm

172. International Agency for Research on Cancer. (1997) IARC Monographs on the Evaluation of Carcinogenic Risk to Humans. Vol. 69. *Polychlorinated Dibenzodioxins and Dibenzofurans.* IARC, Lyons.

173. World Health Organiation. (1996) Levels of PCBs, PCDDs, and PCDFs in human milk. WHO European Centre for Environment and Health.

174. Warner MB *et al.* (2002) Serum dioxin concentrations and breast cancer risk in the Seveso Women's Health Study. *Environ Health Perspect* **110**: 625–628.

175. Steenland K *et al.* (2003) Ethylene oxide and breast cancer incidence in a cohort study of 7,576 women. *Canc Cases Contr* **14**: 531–539.

176. CDC. (2005) Third National Report on Human Exposure to Environmental Chemicals. Centers for Disease Control and Prevention Atlanta.

177. Dich J *et al.* (1997) Pesticides (heptachlor) and cancer. *Can Causes Contr* **8**: 420–443.

178. National Cancer Institute. (2005) State cancer profiles. www.statecancerprofiles.cancer.gov

179. US EPA. (1994) Federal Register Notice (59FR 18100). Voluntary cancellation of the registrations of simazine for use in swimming pools, hot tubs, and whirlpools.

180. US EPA. (2000) Atrazine Third Report of the Hazard Identification Assessment Review Committee. Office of the Pesticide Programs. www.epa.gov/pesticides/reregistration/atrazine/3rd_hiarc.pdf

181. Moses M. Pesticides and breast cancer. PAN. www.pan-uk.org/pestnews/issue/pn22/pn22p3.htm

182. Rayner JL *et al.* (2005) Adverse effects of prenatal exposure to atrazine during a critical period of mammary gland growth. *Toxicol Sci* **87**: 255–266.

183. Hayden C *et al.* (1997) Systemic absorption of sunscreen after topical application. *Lancet* **350**: 853–864.

184. Klann A *et al.* (2005) Estrogen-like effects of ultraviolet screen 3-(4methylbenzylidene)-camphor (eusolex 6300) on cell proliferation and gene induction in mammalian and amphibian cells. *Environ Res* **97**: 274–281.

185. Schlumpf M *et al.* (2001) *In vitro* and *in vivo* estrogenicity of UV screens. Environ *Health Perspect* **109(3)**: 239–244.

186. Kim IY *et al.* (2004) Pthalates inhibit tamoxifen-induced apoptosis in MCF-7 human breast cancer cells. *J Toxicol Environ Health* **67**: 2025–2035.

187. Gray LE *et al.* (1999) Administration of potentially antiangiogenic pesticides (procymidone, linuron, ipridione, chlozolinate, p,p'-DDE, and ketoconazole) and toxic substances (dibutyl- and diethylhexyl phthalate, PCB 1169, and ethane dimethane sulphanate) during sexual differentiation produces diverse profiles of reproductive malformations in the male rat. *Toxicol Ind Health.* **15**: 94–118.

188. Liu S *et al.* (2004) Transformations of MCF-7 human breast epithelial cells by zeranol and estradiol-17. *Breast J* **10**: 515–521.

189. The European Commission. Brussels; Feb. 2, 2000. www.gdrc.org/u-gov/precaution-4.htmal

190. Hankinson S *et al.* (2005) Circulating concentrations of insulin-like growth factor-1 (IGF-1), IGF-II, IGF-binding protein-3 and breast cancer risk. *Br J Canc* **92**: 1283–1287.

192. Schernhammer EsS *et al.* (2005) Circulating levels of insulin-like growth factors, their binding proteins, and breast cancer risk. *Canc Epidemiol Biomarkers Pharmacol* **14**: 699–704.

193. Resnicoff M, Baserga R. (1995) The insulin-like growth factor 1 receptor protects tumor cells from apoptosis *in vivo*. *Canc Res* **55**: 2463–2469.

194. Xian C. (1995) Degradation of IGF-1 in the adult rat gastrointestinal tract is limited by a specific antiserum of the dietary protein casein. *J Endocrinol* **146**: 215.

195. Liu S *et al.* (2002) Involvement of breast epithelial–stromal interactions in the regulation of protein tyrosine phosphatase gamma (PTP gamma) mRNA expression by estrogenically active agents. *Breast Canc Res Treat* **71**: 21–35.

196. Liu S, Lin YC. (2004) Transformation of MCF-10a human breast epithelial cells by zeranol and estradiol-17. *Breast Canc Res Treat*

197. Cho E *et al.* (2003) Premenopausal fat intake and risk of breast cancer. *J Natl Canc Inst* **95**: 1079–1085.

198. Leffers H *et al.* (2001) Oestrogenic potencies of zeranol, oestradiol, diethylstilbesterol, bisphenol-A and genistein: implications for exposure assessment of potential endocrine disruptors. *Hum Reprod* **16**: 1037–1045.

199. Erren TC. (2001) A meta-analysis of epidemiologic studies of electric and magnetic fields and breast cancer in men and women. *Bioelectromagnetics*. **Supplement 5**: S105–S119.

200. Steingrabber S. The falling age of puberty in US girls. Breast Cancer Fund. www.breastcancerfund.org/assets/pdfs/publications/falling-age-of-puberty

201. Early puberty in girls. Explore Health (49,168)=women'shealth-femalehormonalissues (69).

202. McDowell MA *et al.* (2007) Has age at menarche changed? Results from National Health and Nutrition Examination Survey (NHANES) 1999–2004. *J Adolesc Health* **40(3)**: 227–231.

203. Shuttleworth FK. (1937) *Sexual Maturation and the Physical Growth of Girls Aged Six to Nineteen*. Monograph for the Society for Research in Child Development. Vol. 3, No. 5.

204. Harlan WR *et al.* (1980) Secondary sex characteristics of girls 12–17 years of age: the US Health Examination Survey. *J Pediatr* **96:** 1074–1078.

205. *Op. cit.* No. 202.

206. Anderson SE Must A. (2005) Interpreting the continued decline in the average age at menarche: results from the two nationally represented surveys of US girls studied 10 years apart. *J Pediatr* **147**: 753–760.

207. *Op. cit.*, No. 200.

208. Marshall NA, Tanner JM. (1969) Variations in the pattern of pubertal changes in girls. *Arch Dis Childhood* **44**: 291–303.

209. Herman-Giddens ME. (2007) The decline of the age of menarche in the United States: Should we be concerned? *J Adolesc Health* **40**: 201–203.

210. Euling SY *et al.* (2005) Environmental factors and puberty timing: summary of an expert panel workshop. *Toxicologist* **84**: S-1.

211. Kaplowitz P. (2006) Pubertal development in girls: secular trends. *Curr Opin Obstet Gynecol* **18**: 487–491.

212. Ebling E. (2005) The neuroendocrine timing of puberty. *Reproduction* **129**: 675–683.

213. *Ibid.*

214. Papathanasiou A, Hadjathanasiou C. (2006) Recocious puberty. *Pediatr Endocrinol Rev* **3** (**Suppl 1**): 182–187.

215. Murcia GJ *et al.* Puberty and melatonin. *Anales Espandes de Pediatria* **57**: 121–126.

216. Terasana E. (2005) Role of GABA in the mechanism of the onset of puberty in non-human primates. *Int Rev Neurobiol* **71**: 113–129

217. Grumbach MM, Styne DM. (2003) Puberty: ontogeny, neuroendocrinology, physiology, and disorders. Laren PR *et al.* (eds.) *Williams Textbook of Endocrinology*, 10th edition. Saunders, Philadelphia: pp.1115–1286.

218. Ibanez L *et al.* (2006) Early puberty–menarche after precocious pubarche: relation to pre-natal growth. *Pediatrics* **117(2006)**: 117–121

219. Neville KA, Walker JL. (2005) Precocious pubarche is associated with SGA, prematurity, weight gain, and obesity. *Arch Dis Childhood* **90**: 258–261.

220. Barker DJ. (1990) The fetal and infant origins of adult diseases. *Br Med J* **301**: 1111.

221. Ritz B, Yu F. (1999) The effect of ambient carbon monoxide on low birth weight among children born in Southern California between 1989 and 1993. *Environ Health Perspect* **107**: 17–25.

222. McMillen IC, Robinson JS. (2005) Developmental origins of the metabolic syndrome: prediction, plasticity, programming. *Physiol Rev* **85**: 571–633.

223. Behrman RE, Butler AS (eds.). (2006) Preterm birth: causes, consequences, and prevention. Report from the Institute of Medicine's Committee on Understanding Premature Birth and Assuring Healthy Outcomes. National Academies Press. Washington, D.C.

224. Biro FM. (2005) Stone-Age genes, Space-Age times. Presentation at the Breast Cancer and Environmental Risk Factors Scientific Symposium (East Lansing, Michigan; Nov. 2005).

225. Kaplowitz P. (2001) Earlier onset of puberty in girls: relation to body mass index and race. *Pediatrics* **108**: 147–153.

---

226. Kaplowitz P. (2006) Pubertal development in girls: secular trends. *Curr Opin Obstet Gynecol* **18**: 247–255.
227. Davison KK *et al.* (2003) Percent body fat at age 5 predicts earlier pubertal development among girls at age 9. *Pediatrics* **111 4 pt1**): 816–821.
228. Lee DH *et al.* (2009) Weight status in young girls and the onset of puberty. *Pediatrics* **119**: 24–30.
229. Slyper AH (2006) The pubertal timing controversy in the USA, and a review of possible causative factors for the advance in timing of onset of puberty. *Clin Endocrinol* **65**: 1–8.
230. Berkey CS *et al.* (2000) Relation of childhood diet and body size to menarche and adolescent growth in white girls. *Am J Epidemiol* **152**: 446–452.
231. *Op. cit.*, No. 229.
232. *Ibid.*
233. *Op. cit.*, No. 228.
234. Lee DH *et al.* (2006) A strong dose–response relation between serum concentration of persistent organic pollutants and diabetes. Results of the National Health and Examination Survey. 1999–2002. *Diabetes Care* **29**: 1638–1644.
235. Parta M. (2006) Persistent organic pollutants and the burden of diabetes. *Lancet* **368**: 558–558.
236. Keith SW *et al.* (2006) Putative contributors to the secular increase in obesity: exploring the road less traveled. *Int J Obes* **30**: 1585–1594.
237. Bergstrom E *et al.* (1995) Serum lipid values in adolescents are related to family history, infant feeding, and physical growth. *Atherosclerosis* **117**: 1–13.
238. Kimbro RT *et al.* (2007) Racial and ethnic differentials in children's overweight and obesity among 3-year-olds. *Am J Publ Health* **97**: 208–305.
239. Kimm SY *et al.* (2002) Decline in physical activity in black girls and white girls during adolescence. *NEJM* **347**: 709–715.
240. Grumbach MM, Styne DM. (2003) Puberty, ontogeny, neuroendocrinology, physiology, and disorders. In: Larsen PR *et al.* (eds.), *Williams Textbook of Endocrinology*, 10th ed. Saunders, Philadelphia pp. 1115–1286.

241. Georgopoulos KA *et al.* (2004) Growth, pubertal development, skeletal maturation, and bone mass requisition in athletes. *Hormones (Athens)* **3**: 233–243.

242. *Op. cit.*, No. 240.

243. Ellis BJ *et al.* (1999) Quality of early family relationships and individual differences in the timing of pubertal maturation in girls: a longitudinal test of an evolutionary model. *J Pers Soc Psychol* **77**: 387–401.

244. Bogurt AF. (2005) Age of puberty and father absence in a national probability sample. *J Adolesc* **28**: 541–546.

245. Brown JD *et al.* (2005) Mass media as a sexual super peer for early maturing girls. *J Adolesc Health* **36**: 420–427.

246. Davison KK *et al.* (2006) Cross-sectional and longitudinal associations between TV viewing and girls' body mass index overweight status, and percentage of body fat. *J Pediat* **149**: 32–37.

247. Salti R *et al.* (2006) Age-dependent association of exposure to television screen with children's urinary melatonin excretion. *Neuroendocrinol Lett* **27**: 73–80.

248. Parent AS *et al.* (2003) The timing of normal puberty and the age limits of sexual precocity: variations around the world, secular trends, and change after migration. *Endocr Rev* **24**: 668–693.

249. Aksglaede I *et al.* (2006) The sensitivity of the child to sex steroids: possible impact of exogenous estrogens. *Hum Reprod Update* **32**: 341–348.

250. *Ibid.*

251. Blanck HM *et al.* (2000) Age at menarche and turner stage in girls exposed *in utero* and postnatally to polybrominated biphenyl. *Epidemiology* **11**: 641–647.

252. Kunz GJ *et al.* (2004) Virilization of young children after topical abdrogen use by their parents. *Pediatrics* **114**: 282–284.

253. Regan WJ, Ragan NB. (2003) Evidence of effects of environmental chemicals on the endocrine systems of children. *Pediatrics* **112**: 247–252.

254. *Op. cit.*, No. 249.

CHAPTER 5

Yin and *Yang* — Prostate Cancer

I want to be a small deer running under the sky through
the green grass
Don't make me go into the thick jungle, or I will
become a fierce wolf
Who can foresee the tricks and snares of life?
Deception is disguised by sweet tongues
I was an unwitting deer, wandering far from my field of
fresh grass
My face was the face of a wolf in deep caves, in shad-
ows, dark and still
Then a call startled me awake, and I remembered that
once my eyes had been clear, the eyes of a deer
At the end of the road, I fell down when a bullet struck
my blood-filled chest
If you look under the wolf's skin, you'll find the red
heart of an innocent deer
> — *Vietnamese poet Lum Ti Mi Da*

The plunder from the spoils that the soldiers took was
675,000 sheep, 72,000 cattle, 61,000 donkeys and
32,000 women and girls who had never been with a man.
> — Numbers 31:32–35

Introduction

What is it that constantly leads us down the path of destruction and
cruelty? When we look at the history of mankind as written in modern history books, it appears to be largely a struggle for power
among men and the nations they rule. But, beginning in the last half
of the 20th century, new voices began to weave together evidence

from art, archeology, religion, social science, history, and many other fields of inquiry that reveal new patterns of our cultural heritage that are more accurate and complete. This evidence shows that war, including the war of the sexes, is not biologically or divinely ordained.[1]

The agrarian Old European Neolithic societies planted some of the first gardens on the Earth. They were primarily partnership societies where the establishment of the concept of the Great Chain of Being originated in the West.[2] Social relations were based primarily on the principle of linking rather than on ranking. These partnership societies were nonhierarchical, with the "Mother" principle at the center not as the head of a ranking system where Amazonian-like women ruled over men but as the hub of an interrelated sphere in which all were equal. In what is known anthropologically as Old Europe, the Neolithic and early Minoan and Crete cultures were peaceful and prosperous. The social, technological, and cultural evolution of humanity moved forward during this period without male or female dominance, or violence, or a hierarchical system.[3]

Cultural transformation theory proposes that in Western civilization's development the original direction of cultural evolution was toward partnership and equality but that, following a period of chaos from volcanic eruptions and tidal waves in the hub of Old European cultures around the eastern Mediterranean, catastrophes caused immense physical and cultural disruption, and there occurred a fundamental shift. This shift has been well documented and, as defined by Riane Eisler in *The Chalice and the Blade Our History Our Future*, was from a partnership model to a dominator model perhaps brought in by nomadic tribes from the steppes.[4]

It may not be a fair analogy but the modern day invasion by China of Tibet, a country of nonviolent Buddhists with no army to speak of and a long history of cultivated peacefulness and the sacredness of life, is perhaps an apt example of what happened to the weakened societies along the eastern Mediterranean. The cataclysmic turning point during the prehistory of Western civilization replaced the concept of life-generating and nurturing powers of the universe, the feminine interior principle, with invaders who worshipped the power to take rather than give life as a way of establishing and enforcing domination, what has come to be known as the male domination principle, an extreme expression of the exterior principle (as opposed to the interior and listening traditions and the receptive).[5] The partnership societies took the Iron Age and made tools. The dominator societies took the Iron Age and made weapons. It was at this point that the interior circular meaning approach to life began to be separated from and appropriated by the exterior linear approach to life. It is difficult to know how or why this happened, and certainly laying blame at the feet of the East, the same East that gave us most of the meditation traditions, is not constructive or probably even true.

The interior aspects of life are considered to be those that give meaning to action.[6,7] They are those aspects that evolve out of wisdom and often religious or spiritual insights derived from a faith, and some would say experience, that there is something bigger than what we can see and measure. These aspects of life are interior because one must look inwardly to settle the mind and open receptivity to their truths,[8] the opposite of modern science, which relies upon the mind and the external observation skills for its conclusions. This receptivity is what leads some people to feel that the inner traditions seeking peace, beauty, wisdom, and meaning are all part of the feminine tradition as expressed in the early perennial cultures.[9] The exterior aspects of life refer only to those truths that can be observed and measured, and hopefully, in the best of all possible scientific worlds, measured completely out of relationship with anything else. It is thought that relationship to anything outside of itself is what muddies the waters of objective truth. Truth in this sense is supposed to be so objective that it tells us only what is and not what should or could be. Truth is value-free and neither good nor bad. The scientific model has become the spokesperson for "the" truth. The religious traditions have become the spokesperson for "genuine" wisdom.[10]

The gradual replacement of interior-oriented partnership societies with exterior-oriented dominator societies has taken many millennia to achieve and has continued to this day. The concept of empire as the primary example of a dominator society has driven almost all of modern life. The root of the philosophy for social systems devised from a dominator model of consciousness is one that we still dig for in the hope that we might understand ourselves. From day one, starting millennia ago, males and females have been taught to equate true masculinity and power with violence, dominance, and superiority, and ultimately to foster the concept that meaning and receptive values are not part of and do not drive the goals and expression of a successful life.[11] This shift during our earlier history was not only in social structure but also in the manifestations of a dominator philosophy as seen in technology. The technological emphasis throughout most of recorded history has been the application of technology to destroy and dominate, the technology of "progress," a concept that expresses the philosophy of the dominator model. The plow versus the drill in agriculture; wellness, food as purification and rehabilitation versus antibiotics and the "attack array" in medicine; biodiversity and sustainability versus monoculture and resource mining in economics; the Commons versus private ownership in all resource management including the resource of knowledge; consensus versus hierarchy in governance: all are examples of the millennia-long shifts from partnership to domination. This emphasis has reached a conclusion in modern times that threatens to end not just one culture or people or nation or species, but the entire world.

The modern struggles of male versus female, capitalism versus socialism, technology versus nature, science versus religion, and so on are all struggles that have their seeds in the partnership versus dominator models for life and the gradual loss of a connection between the interior and exterior aspects of life. Our evolution as a species has not been consistently evolving toward a higher level. There have been many massive regressions, such as the Greek Dark Age and the Dark Ages in Europe, and many comparable dark times in Asia. In the 100 years of the 20th century, there were 250 wars, each with the possibility that it could end life on the Earth as we know it.[12] It is difficult to see our current situation as an opportunity for evolution rather than as one for our demise.

One manifestation among many and a resultant example of the end stage of the dominator model is the modern cancer epidemic and the "war on cancer." As of 2005, one in every two men and one in every three women are being diagnosed with cancer in their lifetime in the US — the most affluent country in the world.[13] Many people are dying. The loss of our brothers and sisters, children and parents to cancer is emblematic of a larger struggle that has been going on for at least the last two centuries. The number of species lost is uncountable; and the degradation of whole ecosystems is obvious even to the untrained eye. The thread that seems to run through the stream of history since the prehistoric loss of the partnership model is the thread of domination as a means of power and as the purpose of life: domination over all of life, no matter the loss of living beings, whether they be human or otherwise, is the *modus operandi*. And, ultimately, this model is an example of the separation of *Yin* and *Yang*, interior and exterior, mind from heart, meaning and values from action and goals.[14]

Although the foundations of democracy are in Greek city states, even by that early time the partnership cultures were gone. Women did not have the right to vote in democratic early Greece. The feminine principle of interior and relational truths did not have equal inputs into how society would define and order itself — at least the feminine principle as expressed by women. Centuries had already gone by during which the social structures of society in the West first literally murdered all that was from the "Mother" and the interior traditions. This philosophy continued throughout European history, with the Roman Christian church as the main perpetrator,[15] and all forms of nature-based wisdom groups became the lightning rod. After the threat of death was firmly established in a culture and those who were dominated had submitted to the dominator authority, the device of ridicule and trivialization was used to keep the feminine principle down, whether it lived in women or in men, in healers, in wisdom traditions, in Earth-based peoples, in societies still founded on a circular versus a linear tradition. It is still used today. One example is that of Nazi Germany and the extermination of the Jews and many others in Europe.[16] Another example is that of modern science, which states that the only real truth that exists is that defined by science — in particular, Western science.[17,18] The result today is that the systematic omission of women and feminine activities and the interior principles from all accounts of our human past has ultimately led to the almost-complete loss of any concept of partnership societies where the interior truths are as important as the exterior truths.

Soul Murder

Freud believed that destructiveness and the abuse of power are part of our inherited biological nature. He viewed our attempts at civilization, at transcending our murderous human nature, as heroic and tragic.[19] If he had been born in a different age than the Victorian and had been a fly on the wall in the Old European Neolithic, it is very possible that he would have developed different theories about why we are the way we are, have been, and are becoming. The modern 20th century psychoanalytic term "soul murder"[20] may be closer to what we experience in varying degrees in a dominator society that works to maintain a hierarchical system of power, dominance, and the right to live, a system that requires its participants to separate themselves from an interior life of meaning and values in order to maintain dominance at the expense of others, even when it causes harm to all.

The term "soul murder" was first used in the very early 1900s, about a child who had been kept in a cellar and separated from all communication with the outside world from birth until about age 17. This individual was turned loose as a teenager and was found wandering the streets of Nuremberg. He functioned at the level of a 2- or 3-year-old but in the body of a young man. He had to be taught to walk upright because he had never seen humans walk, and to speak because he had never heard a word. He had an intensely passionate desire to learn but his only human contact was with the "Man who was always there," apparently his father or some caregiver who had no relationship with him except to shove food to him, somewhat like a person feeding a caged wild animal. This child had no indignation toward his keeper, because he had no sense that his life was any different from the life of anyone else. In fact, he did not know that there was anyone else. There proved to be no way of making up for the emotional deficits of his solitary early existence, and as he became aware of his deprivation to the extent that he could, he regressed into a kind of obsessive–compulsive automaton. This loss of an understanding of self and of a conscious experience of the soul — formed through relationship — has come to be called "soul murder" or "psychic murder."

Soul murder occurs not only as a result of profound neglect but also from parental abuse of a child who must somehow split from self in order to survive the abuse and continue to love the parent, usually the only human being with whom the child has a connection and who provides sustenance and the basic relationship of belonging.[21] Abuse almost always comes in the form of overstimulation either from physical beatings or sexual abuse accompanied by abuse of the soul resulting from a lack of recognition on the part of the abuser of the human being across from them. It is this overstimulation and lack of recognition of the child as a separate human being that is so unbearable that the child is forced to leave the body through a psychic split, almost a form of autohypnosis. This split is another form of a cellar. The torture of the child in Nuremberg was through lack of stimulation, a very rare occurrence. Soul murder occurs through the lack of recognition of and connection to a child as an individual human being, a human being with creative, remarkable, and unique characteristics personal only to them that make them valuable and lovable. The truth is that the adult perpetrator probably experienced similar abuse as a child.[22]

Children who are raised with varying degrees of soul murder, what German psychiatrist Alice Miller calls "poisonous pedagogy,"[23] come to not notice, even as adults, when they are being taking advantage of by others in authority. In the first two years of life children are molded, dominated, scolded, taught without the possibility of repercussions or revenge being directed to the parent or person of authority. A child of this age can defend themselves only if they are allowed to express pain and anger. If parents or other caretakers cannot tolerate these reactions and forbid them by means of looks or other pedagogical methods, the child will learn to be silent even when being dominated or abused. If there is no way of reacting appropriately to hurt, humiliation, and coercion, then these experiences cannot be integrated into the personality, and the feelings they evoke are repressed. The need to express them remains unsatisfied, without any hope of being fulfilled. This process begins in the very first days of life. In many ways what is being described here is the making of a slave. And it is a manifestation of the separation, the psychic split that occurs when an individual is forced to turn away from the interior side of life which would give them access to themselves and to live only on the exterior side of life in order to survive. In varying degrees we all suffer from these experiences as we learn via osmosis what is the nature of the culture in which we grow. Without this knowledge of acceptable and unacceptable, we would never know how to survive and become part of a family or tribe.

Human destructiveness is a reactive and not an innate phenomenon, as Freud believed.[25,26] When we indignantly refer to something in human behavior as inhuman, we lose the opportunity to understand anything about its and our own nature. "The risk will then be greater, when we next encounter it, of once again aiding and abetting it by our innocence and naivety." (Alice Miller in *For Your Own Good*). Judgment is, in fact, an effort to avoid encountering these behaviors within our self.[24] And if we were able to do so and have compassion for the perpetrators and ourselves, then the knowledge derived could literally save the world. When Miller looked at Adolph Hitler's life from the point of view of a compassionate German psychiatrist interested in how the Second World War ever came about, her main questions were how he became so possessed by hatred and how he was able to involve so many other people in his hatred. The example of Hitler's childhood allows us to study the genesis of hatred and poisonous pedagogy, the consequences of which caused the suffering of millions. Hitler's entire life is an example of domination and of his evolution into a dominator within an enabling dominator culture. And it is emblematic of the split that all men endure from birth onward. This split enables the separation of mind and heart, which in turn enables the domination of our environment, even when it causes illness and destroys life. The following is taken from Miller's works.

Hitler

Hitler grew up in a household that was the prototype of a totalitarian regime.[27] His father was the undisputed and often-brutal head, and his mother was like the security police, carrying out the dictator's wishes, including instilling fear and meting out punishment. The children in this household were the oppressed. This hierarchy was put in place within all of the structures of the Third Reich, including the concentration camps. In the Austria/Germany of that time, the totalitarian system was the template for most households — an extension of a dominator society structure. In varying degrees, it remains the system under which many of the world's families operate. However, the brutality of Hitler's upbringing made him into what today we would call a battered child,[28] a child on whom soul murder had been carried out, a child who could become as an adult what amounts to a serial killer and a psychopath. The beatings began when he was three or four, the idea being that wickedness must be driven out so that goodness might grow undisturbed. This Victorian concept of inherent evil in a child that must be violently forced out[29,30] is a concept repeated throughout history by dominator cultures as they took over the partnership cultures, eliminated women from positions of equality, and formed hierarchical institutions, like the Roman church, of domination by strength.[31] All of the expressions of a partnership society that would have believed in the innocence of children were made small and wrong, evil and worthy of surgical excision, brutality, and even death. In many ways this is how colonialism works. And the philosophy of colonialism has remained to this day in international relationships between the developed countries and the Third World, between the "civilized world" and "ignorant and even savage" indigenous peoples.

Although Hitler's ancestry is questionable and his father may have been part-Jewish,[32] his anti-Semitic attitude toward Jews as bad and evil was no doubt rooted in experiences lived through in the obscurity of his childhood. His father called him by whistling for him as though he were a dog. He was tyrannized and brutalized by his father. Jews in the Third Reich were treated similarly. It is Alice Miller's contention, as a psychoanalyst, that the trauma of Hitler's family life was transferred onto the entire German nation. Racial laws forced every citizen to trace his or her descent back to the third generation, the generation where in Hitler's life the bad seed of a possibly half-Jewish grandfather was said to have come in. And based on those results, each citizen was to bear the ensuing consequences. The wrong ancestry meant disgrace and degradation; later it meant death — and this during peacetime in a civilized country. Even during the persecution of the Jews in the Spanish Inquisition, they were offered the chance to survive if they accepted baptism. In the Third Reich, on the basis of descent alone a Jew was condemned to death. The Jew had no way to escape; the child Adolph could not escape his father's soul-murdering brutality. The Jews also may have served the same function in the Third Reich as it attempted to recover from the disgrace of the Weimar Republic at their expense. Hitler went through a childhood experience of soul murder and projected this experience onto his nation in an attempt to resolve the experience without having to re-experience the pain of it by consciously remembering the reality and the psychic material of the interior emotion and humiliation and profound suffering of the small innocent child.[33]

Adolph the child could not escape the daily beatings he received. All he could do was deny the pain; this meant denying himself and identifying with the aggressor. No one could help him. In his early life there was no one on his side, no one who loved him unconditionally. This state of constant jeopardy is reflected very clearly in the fate of the Jews in the Third Reich. Anyone wearing an SA armband could attack a Jew walking down the street and do anything to them that their internal fantasy dictated. The Jew and Hitler the child shared the same fate. The brutal dictator was found in many German soldiers who were raised under the same pedagogical theory as was Hitler — the theory that childhood was rampant with an evilness that must be broken. Hitler's experience of this pedagogical ideology was extreme but close enough to the same way that many were raised at that time to be a link between the dictator and the dictated-to. This ideology was the extreme of a hierarchical dominator ideology. When Hitler succeeded in transferring the evil he felt within himself to the Jew, he succeeded in breaking out of his isolation. People harbor a forbidden hatred and are eager to legitimize it; since Jews have been persecuted for 2000 years by the highest authorities of church and state, they are a convenient lightning rod for the ongoing problem of dominator cultures — the need for a scapegoat for the rage brought on by the nature of domination itself, often beginning in childhood and fostered by societal norms of hierarchy and dominance. Currently the West, particularly the United States, sometimes for good reasons, is the lightning rod for this hatred in the world. However, holocausts are part of written history and continue even today in places like Cambodia, Sudan, Bosnia, Palestine, the North America of the 16th–20th centuries, and so on.[34,35] These are injuries to all of life but in particular to the *Yang* side of life, which are then transferred to the *Yin* side of life — a vicious circle.

The recurrent experiences of psychological humiliation, beatings in contact sports, getting tough, "boys don't cry," and depending on self with often no helping hand are all examples for boys.[36] They are examples of living in a hell that no one considers to be a hell. Boys do not become men through positive affirmations but through learning what they are not — not female, not vulnerable, not weak, not caring, not humane. When coupled with the idea that one is inherently superior, it can be immensely confusing and provide the basis for making a narcissist. It is a continuous conditioning that is repeatedly encountered starting from birth for male children in many cultures with a hierarchical and dominator mentality. These experiences can be forgotten or coped with only with the aid of splitting off and repression. "The jubilation characteristic of those who declare war is the expression of the revived hope for finally being able to avenge earlier debasement, and presumably also of the relief at being able to hate and rage" (Alice Miller). The adolescent's heroic willingness to fight in wars just as life is beginning and to die for someone else's cause may be a result of the fact that during puberty the warded-off hatred taught in early childhood becomes reintensified. Adolescents can divert the hatred from their parents and their societal dominator paradigm if they are given a clear-cut enemy whom they are permitted to hate freely and with impunity while they fight for domination. Being taught to kill is sometimes not a far cry from learning to "waste" one's opponent in sports. These gladiator sports are examples of soul murder where a young man must split his soul self from his societal self and allow injury in the interest of climbing upward in the hierarchy — hence the majority of black athletes in the professional gladiator sports. And often the climb itself appears to be the only purpose of life.

Hitler was mistreating the Jew just as he himself had been mistreated as a helpless child. At age 11 he was nearly beaten to death. One way that he came to separate himself from the internal rage, fear, shame, and powerlessness that he felt was to identify with the aggressor, his father, and proclaim to his mother after the beatings that he had withstood "130 hits without crying or making any sound." For Hitler, the extermination that took place in Europe was really an attempt to exterminate his own former weakness and to avoid the pain of intense sorrow — the sorrow expressed by the poem of the Vietnamese woman at the head of this chapter for the innocent heart of the child forced to wage war.

Children very often fantasize that they must save or rescue their mother so that she can finally be the mother to them whom they needed from the beginning.[37] This of course is not possible. A child should never have to save their mother from the rage of the father or any other perpetrator. Women frequently become oppressors themselves in a hierarchical system run by hatred and fear. And, separate from the terrible reality of child abuse and its repercussions, the truth remains that women are complicit in this problem. Somewhere the cycle must be broken, and the burden lies on us all. We cannot raise our children to believe that war is necessary, whether it be at home or in one's society or world. These are sins of the culture handed on from generation to generation for millennia. At the same time, we cannot continue to believe that destruction of the environment is necessary and acceptable.

The persecution of the Jews made it possible for Hitler to "correct" his past on the level of fantasy and the subconscious, to take revenge on his father (who was suspected of being part-Jewish), to win his mother's love and freedom by saving Germany from the shame of World War I, to reverse roles with his oppressor father and become the dictator himself, and to persecute the weak child within himself so that he did not have to experience the pain and grief about his childhood.[38] Today our prisons are full of young men who have murdered others as a tragic outcome of a hopeless childhood with no hope whatsoever for the future. These imprisonments are more about poverty; and the real evil is in the society that allows poverty to occur in a world awash with money where the hierarchical system of domination allows only a few to succeed.

Even Hitler, who has killed more human beings than anyone else in history, was not born a criminal. None of us are exonerated from our own cruel acts but even the cruelest of us deserves empathy. Those who persecute others are fending off knowledge of their own fate as victims. Sadism is an offshoot of being tormented and humiliated. The Fourth Commandment is a perpetuation of the poisonous pedagogy handed down through generations of dominator societies; it continues to make possible the protection of people, who, in the secret society of the home, abuse and torture because they themselves were, and they cannot face the painful vulnerability of this truth. We continue to protect those in power who are to inflicting the same agonies on others in the name of freedom for us at home, or in the name of progress. The ubiquitous nature of this issue is not an excuse to absolve us from examining it. The Nuremburg trials never delved into the deeper realities of the German psyche that drove World War II. Although these trials were legal proceedings, there now needs to be an inclusive examination, across disciplines, of the problem of violence — an examination of the interior meaning and the exterior expression of that particular violence. If we had asked "Why?" during those trials, it is very possible that we would have seen ourselves. Perhaps that is why we did not ask.

"Living out hatred is the opposite of experiencing it. To experience something is an intra-psychic reality; to live it out, on the other hand, is an action that can cost other people their lives. If the path to experiencing one's feelings is blocked by the prohibitions of poisonous pedagogy or by the needs of the parents (or a society), then these feelings will have to be lived out" (Alice Miller). This is the cycle in which we are caught and have been for several thousand years.[39]

Rage and violence is not a factor of testosterone.[40] Violence is an expression of rage, and rage is the consequence of the frustrating experience of limitation. The abusive and humiliating limits that human cruelty can inflict are a universal impetus for grief. Rage and concomitant anger needs to be grounded in compassion and a sense of humanity on the positive side. If it becomes destructive, then the result is egocentricity and brutalizing vengeance. Rage can be used as a positive force for change. Current childcare practices hinder the development of positive constructs for management of rage, especially in boys. In many ways, we have not come any further since the dark days of Hitler's Victorian childhood. Physical punishment and deliberate humiliation, especially of boys, remains common, legal, and acceptable. And this bullying business has begun to permeate childhood for girls as well. The price of equality seems to be that we are all suffering from the same disease not from opposite sides of the coin but now even from the same side.

The premise of this chapter is that all boys are raised more or less in a spirit of dominance and supremacy as a primary value. What this means for girls was spoken of in the previous chapter. The subtle but overpowering expectation given by societies at large is that boys are superior and at the top of the hierarchy of a dominator society. They are superior because they are bigger and stronger, louder, more demanding, tougher, unemotional, and competitive — all values of any hierarchical society. Boys are not necessarily taught prosocial values and behavior, including nonviolent conflict resolution. If a boy is bullied for being a sissy, the response is to teach that child how to fend for himself by standing up to and fighting off the bully. Adults do not step in as a rule and teach nonviolent techniques to the bully (who is probably being bullied or forced to submit at home) and the bullied. Both would benefit, because together they carry the same problem within themselves.

Boys are often humiliated, made to feel tiresome and wicked. They are taught not to cry when hurt and, as a result, often hit instead. Being taught nonviolent ways of getting what one wants teaches communication skills and instills in a child an investment with others and with human values.[41] If children learn to listen to one another, it is often because adults listen to them. Adults need to take responsibility for protecting children from violence done to them and for preventing violence. Adults, especially male adults, need to take responsibility for the violence within themselves by understanding its roots and resolving them. This new psychic milieu will provide an example to all children that domination is unnecessary and war and all other forms of destructiveness are a sickness, a manifestation of the separation of heart, mind, and spirit.

Rage is often disowned and unconscious, hiding behind a veneer of civilized rationality. The denial of tyrannical ideology is projected onto particular groups, who become demonized.[42] Children learn this early on and seek the dominant groups to be part of in an effort to belong, even if belonging is uncomfortable. Black males in the United States are largely the scapegoat and carriers of rage for many societies today. In the US, our prisons are filled beyond brimming with young black men. The most violent sports, like football, are peopled particularly by young black men who are trying to find a place in the hierarchy. The reality of discrimination in schools, in employment fed by a reactionary cultural identity focused on drugs, violence, criminality, and macho hipness, are all fueling a down-ward cycle. Black males as demons become the fact of violence and antisocial behaviors.[43] But these are social creations fueled by the projection for centuries now of a mainly white society in the US that has denied its own destructive rage as we all struggle to survive. The enactment of slavery is the ultimate example of a society that has split from its own essential heart by living only in the rationalities of the mind to lend an excuse for this evil. Slavery continues in the US for all people who are not white and for the poor of all colors, and for women and children, and for the land. Nonwhite peoples and immigrants do the low-wage work that no one else wants in exchange for a chance to live. We do not call it slavery; we call it poverty.[44] The dominator culture persists.

The valuing of power and dominion over intimacy and cooperation is reflective of a certain type of male identity that has suffered moral trauma and pervades most of the world's cultures.[45] This is especially true for working-class or lower-class men who have lost access to the patriarchal dividend in all of its various cultural manifestations. Men who have succeeded according to the societal measures of their milieu at least can partake of the fruits they are taught are their due. For men who cannot access these fruits, often because there is no expectation that they will, no inheritance, or for whatever other reason, the result is humiliation and frustration in varying degrees. The stress experienced as a result comes out in work and relationships and in the human body. These men, the majority, are seen as powerless, the working-class bloke, a peasant, a farmer. And the result of this is a loss of connection to self and others in an effort to survive the pain of there being no hope for a better life. Nonviolent empowerment is more difficult to embody when there is a disconnection from self and others. Almost all wars are mainly fought by males who are suffering from an inability to connect to life because they are young and as yet unconnected, and/or because they have failed to make these connections to others and to their own self and there is no expectation that they will. These young men are looking for a place to belong and to express themselves in whatever ways they can. Often, they are looking for a path to survival that does not exist for them within their own milieu and society. Currently, Native Americans enlist in the military more often per capita than any other group. African-American males come in second.

Males who are violent are in constant defensive mode. There is a disconnection from self and others. Women, who are relational, are a danger to them, because they may be forced to feel their pain. Love and emotional comfort may force them to let down their guard and feel their pain in the process of being open.[46] The only relationship that can be imagined is one of sexual rape, and not sexual intimacy. Most behavior is impulsive. There is an excessive quality about work; relaxing is an impossibility unless one is aided by drugs or alcohol. Material goals are the only goals the individual has. These material goals lead to the rape of the Earth. It is always poor men who do the actual ripping-away of the skin of the Earth. It is always men of means who instruct them to do so. Either way, it is a lonely life. Men in prison who can access a process by which they can reparent themselves and form a new family, where nonviolence becomes a pathway to change and self-empowerment, where nonjudgmental self-criticism can be learned as a means of finding one's true self, where mediation and other life skills can be seen as tools of strength, all do better and do not re-offend when released. Poverty and societal enslavement are the roots of these problems for males and are expressions of the hierarchical outcomes of a dominator society. Poverty, hierarchical societies, and war all go hand in hand. However, even males who manage to succeed also suffer from the stress of trying to live in a hierarchy where the interior truth of meaning and dignity and love and beauty is completely overwhelmed by the exterior truth of "making it" and the guilt of walking on others' bodies in order to get there.[47] Splitting is the only way of surviving.[48]

All of these issues are expressions of injuries to the *heart–liver–kidney* axis — all impacted energetically in prostate cancer. "To feel is to leave yourself open," says Tom, a man in an anger management class in Australia. To be open, these energetic interconnections must be strong and functional. Men's use of violent and controlling behavior can indicate a lack of empathy for others but it also indicates a lack of empathy for self. Just as Hitler projected his pain onto others, many men in our time are doing the same, including onto the environment. The fortress mentality of violent men is a cover for emotional pain. The pathway to finding a new male identity and a new meaning for the *Yang* of life is the work of repairing the axis of the *liver, kidney, spleen,* and *heart.*[49,50] We are at an evolutionary point in human life on the Earth that requires that we find a way to put the interior meaning of life together with the exterior expression of the truth. This point in evolutionary time is the equivalent in consciousness of discovering fire — for our demise or an opportunity to push the evolution of humanity forward.

Chinese Medicine

Cancer is a problem where these issues come together in a perfect storm of interior realities and exterior manifestations. Prostate cancer has its own peculiar set of risks that are emblematic of the struggle.

Androgens, stress, diet, race, and obesity are thought to play roles in the pathogenesis of this cancer.[51] Several studies have been done to evaluate interrelationships between the PSA level, serum testosterone, serum cholesterol, HDL, triglycerides, BMI, and race in men with and without prostate cancer.

Significantly higher levels of serum testosterone were found in black men in the US with prostate cancer than in black men without prostate cancer.[52] The same variants were found in white men with prostate cancer and white men without prostate cancer. HDL was higher in black men than in white men, and triglycerides were higher in white men than in black men. Cholesterol was similar in all groups but the BMI was highest in white men with prostate cancer. There was a significant association between the BMI and the pathological stage of prostate cancer patients in black and white men.[53] All of these issues have relationships to *liver, heart, spleen,* and *kidney* function in Chinese medicine.[54] And all of these issues are emblematic of the split required for modern men (and women — with different results) to survive in a complex world where destruction and domination is a daily phenomenon.

The occurrence of prostate cancer in black men in the US is about twice that of white men, and more black men die from their disease than white men die from prostate cancer.[55] Black men in the US have higher ditestosterone levels than white or Asian men. Testosterone levels of this type are considered a risk factor for prostate cancer, and the higher level in black men in the US is one reason why race is considered a risk factor for prostate cancer. Being Asian appears to be protective, partly because Asian men have lower testosterone levels. These issues are significant and studies have been done to determine if testosterone levels have a genetic or an environmental basis.[56] At the moment, it appears that racial variation in testosterone levels may be dependent on sociocultural factors, such as diet and stress. Testosterone levels are linked to cortisol levels in various ways.[57] Cortisol is an adrenal hormone that is elevated due to stress. Violence within inner-city neighborhoods has been found to raise cortisol levels and testosterone levels. Higher cortisol levels depress immune function.[58] These issues are immensely important in helping our patients avoid a diagnosis of prostate cancer, and point to a possible link between one's class and status in society and the stressors these realities place on an individual. Men of the Negroid race and other black races outside the US do not have higher testosterone levels. The highest rates for prostate cancer in the US are in Oakland, California, among the African-American population. The US currently has the highest rate of prostate cancer in the world. Others running a close second include the Tyrol region of Europe. Some of the lowest rates are among men in India, China, and certain countries in South America, according to the WHO.

Research shows that angry, hostile men are not suffering from testosterone excess.[59,60] They are suffering, however. Some studies have shown that the angriest men in the studies tended to be the most overweight, they also had the lowest levels of good HDL cholesterol, and younger men with a cluster of risk factors for diabetes and heart disease tended to be the most aggressive.[61] The most angry and hostile men in the studies had sex hormone levels similar to those seen in the least aggressive men. One of the groups with the highest rates of hypertension in the US is young black men. The links between HTN,[62] diet,[63,64] stress, race, and prostate cancer are just beginning to be teased out.[65]

There are also links between estrogen from birth control pills in water and prostate cancer.[66] In addition, a total of eight different organochlorine pesticides have been found to have a likely association with prostate cancer.[67] And the following exposures have been found to require further studies: cadmium, dioxin, and calcium intake.[68]

The suggestion is, therefore, that within the context of the system of Chinese medicine the disease of prostate cancer is one of *liver* and *heart constraint*, acquired *kidney* and *Source Qi deficiency*, *toxin* exposure, and *damp phlegm* caused by *spleen* and *kidney deficiency* leading to an injury to the *San Jiao*. The constraint placed on all males by a dominator culture that teaches males to be disconnected from their own true hearts sets up a series of cascading injuries that affect them essentially the same way but also differently, depending on their status in our culture. The *liver, heart,* and *kidneys* are inseparable components of a dynamic mind–body system. Just as women have an inner connection between the *heart* and the uterus, men have an inner connection between the *heart* and the reproductive system (including the prostate). These components are a unified network designed to foster homeostasis, information flow, and psychophysical regeneration. Men have been forced to split from the internal process of communication between these components, a process that is really part of an internal healing system. The result is that most men, especially men who must struggle to succeed in a hierarchical and dominator society, or do not have the personality to compete within it, and who remain at the bottom, are severely injured because they do not have access to a valid expression of themselves in the world (*liver Qi constraint*) and to their own healing power (*heart* and *kidney* communication).

Just as women have an internal channel between the *heart* and the *uterus* that must be in place for a connection in sexual intimacy, men have an internal channel between the *heart* and the sexual reproductive organs. If this channel is broken or injured, sexual intimacy and bonding is injured. Men who rape have this injury. The *liver* channel runs through the testes and the sexual reproductive organs in men. Injury to this channel occurs when men are constrained by a lack of self-esteem and have instead an abundance of unconscious self-hatred, especially when it comes to vulnerability. When a human being cannot envision a life for self that can be fulfilled, the resulting injury harms the *liver* and all that it governs, including the channel and the organs associated with it via the *shen* and *ko cycles*. The stress of being unable to express one's one will (*zhi*) in life slowly drains away the *Qi* of the *kidneys*. All of these units within the system of Chinese medicine are harmed when any human being cannot be who they truly are.

The *heart*, as a purely energetic reality, is a void floating within the body as a part of the "great void," the *Tao*, the dwelling place for the spirit that requires this solitude to be at rest. The art of the *heart* of Chinese philosophy is the way to obtain and conserve this void, because it is a way to allow the spirit to be present and to impart spiritual essences and power to the blood and, therefore, all of life.

The character for the *heart* is the only character for a visceral organ that does not contain the radical for flesh. This implies a special position for the *heart*. Humans who can live from the *heart* are manifesting the *"zhu,"* or the active aspect of the *heart*. The character *"zhu"* is a lamp stand with a rising flame, and by extension is a human spreading the light of the spirit from an unobstructed *heart*.

The mind has a strong connection to the *heart*. It is a relatively outer level of being whose functioning comprises the *Yang* organs and their relationship to the sensory orifices. The *shen* is that aspect of self that is capable of introspection. It conveys the spirit within the *heart* to the outer world. The spirit of the *heart*, or the *shen*, arises from the *kidney Jing* and expresses one's true deep nature — the truth of a person. The alignment of the mind and *heart* with the *Tao*, or whatever one wishes to call it, allows life events to be accurately perceived.

Since before the Old Testament account of the spoils of war, newborns have been surrounded by the essential mistruths being lived out in dominator cultures around the world, absorbing via osmosis and early training this interpretation of who we are. The chain of this injury is passed on again and again for generations and in varying degrees. Right from the very beginning of life, we *learn* who we are rather than discovering our true selves. Learning implies the process of procuring data and analyzing and integrating them. When there is aberrant functioning of this faculty, there is a separation between *Yin* and *Yang*, and this allows the mind to rule our lives rather than serving our lives. The aberrant functioning needed to engage in actions that cause slavery, abuse, domination, war, poverty within the milieu of plenty, and many other forms of violence, is an expression of a cultural split between *heart* and mind. The separation of *heart* and mind is a fundamental tearing-apart of the fabric of life. Males in particular are asked on a daily basis to make this split in their being. The price is high. And as more women become involved in the hierarchical struggles that dominator societies purvey, the cost becomes high for them as well. *Heart* disease in the conventional medical sense used to be a disease mainly of men but is now also a disease of women. Modern psychotherapeutic models often work to address the early context of the learning process of who we are in order to enable a discovery of who we truly are without this early programming. They work to reconnect the mind with the *heart.*

Shen (*Heart*) and *jing* (*Kidney*) have a deep relationship because the *heart–kidney* axis is the central axis of spiritual stability and power within. This axis is contained within and continues through all of the other *Yin* and *Yang* relationships of the *zang–fu.* The *shen* and *ko* cycles of the five-phase relationships are emblematic of this relationship and how the loss of internal communication between *heart* and mind can ultimately undermine the spiritual essence of an individual and a culture. By restoring communication between *Yin* and *Yang,* one can touch the depth of all separation and reassert balance between *shen* and *jing.* Where the spirit goes, the will can follow. The habituated truth of male dominance and all that it means can be repaired. We can heal ourselves even when there is material damage to the *heart* and the circulatory energetic mechanism of the body. The following material diseases are all indicative of various energetic injuries that occur as a result of *heart, liver,* and *kidney* imbalances and *phlegm damp* accumulations from *spleen* and *kidney* injury. These diseases are almost always underlying prostate *cancer* and provide a terrain in which prostate diseases can occur. Part of treating these conditions and preventing prostate *cancer* means attending to the psychoemotional imbalances and injuries that precluded material damage to the organs involved.

Hypertension

Hypertension (HTN) is the most prevalent example of the tension that results from a mind-and-*heart* split. Certainly, it is not a cause of prostate *cancer,* but it is a manifestation of a lifestyle and of internal injuries resulting from that lifestyle that commonly contribute to or are considered risk factors for prostate cancer — obesity, high cholesterol, and the diet that causes these conditions, and aging due to loss of vitality from a sedentary lifestyle. The *liver, heart, spleen,* and *kidney* are all scenes of the crime and all are harmed in HTN. By treating and changing a patient's relationship to this diagnosis,

Chinese medicine can not only cure the HTN but also teach a patient the skills to prevent prostate cancer. They are all linked through stress, dietary choices, exercise habits, coping mechanisms, and living in one's whole body rather than only from the neck up.

The environment and a number of environmental factors have been specifically implicated in the development of HTN, including salt intake, age, race, gender, smoking, serum cholesterol, glucose intolerance, weight, obesity, occupation, family size, and crowding. Many of these same issues are risk factors for prostate cancer. And it is important to note that blood pressure increases with age in affluent societies and traditionally decreases with age in nondeveloped (i.e. Third World or nonaffluent) societies or primitive cultures.[69]

- The WHO defines HTN as:[70]
- Normal — less than 140/90;
- HTN — 160/95;
- Borderline HTN — 141–159/91–94.

There are several types of HTN, including essential and secondary. Essential HTN may have hereditary and genetic factors, and the kidneys and renin activity probably play a role. Renin is an enzyme produced by the kidneys which acts on angiotensin to form a pressor (stimulatory) substance called angiotensin I. It is elevated in some forms of HTN.

Secondary HTN forms are related to alterations of hormonal secretion and/or renal function. Renal HTN is caused by loss of the kidneys' ability to handle sodium and fluids, leading to volume expansion, or by an alteration in renal secretion of vasoactive materials that results in a change in the arteriolar tone.

Endocrine or adrenal HTN is the outcome of a variety of adrenal cortical abnormalities, including primary aldosteronism. The most common cause of endocrine HTN is that resulting from the use of estrogen-containing oral contraceptives.[71] However, in young black males adrenal HTN may be due to chronic and persistent stress combined with a high-salt diet. Aldosterone causes sodium retention by stimulating tubule exchange of sodium for potassium; hypokalemia is a prominent feature in most patients with primary aldosteronism. The effect of sodium retention and volume expansion in chronically suppressing plasma renin activity is critically important. Also, the change in the arteriolar tone in Chinese medicine is reflective of injury to the *heart–liver–kidney* axis. The fact that black men have an incidence of prostate cancer twice that of white men, a higher rate of HTN, hypercholesterolenemia, and diabetes is emblematic not of genetic predispositions, although this does play a small role, but of chronic and persistent "fight or flight" stress.[72]

Patients with HTN die prematurely. It causes *heart* attacks, *brain* attacks (stroke), and renal failure. Cardiac compensation for the excessive workload imposed by increased systemic pressure initially causes left-ventricular hypertrophy. Ultimately, the function of this chamber deteriorates, it dilates, and the signs and symptoms of *heart* failure appear. Angina pectoris may also occur, because of accelerated coronary arterial disease and/or increased myocardial oxygen requirements as a result of the increased myocardial mass that ends up exceeding the coronary blood supply output. The heart is enlarged and has a prominent left-ventricular impulse. There may be a faint murmur of aortic regurgitation. Presystolic heart sounds can appear. A summation gallop rhythm may be present. ECG changes are present: evidence of ischemia or infarction may be observed later. Death occurs as a result of congestive heart failure or myocardial infarction.[73]

The neurological effects of longstanding HTN are retinal changes and CNS changes. The retina is the only tissue in which the arteries and arterioles can be examined directly. Although Chinese medicine views the nail beds and the tip of the tongue with high-intensity magnification and white light for signs of blood stasis, this technique shows primarily the movement of RBCs through the microcapillaries and not the status of the vessels systemically as they are impacted by HTN. The retina can be viewed for ongoing changes in the vascular network. Increasing severity of HTN is associated with focal spasm and progressive narrowing of the arterioles. In the retina there may be fields of blurred vision and, if papilledema is present, can lead to hemorrhages in the macular area. Occipital headaches, most often in the morning, are among early CNS symptoms. Dizziness, light-headedness, vertigo, tinnitus, and dimmed vision are all due to vascular occlusion or hemorrhage.[74]

Renal vascular lesions result in decreased glomerular filtration and tubular dysfunction. Proteinuria and microscopic hematuria occur because of glomerular lesions. Approximately 10% of deaths secondary to HTN result from renal failure.

Young black males are currently the highest-risk group for HTN in the US.[75] Seeing HTN in young men denotes a public health crisis. HTN is also becoming more prevalent in children, primarily because of obesity and lack of exercise.[76] As the greater omentum expands (abdominal fat) with fat cells, this applies pressure on the kidneys and causes kidney dysfunction. This is one reason why weight control is so very important. Children with HTN have also been found to have atherosclerosis, a disease of the elderly. And type II diabetes in children is a major health crisis.[77] HTN in young black men in the US is the result of vascular tension caused by societal stress and poor nutrition. HTN in obese children is caused by improper diet and lack of exercise. HTN, in general, can be treated by re-establishing communication between the heart — the spirit — and the mind. When these are connected, an individual can live *in* the body and make healthy rather than unhealthy choices because the feedback mechanism of the mind and heart and body is intact. This is immensely important because, in men, these diseases place one at risk for prostate cancer. The same diet that prevents heart-related diseases also prevents prostate cancer. These issues are societal and require everyone to be aware of and support all members of our society, including people of other races and our children.

Parents need to lead by example and provide living testimony to their children by eating right themselves and staying active. We all need to recognize that young men of all races in our culture are in crisis. They need our attention and help. Adults with HTN need to reassess their entire life structure and see if it is working. By reconnecting the heart and the mind, one then lives in the body. Living in the body means that one feels what is happening and, therefore, can recognize what is not working properly. The mind does not start at the neck and go up from there. The mind is in every cell of the body.

The *shen* is also in every cell of the body. Mind and *heart* are not far from each other, unless we stop living in the body and shut down to all of the messages, interior and exterior, that occur in every moment. Injury happens when we do not listen.

HTN is included in the categories of *xuan yun* (vertigo) and *tou tong* (headache). It occurs when there is a lack of coordination between *Yin* and *Yang* that is caused by injury due to the seven emotions, improper diet, and internal injury. The primary pathogenesis for HTN is divided as follows:[78,79]

(1) *Hyperactivity of liver Yang*

Long-term emotional *stasis* can lead to *liver Qi* stasis and the formation of *liver fire*. This manifests as headache, dizziness, tinnitus, restlessness, and a flushed face. Overexertion or general systemic deficiency may cause blood consumption or *Yin deficiency* and gradually leads to a *deficiency* of *Yin* and an inability of the *Yin* to anchor the *Yang*. This leads to hyperactive *Yang*, which in turn consumes *Yin* and other bodily fluids. This results in usually milder forms of HTN.

(2) *Deficiency of liver and kidney Yin*

There is a close relationship between the *liver* and *kidneys*, and a mutual supply of nutrients. The *liver* stores the blood and the *kidneys* store the *essence*. The blood and the *essence* are able to transform each other. Deficient *kidney Yin* usually causes *liver Yin deficiency* and vice versa. This leads to *liver* and *kidney Yin deficiency*, which in turn leads to HTN.

(3) *Yin deficiency leading to hyperactivity of Yang*

Disharmony between *Yin* and *Yang* is a morbid condition that is due to the consumption of *essence*, blood, and bodily fluid. When the *Yin* and the *Yang* are in disharmony, the *Yin* is unable to inhibit the *Yang* and it causes hyperactivity or rising of the *Yang*, which further consumes the *Yin* and *Jin Ye*. In this presentation there will be concomitant appearance of *liver* and *kidney Yin deficiency* accompanied by *liver Yang rising*. The *liver Yang* rising syndrome has progressed to a more systemic and deeper level of *kidney deficiency*.

(4) *Heart Yin deficiency*

The *heart Yin* is the nutrient part of fluid of the *heart* and is also a component of blood (serum). Therefore, it has a close relationship to the *heart* physiologically and pathologically. It is also related to the lung *Yin* and *kidney Yin*. *Deficiency* of *kidney Yin* may cause water to fail to inhibit fire, which will gradually lead to an *excess of fire* and result in *heart Yin deficiency*. The common features are palpitations, insomnia, memory loss, and HTN.

(5) *Deficiency of both Yin and Yang*

This condition is commonly seen in the later stage of HTN. It occurs as a result of prolonged HTN with improper or no treatment. Chronic *kidney deficiency* leads first to *Yin deficiency* and then to *Yang* deficiency. This type can be seen in menopausal HTN as well, where both the *kidney Yin* and the *kidney Yang* are *deficient*.

(6) *Qi and Yin deficiency*

This is moderately severe HTN in terms of injury and length of disease. Both the *Yin* and the *Qi* are damaged. Deficient *Qi* may cause hypofunction of the organs and a lowering of metabolic activity due to insufficient *Yang*. This fails to warm and nourish the organs and manifests as pallor, dizziness, tinnitus, palpitations, shortness of breath, and spontaneous sweating. *Yin deficiency* may simultaneously cause hyperactivity of *fire*, which manifests as five-center heat, dry mouth, dark concentrated urine, constipation, headache, and a dry tongue with little coating.

(7) *Maladjustment of the chong and ren channels*

This form of HTN may result from *liver* and *kidney Yin deficiency*, especially in the elderly and in perimenopause when the menses are irregular. The downward flow of blood during normal menses is a vehicle for releasing many *toxins* and *heat* related to sexual inter-course and also the *hun* aspect of the *liver*. The downward flow of blood is a normal part of the overall circulation of blood in the body and not just menstrual blood. When this releasing flow is lost as part of menopause, there is a tendency for blood and heat products to stagnate in the chest. This can contribute to perimenopausal and menopausal HTN. It is important for women to understand this and make adjustments in their lifestyle to manage this natural tendency. The transition of menopause occurs over a period of time and gives women a mirror in which they can see reflected those things that have and have not been working for them in life.

All of these forms of HTN and, for that matter, every condition or form of disease give us an opportunity to make changes in our lives and help our patients to make changes in their lives. Suffering can be an opportunity and not a sentence written in stone.

Treatment

(1) *Liver Yang rising*

• Symptoms — dizziness, headache, a feeling of pressure in the head, irritability, temperamental, red eyes;
• Tongue — red, with a yellow coating;
• Pulse — taut and forceful;
• Treatment principle — calm the *liver* and anchor the *Yang*;
• Rx — *Tian ma gou teng wan.*

(2) *Liver and kidney Yin deficiency*

• Symptoms — headache, vertigo, tinnitus, dry eyes, irritability, palpitations, insomnia, poor memory, five-center *heat*, weak legs and/or knees;
• Tongue — red, with little fur;
• Pulse — fine or thread;
• Treatment principle — nourish the *Yin* and anchor the *Yang*;
• Rx — modified decoction of *Liu wei di huang wan.*

(3) *Yin deficiency with hyperactive Yang*

* Symptoms — same as *liver* and *kidney Yin deficiency* with hyperactive *Yang*;
* Treatment principle — nourish the *Yin* and anchor the *Yang*;
* Rx — *Qi ju di huang wan.*

(4) *Heart Yin deficiency*

* Symptoms — irritability, palpitations, mental weariness, nocturnal emission, memory loss, dry stools, sores in the mouth;
* Tongue — red, with little fur and possible sores;
* Pulse — thready and rapid;
* Treatment principle — nourish the *kidneys* and tonify the *heart*, enrich *Yin* and blood, and reduce *fire*;
* Rx — *shu di, dan shen, dang gui, ren shen, fu ling, tian dong, bai zi ren, he shou wu, jie geng.*

(5) *Deficiency of Yin and Yang*

* Symptoms — dizziness, tinnitus, memory loss, palpitations, fatigue, sore low back and knees, cold extremities in *Yang deficiency*, five-center *heat* with more *Yin deficiency*.
* Tongue — *Yin* deficiency — red tongue; *Yang deficiency* — more pale;
* Pulse — *Yin* deficiency — rapid and fine; more *Yang deficiency* — deep and thready;
* Treatment principle — nourish and restore the *Yang*;
* Rx — *Er xian tang.*

(6) *Deficiency of Qi and Yin*

* Symptoms — fatigue, a low voice, intolerance of *cold*, a poor appetite, loose stools, a puffy face, extremity edema;
* Tongue — pale and tender (as in *liver blood deficiency*);
* Pulse — deep and thread;

- Treatment principle — tonify the *Qi*, nourish the *Yin*, tonify the *spleen*, and transform *dampness*
- Rx — *Si jun zi tang* with *wu li san* and *fu ling*.

(7) *Disharmony between the chong and the ren*

- Symptoms — headache, dizziness, restlessness, insomnia, hypochondrium area distenstion, general malaise, fluctuation of blood pressure, all worse prior to and during the menses;
- Tongue — varied;
- Pulse — taut and thready or wiry and forceless;
- Treatment principle — regulate the *chong* and *ren*;
- Rx — modified *Xiao Yao San*.

Acupuncture Points

(1) *Liver fire* — LI 11, Lv 3, Gb 20, *Taiyang* with reducing or even method;

(2) Excess *phlegm* and *dampness* in *Qi*-deficient type — St 40, CV 12, P 6, Bl 20;

(3) *Yin* deficiency with *Yang* rising — LI 11, Lv 3, Bl 23, Bl 18, K 3, Sp 6, with reinforcing method;

(4) To calm *liver Yang* — Gb 20, Du 20, Gb 5, Gb 43, Lv 2, draining method;

(5) To replenish and regulate *Qi* and blood — Du 20 (reducing), CV 6, Bl 18, Bl 20, Bl 23, St 36, reinforcing method;

(6) To tonify the *kidneys* — Du 20, Bl 23, Sp 6, CV 6, K 3, K 10, CV 4, reinforcing methods;

(7) General points — LI 11, Gb 20, Bl 10, St 36, Lv 3, LI 4, *taiyang*;

(8) Headache, dizziness, a feeling of distenstion in the head — *taiyang*, Gb 20, LI 4, Lv 3;

(9) Tinnitus — SJ 5, SJ 17, Gb 41.

Auricular medicine — *kidney*, adrenal, infra-antihelix crus end, *brain*, *shenmen*, *heart*, *liver*, groove for lowering blood pressure, ear apex.

Scalp — foot motor sensory area — bilateral, thoracic area, and vasomotor area.

Japanese bleeding technique. Prick the Du 15 area many times with a lancet. When small drops of blood appear over the area, apply strong cupping over Du 15. Often the cup will fill with very dark blood. Sterile hygiene must be used for managing the blood-filled cup. In any bleeding technique, take the blood pressure before and after treatment. It is important to prevent the blood pressure from crashing. This is a strong technique with rare side effects but crashing can occur if the patient has very high blood pressure, for example 200/110. Hypotension should be watched for, and the indicators are the same as for shock. Patients with blood pressure over 200/110 are at risk for a brain attack (stroke). This technique may be appropriate for them.[80]

Japanese naso technique. With one needle, lightly prick the naso area on both sides. This area is above the scalenes and sternocleido-mastoid muscles which cover the carotid artery. In a hypertensive patient it can be very tight and tense. Light needling all over this area releases the musculature and the vessels below. It releases tension in general and helps to stabilize the blood pressure.[81]

Blood pressure control points include the metatarsal joint crease under the third toe. Use moxa only for both high and low blood pressure. Also, the left *hua tou* point around Du 11 (T 5). And SI 11 on the left scapula. The scapula is a diagnostic area for heart disease; if it is puffy here, there is a poorer prognosis. Moxa is good here even in HTN. If the patient cannot feel it to begin, it is a sign of improvement if eventually they can feel it. Always palpate the front *mu* point of the heart at CV 15 in patients with reported heart diseases. CV 15 can become a monitoring point for the efficacy of treatment. Tightness and tenderness at this point are indicators for excess conditions. Flaccidity, or a hole at this area and point, is an indicator for deficiency conditions. Palpation pre- and posttreatment at this point should be done to monitor treatment.

Patients with pear-shaped bodies carry more weight in their lower extremities and have a tendency for hypotension. Patients with apple-shaped bodies carry more weight around the midriff and have a tendency for hypertension.

Dietary advice. Hawthorn berries are available in many health food stores and co-ops. Eating 9–15 g of a morning cereal or a blender drink will help lower blood pressure. Chrysanthemums are very refreshing and gentle. They are especially good for treating eye conditions caused by flaming *liver fire.* A steeped tea is excellent. Celery acts as a *Yin*-nourishing vegetable and a diuretic. Extracted into juice in the amount of about 250 g helps lower blood pressure and move stools. Onions juiced or sautéed have been used for centuries to help prevent blood pressure. Also, garlic, a relative of onions in the *Allium* family, can be used raw, stewed, or baked, or cooked in congee to lower blood pressure and regulate cholesterol levels, thus preventing atherosclerotic plaque. *Capsella,* or shepherd's purse, is a ubiquitous weed that grows all over the US. It can be used in salads to lower and control blood pressure. Many seaweeds, like *Thallus eckloniae,* reduce blood pressure. They are staples of the indigenous peoples on every sea coast of the world. Straw mushrooms (*Volva fungorum*) can be used just like button mushrooms or Crimini's, with the additional effect that they not only taste good but lower blood pressure.

Blood-Pressure-Lowering Medications

Nondrug therapies can be used to control borderline-to-mild HTN. The Multiple Risk Factor Intervention Trial (MRFIT) has shown that drugs offer no benefit in protecting against heart disease in borderline-to-moderate HTN.[82] Most of the studies done on HTN and blood-pressure-lowering medications did not compare pharmaceuticals with natural medicine alternatives. However, the yearly sale of antihypertensive drugs is greater than US $15 billion.

Drugs that are used to treat HTN are divided into four steps:[83]

- A step-one drug is a thiazide diuretic without a beta blocker;
- A step-two drug is a thiazide diuretic with a beta blocker or calcium channel blocker or ACE inhibitor (angiotensin-converting enzyme);

- A step-three drug uses three drugs;
- A step-four drug uses four drugs.

There are other types of blood-pressure-lowering drugs, including those that act on the brain, like clonidine (Catapres), methyl-dopa (Aldomet), and reserpine (Serpasil).

Diuretics lower the blood pressure by reducing the volume of fluid in the blood and body fluids by promoting the elimination of salt and water through increased urination. There are three major types: thiazide, loop diuretics, and potassium-sparing diuretics. Thiazide diuretics can be used at lower doses and are safer. They can also be used in milder forms of HTN. In addition, they potentiate the effectiveness of other blood-pressure-lowering drugs and are used in combination within one pill with beta blockers, vasodilators, or ACE inhibitors. Thiazide diuretics cause the loss of potassium and magnesium, each of which is a mineral shown to exert blood-pressure-lowering effects and prevent heart attacks. The drugs used in these antihypertensives also increase cholesterol and triglyceride levels, increase the viscosity of the blood, raise uric acid levels, and increase platelet aggregation. All of these side effects are risk factors for cancer. Thiazide diuretics also worsen blood sugar control, which makes them difficult for diabetics to use safely.

Beta blockers block the binding of adrenaline on the cellular receptor known as the beta receptor.[84] This results in a reduced heart rate and reduced force of contraction of the heart. It also helps in the relaxation of the arteries. Commonly used beta blockers include propanolol (Inderal), metaprolol (Lopressor), and nadolol (Corgard). These drugs are also used to treat angina and some types of arrhythmias. The reduced amount of blood being pumped in a more relaxed arterial system means that it is difficult to get enough blood to the extremities and the brain. Common symptoms are cold hands and feet, nerve tingling, impaired mental functioning, fatigue, dizziness, and depression. Going suddenly off of a beta blocker will result in a withdrawal syndrome. This can result in an increased heart rate, a dramatic rise in blood pressure, and headache.

Calcium channel blockers are the newest form of antihypertensive drug.[85] They work by blocking the normal passage of calcium through certain channels in cell walls. Since calcium is required for nerve transmission and muscle contraction, the effect of blocking the calcium channel is to slow down nerve conduction and inhibit the contraction of muscle. In the *heart* and vascular system, blocking calcium channels results in reducing the rate and force of contraction, relaxing the arteries, and slowing the nerve impulses in the *heart*. Commonly prescribed drugs in this category include Cardizem, Cardene, Procardia, and Verelan. There are some better-tolerated side effects, which include constipation, allergic reactions, fluid retention, dizziness, headache, fatigue, and impotence. More serious side effects include angina and heart failure.

ACE inhibitors prevent the formation of active angiotensin.[86] This reduces the fluid volume in the blood and relaxes the arterials. ACE inhibitors actually improve *heart* function and increase blood and oxygen flow to the *heart, liver,* and *kidneys.* They include Capoten, Vasotec, and Prinivil. There are some side effects, which include dizziness, headache, and ligh-theadedness. These drugs also cause the body to retain potassium, which can lead to *heart* and *kidney* problems.

All of the above drugs carry side effects.[87]

The potassium and sodium balance is extremely important. Most of us tend to eat a diet high in sodium and low in potassium — leaving most people with a potassium-to-sodium ratio of less than 1:2. In other words, most people eat twice as much sodium as potassium. The recommended ration is greater than 5:1 potassium to sodium. Beneficial foods with good potassium-to-sodium ratios are:

- Apples — 90:1;
- Bananas — 440:1;
- Carrots — 75:1;
- Oranges — 260:1;
- Potatoes — 110:1.

Sugar elevates blood pressure. It is the preferred substrate of cancer cells.[88] Not only does sugar help cancer cells proliferate but also the insulin spikes relative to blood sugar levels.[89] Omega-3 fatty acids lower blood pressure. Men who eat high levels of omega-3s from fish and other sources have lower levels of heart disease and prostate cancer. The short-term effects of caffeine from coffee, tea, chocolate, and colas show an increase in blood pressure. Phosphate drinks like fizzy colas leach zinc, a mineral element needed for good prostate health.

Alcohol even in moderate amounts elevates blood pressure. Alcohol consumption has been negatively linked to breast and prostate cancer. Smoking is a well-documented contributor to all forms of heart disease, including HTN, and almost every cancer. Stress may be one of the greatest contributors to HTN, as we have seen. Vitamin C and calcium and magnesium supplementation offers protection against heart disease of any kind. CoQ10 is also cardio-protective. Many antihypertensives cause weight gain around the midriff. Since this is one of the causes of HTN, the best treatment for HTN is natural treatment and lifestyle changes.

Coronary Artery Disease

Coronary artery disease (CAD)[90] is a heart disease caused by myocardial ischemia, which is in turn caused by an oxygen deficit, and this is in turn caused by coronary atherosclerosis.[91] It is the most common cause of weakened heart pumping, enlargement of the ventricles, · and symptoms of heart failure. Bypass surgery to go around or open the arteries that feed the heart muscle itself with stents is one of the most common surgeries in the US.

Muscle damage resulting from ischemic cardiomyopathy leads to zonal damage of the heart. This is different from the global damage seen in congestive heart failure. This regional damage is relative to the artery involved and the region it nourishes. When the muscle is damaged in that area, it leads to inefficient pumping. The heart muscle is scarred due to CAD. This scarring is irreversible and is a material form of *blood stasis*. Heart muscle may be weakened less commonly by constant poor circulation to the heart without heart attacks. This is called "hibernating myocardium" and is considered reversible. Differentiating between the two is important, because it change strategies in treatment.

CAD is divided into five categories, according to clinical characteristics:

(1) Primary sudden cardiac arrest,
(2) Angina pectoris,
(3) Myocardial infarction (MI),
(4) Heart failure due to CAD,
(5) Arrhythmia.

These categories in Chinese medicine refer to:[91]

- *Xiong bi* — chest *bi* or obstruction of *Qi* in the chest, which may or may not be cardiac arrest;
- *Xiong tong* or chest pain, usually related to angina;
- *Zhen xin tong* or MI;
- *Jue xin tong* or precordial pain with cold limbs — the mild form is with pectoral pain, and the serious form is *zhen xin tong* or true heart pain.

In CAD, the disease is in the *heart* but is related to the *spleen* and *kidneys*. Its general mechanism is deficiency with excess symptoms. These are differentiated according to diagnosis but clinically are seen together and treated together. Risk factors for this disease are traditionally HTN, hyperlipemia, overweight and obesity, diabetes, and cigarette smoking.

Differential Diagnosis

(1) Angina: episodic retrosternal pain, a smothering sensation, choking, pain radiating to left shoulder, arm and jaw, and cold sweating for 1–5 min around an episode. These episodes can be brought on by overwork, exertion, a heavy meal, cold exposure, and emotions. Angina is further divided into types: incipient, stable, and increscent. An ECG will show various degrees of transient ST segment depression and inversion or flatness of T wave arrhythmia.

(2). A MI is the result of chronic myocardial ischemia leading to myocardial necrosis. It can be complicated by arrhythmia, heart failure, and cardiogenic shock. Premonitory symptoms include frequent angina episodes which can be longer and more severe with nausea, vomiting, and arrhythmia. Nitroglycerin sublingual is a common treatment. An MI presents with retrosternal pain, a sense of oppression and doom, radiating pain to the left, sweating, anxiety, pallor, confusion, shock, and a thready pulse. The ECG will show elevation in ST segments, inversion T waves, and pathologic Q waves. The CPK and MB isoenzymes are indicative biomarkers. SGOT and LDH are of diagnostic value; leukocytes and sugar serum myoglobin are prognosticators.

Chinese Medicine Patterns

(1) *Obstruction by cold of the chest Yang*

- Symptoms — an oppressed feeling in the chest, paroxysmal chest pain with palpitations and shortness of breath, worse with cold and brought on by cold exposure, and cyanosis;
- Tongue — white greasy coating, and perhaps a dark or purple body;
- Pulse — tight;
- Treatment principle — warm the *Yang* of the chest, move blood, and reduce pain;
- Rx — *Gua lou ban xia jia wei;*
- Points — Bl 17, Bl 43, Bl 11, P 7, CV 17, St 36, warm needle technique;
- Moxa on CV 8.

(2) *Blood stasis in the heart and vessels*

- Symptoms — twinges in the chest radiating to the shoulder and back or neck and jaw, a chest stifling sensation (men), shortness of breath;
- Tongue — deep-purple, with ecchymoses;
- Pulse — tight and/or choppy;

- Treatment principle — promote the flow of *Qi* and blood, and regulate the blood;
- Rx — *Dan shen tang* with *tao hong si wu tang*;
- Points — same as No.1, since *Yang*-deficient *cold* stasis also leads to *blood stasis*.

(3) *Deficient Qi and Yin*

- Symptoms — indistinct pain in the precordium, lassitude, palpitations, shortness of breath, spontaneous sweating, dry mouth;
- Tongue — red, with little or no coating;
- Pulse — tight and weak;
- Treatment principles — tonify the *Qi*, nourish the *Yin*, and move the blood;
- Rx — *Sheng mai san* with *dan shen* and *yu zhu*;
- Points — St 36, Sp 6, Bl 43, Bl 15, Bl 14, Bl 23, Bl 17, Sp 10, CV 6, Ht 6.

(4) *Stasis due to cold*

- Symptoms — chest pain which radiates to the back and is worsened by cold, palpitations, a choking, sensation in the chest, cold limbs, frequent clear urination;
- Tongue — pale, a dark hue, no coating;
- Pulse — deep and slow;
- Treatment principle — disperse the *cold*, warm the collaterals, tonify the *Yang* (especially of the *kidneys*), and move the blood;
- Rx — *gua lou, xiong bi, gui zhi, dan shen, yu jin, chuan xiong,* and *hong hua* 10 g each;
- Points — St 36, Bl 11, Bl 43, Bl 15, K 3, Lv 3;
- Moxa — a warm needle on St 36 and Bl 43.

(5) *Yin deficiency leading to Yang rising*

- Symptoms — chest pain, a red face, palpitations, chest stifling (men), insomnia, excessive dreaming, irritability, headache, vertigo, HTN;

- Tongue — red, with no coating;
- Pulse — thready or wiry and forceful;
- Treatment principle — nourish the *Yin*, anchor the *Yang*, calm the *spirit*, and soothe the *liver;*
- Rx — *shi jue ming* — 30 g, *zhen zhu* — 30 g, *gout eng, xia ku cao, ju hua, gua lou, huang jing, bai shao, gou Qi zi, dan shen,* and *mai dong* — all 10 g each;
- Points — Lv 8, K 10, Lv 14, Bl 23, K 6, CV 4, CV 17 (downward needling), LI 11, St 36, *yintang.*

(6) *Yin and Yang collapse*

- Symptoms — disorientation, restlessness, *cold* extremities, spontaneous sweating, shortness of breath;
- Tongue — scarlet and dry, with a geographic coating;
- Pulse — thready and rapid or deep and minute;
- Treatment principle — rescue the *Yang*, tonify the *Yang*, and tonify the *Qi*;
- Rx — *ren shen* — 5 g, *fu zi, sheng jiang, wu wei zi,* and *zhi gan cao,* 10 g each;
- Points — St 36, Du 20, with direct moxa.

Auricular medicine: *shen men,* infra-antihelix crus end, *brain, heart, kidney, spleen.*

Scalp: *Fu zang shang jiao* points, and *Dao zang xia jiao* points.

Hyperlipemia or Hypercholesterolnemia[92]

Why talk about these cardiovascular conditions when talking about prostate cancer prevention? One reason is that the same diet and lifestyle factors that treat, resolve, or prevent these conditions are the same diet and lifestyle factors that prevent prostate cancer. It is not an unexpected·fact that Lipitor and other cholesterol-lowering drugs help to prevent cancer. What is cancer in its final form? It is *phlegm–dampness, turbid blockage,* and *blood stasis* knotted together with *toxins.* Cholesterol is a form of *phlegm–dampness* and when pathologic is the stuff from which arterial plaques are made. Drugs that reduce this accumulation of *phlegm–dampness* help reduce some cancers as well. The prostate contains glandular tissue that is a target for phlegm dampness, like the lungs, colon, breast ducts, vessels, and some other tissues that are the essence of dampness in their healthy states. When we treat these conditions we are treating not only the target tissue but also the whole human body. When patients make changes to their diet and lifestyle habits, they are treating not only their HTN or high cholesterol but their whole body and, in men, they are lowering their risk of prostate cancer.

The result of the above conditions is *blood stasis*. This is one reason why some men with coronary artery disease and hypertension have erectile dysfunction.[93] There is a direct connection between the blood pumped by the heart and the blood mechanism of creating an erection. Erectile dysfunction is a sign of heart disease. *Blood stasis* is the cause of both. And *blood stasis* is also a terrain for many cancers. The stickiness of higher blood viscosity resulting from blood stasis is also a primary mechanism of metastatic spread of cancer cells. Changing this systemic environment is important in preventing a cancer diagnosis and in secondary prevention of recurrence of a cancer. The ecology of the body must be made healthy and transformed into an ecology that does not support cancers.

It is important to realize, too, that liver constraint can be one cause of blood stasis.[94] The emotional factors like rage and constant frustration impact the vessels of the body, making them stiffer and leathery. This disallows the blood to flow through as smoothly as when we were young, leading to HTN and *blood stasis* and erectile dysfunction. Rage and disconnectedness can be part of the underlying environment of the individual with these conditions.

Blood lipids are an important part of overall health and include cholesterol, triglyceride, phospholipids, and free fatty acid. Hyperlipemia refers to the extension beyond normal limits of one of these lipid factors in the blood. It is the elevation of cholesterol and triglyceride in the plasma and is closely related to atherosclerosis. It is also called hyperlipoproteinemia, because the fat-soluble plasma lipids have come to combine with the protein to become water-soluble compounds to be transported to all parts of the body. In clinical practice, hyperlipemia is classified into two types: primary and secondary. The secondary type is caused by abnormal metabolism of plasma lipids and lipoprotein. This occurs in diabetes, and in diseases of the liver, pancreas, and gallbladder.

Hyperlipoproteinemia can also be divided into five different types:

- Type I is chylomicronemia, which is a rare disorder due to congenital deficiency of lipoprotein lipase, a digestive enzyme.
- Type II is hyperbetalipoproteinemia, which is commonly seen with marked elevation of plasma cholesterol and is a disorder related to atherosclerosis and coronary heart disease. In some patients this is an inherited condition but most commonly it is due to a high-cholesterol diet or secondary myeloma, nephritic syndrome, liver disease, and other conditions.
- Type III is an autosomal dominant disorder in which the plasma concentration of cholesterol and of triglyceride are both elevated. The disease occurs mostly after middle age and patients usually present with obesity and a disturbance of carbohydrate metabolism. There may be a relationship to diabetes.
- Type IV is the most common disorder, in which the endogenous plasma triglyceride is elevated due to a disturbance of carbohydrate metabolism, but plasma cholesterol is not necessarily elevated.
- Type V is very rare and is a combination of types I and IV.

The cholesterol-lowering drug industry is a USD 22 billion industry in the US Vytorin, a cholesterol-lowering drug that is a combination of two different drugs, was recently found to *increase* the laying-down of plaque in the vessels.[95] This finding came out two years after Merck knew of these results from their monitoring of this drug. Like many diseases and conditions of the developed world, hyperlipemia is a preventable disease. Because high cholesterol plays such an important role in cardiovascular disease and the pathogenesis of prostate and other cancers, it is immensely important to treat these conditions in a natural way, including giving patients information that will spur them to change their dietary and lifestyle habits. It is diet and lack of exercise that are the main causes of high cholesterol. These lifestyle issues are changeable and do not require the input of the pharmaceutical industry and the FDA. Part of what drives up the cost of health care is the fact that people look to medicine for cures of conditions that they themselves can prevent through proper diet and exercise. The pharmaceutical industry is a profit-driven industry just like any other. When firms' patents run out on old drugs, they must tweak or change these drugs in some way to maintain profits by preventing those drugs from going generic. Vytorin is an example of such a drug. Aging and cardiovascular diseases are very much a process of loss of vitality due to giving up on living actively. The daily work of maintaining an active mind and body is part of life, and people must ask themselves why they have stopped living fully. Our job as healers/physicians is to teach and engage our patients on this level.

In Chinese medicine, this condition of high cholesterol belongs to categories of *phlegm–dampness*, *turbid blockage*, and *blood stasis*, and is considered related to the *spleen*, *liver*, and *kidney*. The exogenous cause relates to diet and the intake of too much fatty and sweet food, resulting in *spleen deficiency* and the production of *dampness* and *phlegm*. This leads to the material formation of *phlegm–dampness* — in this case plaque. Atherosclerotic plaques on the interior of vessels cause a narrowing of the vessels, and then *blood stasis* as the lumen of the vessel narrows. *Blood stasis* is the result of an enlargement of the heart caused by HTN and atherosclerosis; this leads to an inability of the enlarged heart to pump blood efficiently and the blood becomes static and more congealed. Dietary habits have a basis in the emotions and changing these habits requires a multipronged approach that empowers a patient to begin to explore their personal interpretations of the meaning of food. The internal cause of hyperlipemia is *Yin deficiency* of the *liver* and *kidney* which results in *phlegm heat*, or *liver Qi stasis* which results in *phlegm* turbidity and *blood stasis*. There may be primary and secondary aspects to the disease.

When one is treating the primary aspects, tonifying the *kidney*, harmonizing the *liver*, and strengthening the *spleen* are necessary strategies. When one is treating the secondary aspects, the focus becomes more the promotion of digestion and relieving stasis, eliminating *phlegm* and seeping out *dampness*, clearing *heat*, and dissolving *blood stasis*.

Diagnosis requires a detailed intake in terms of family history, presence of diabetes, gout, liver diseases, renal disease, and CAD. Some patients may not know that they have these conditions, and so it is necessary to know the possible signs and early symptoms of these conditions. This may require a referral for diagnosis. Physical examination should pay attention to yellowish papules or raised skin conditions that are sebaceous in nature, xanthomas, eye conditions that may be related to *phlegm* accumulation (like cataracts and glaucoma), and peripheral vascular disorders like DVT, intermittent claudication, and PAD. The most important tests are assays of cholesterol (LDL, HDL, and the ratio between LDL and HDL cholesterol) and triglyceride levels.

Differentiation and Treatment

(1) *Retention of damp-heat in the interior*

- Symptoms — dizziness, heaviness in the *head*, headache, *fan*, fatigue and listlessness, a bitter taste, a dry throat, overweight or obesity, dry stools;
- Tongue — slightly red, with yellow and greasy fur;
- Pulse — slippery;
- Treatment principle — clear *heat* and transform *dampness*;
- Rx — *Wen dan tang.*

(2) *Liver and kidney Yin deficiency*

- Symptoms — dizziness, tinnitus, blurred vision, irritability, memory loss, weak and sore low back and knees;
- Tongue — red, with little fury
- Pulse — tight and thread
- Treatment principle — nourish the *Yin* of the *liver* and *kidneys*;
- Rx — *Liu wei di huang wan.*

(3) *Phlegm stasis*

- Symptoms — obesity, a long history of overindulgence in fatty and sweet foods, an oily sheen on the face denoting food stasis, heavy distension in the head, frequent spitting of saliva or *phlegm*, a bitter taste, stickiness in the mouth or throat, stuffy pain in the chest and epigastrium, heavy or numb limbs;
- Tongue — a dark body with a thick and greasy coating;
- Pulse — thin or slippery;
- Treatment principle — *Yi shen jiang zhi ling* ("reduce-blood-lipids-and-prolong-life pills")

Acupuncture: (1) St 36 between 7 and 9 am daily with an even technique for two courses; (2) St 40 with needle sensation to toes; a strong technique for 30 min per day for two courses.

There are several herbs that lower blood lipids, and they can be added to the above formulas, as would be appropriate given the pattern. They include *shan zha, jue ming zi, yi mu cao, bai guo ye, da suan, dan shen, gou qi zi, gua lou ren, hai zao, he shou wu, huai hua mi, jin ying zi, ren shen, san qi, yin chen, ze xie, hu zhang,* and *jin yin hua.*

Congee: *he shou wu* — 15 g powdered; *rice or sprouted millet* — 50 g; *gou qi zi* — 10 g; sugar — a small amount. Cook in 500 ml water over slow heat for several hours to make a gruel or *shi fan* (congee). Eat twice daily for breakfast and dinner as one part of the meal. This combination is cardiotonic, reduces blood lipids, and reduces blood pressure.

Congestive Heart Failure[96]

The incidence of prostate cancer rises incrementally with every decade of life. Postmortem studies of elderly men show that a large percentage of men die with prostate cancer present but with no signs or symptoms. The indolent nature of some prostate cancers lets some off the hook. However, many men are not so lucky and, as a result, prostate cancer is a killing disease of older men after the age of 60.

This means that, given everything we have just discussed, more serious cardiovascular diseases can be found alongside prostate cancer. It is never too late to treat. And treating these conditions in men who have no signs of prostate cancer may actually not only help them with their heart disease by prolonging life but also prevent a diagnosis of prostate cancer at the age of 80. Surely this is a gift. And the changes that are made to improve one's status with heart disease will materially improve the quality of life.

Congestive heart failure (CHF) is a pathophysiologic state in which the left and/or right ventricles of the heart fail to pump adequate quantities of blood needed to meet the metabolic requirements of the various organs of the body, especially during stress or exercise. Numerous underlying heart diseases, like CAD, HTN, rheumatic heart disease, congenital heart disease, arterial hypertension, or cardiomyopathy, may cause CHF. Therefore, CHF is not a primary diagnosis of heart disease but rather an expression of the end result of abnormal cardiac function of different degrees resulting from a variety of underlying cardiac diseases.

Clinical manifestations are primarily related to the resultant dysfunction of other vital organs. CHF is commonly manifested by pulmonary congestion, pulmonary edema, pleural effusion, hepatomegaly with ascites, and various abnormalities of kidney function.

Symptoms:

- Dyspnea with elevated pulmonary venous pressures;
- Difficulty in breathing, possibly only during physical effort in the early stage, getting gradually worse as cardiac function deteriorates;
- Dyspnea even at rest in the later stage; shortness of breath even at night;
- Orthopnea;
- Fatigue as a late symptom due to reduction in cardiac output;
- Left ventricular failure (LVF) as manifested by nocturia, sweating, cough, hemoptysis, and cachexia;
- Far advanced LVF will manifest as acute pulmonary edema, which can lead to death.

Physical findings:

- LVF — tachycardia, tachypnes, cool skin, sweating, cyanosis, moist rales, wheezing, cardiomegaly, gallops; the apical pulse of the heart may be displaced to the left, there may be a mitral valve murmur, and there may be pleural or pericardial effusion;
- RVF — elevated venous pressure leading to engorgement of the veins in the neck, hepatomegaly with tenderness, jaundice, extremity edema; in the advanced stage there may be spleno-megaly, ascites, anasarca (all due primarily to liver dysfunction), and a tricuspid valve murmur;
- Biventricular failure — all of the above.

CHF is classified according to functional capacity:

- Class I — asymptomatic patients with documented heart disease;
- Class II — slight limitation of physical activity, because of symp-toms like shortness of breath and chest pain which occur only with extraordinary physical activity;
- Class III — marked limitation of physical activity, because symp-toms appear even with a normal activity like eating;
- Class IV — severe limitation of physical activity, because symp-toms appear even at rest.

Etiology According to Chinese Medicine

(1) Attack of EPIs which invade at the blood level and disturb circu-lation and cause cardiac dysfunction. Examples are infection with *Streptococcus* and rheumatic heart disease (RHD).
(2) *Qi* deficiency of the *heart* and *spleen* due to overwork or anxiety that injures the *heart–spleen* axis, causing *Qi deficiency. Qi defi-ciency* results in poorer *blood* circulation and *blood* stasis.
(3) *Kidney* and *spleen Yang* deficiency occurs with longstanding *Qi deficiency* and leads to *Yang deficiency* of the *spleen* and *kidneys*. If the *spleen Yang* is *deficient*, the *spleen* fails to transport and

transform food and fluids. Accumulation of fluids leads to edema. The pathogenic fluids affect the *heart* and cause palpitations. The accumulated fluids also attack the *lungs,* leading to cough with expectoration of sputum (*tan yin*), shortness of breath, and dyspnea.

Differentiation

(1) *Heart* Qi *deficiency*

- Symptoms — lassitude, shortness of breath, sweating, palpitations that worsen on exertion;
- Tongue — pale, with tooth marks;
- Pulse — weak or irregular;
- Treatment principle — replenish *heart Qi;*
- Rx — Bu *zhong yi qi tang.*

(2) *Qi and Yin deficiency*

- Symptoms — lassitude, shortness of breath, palpitations, five-center heat, dry mouth, thirst;
- Tongue — red, with no coating;
- Pulse — fine and rapid or irregular;
- Treatment principle — tonify *Qi* and nourish *Yin;*
- RX — *Shang mai san* or *sheng mai yin;*

(3) *Blood stasis and fluid obstruction*

- Symptoms — cyanosis of the lips, dark-red cheeks, palpitations, anxiety, shortness of breath aggravated by exertion, edema in the lower extremities;
- Tongue — dark, with.a white and greasy coating;
- Pulse — hesitant or irregular;
- Treatment principle — regulate and move the blood, and eliminate fluids;
- Rx — *Dan shen zhu she ye.*

(4) *Blood stasis due to Qi deficiency*

- Symptoms — a gloomy and gray complexion, palpitations, short-ness of breath, lassitude, stabbing pain in the chest, dilated neck veins, hepatomegaly;
- Tongue — a thin white coating dark body, and dark lips;
- Pulse — uneven or irregular;
- Treatment principle — tonify the *Qi* and move and regulate the blood;
- Rx — *Bu yang huan wu tang;*

(5) *Retention of fluids due to Yang deficiency*

- Symptoms — palpitations, shortness of breath, dyspnea cough with expectoration, edema, lassitude, intolerance of cold, cold limbs;
- Tongue — swollen and pale, with a white coating;
- Pulse — soggy and uneven or minute and deep;
- Treatment principle — warm the *Yang*, promote diuresis, and invigorate the *spleen* and *kidney Yang;*
- Rx — *Gui zhi fu zi tang* or *mao dongqing zhu she ye.*

General points: Bl 15, Bl 14, CV 14, CV 17, P 6, Ht 5, CV 6, Ht 6, Bl 17, Sp 10. These points should be added appropriately to the con-stitutional treatment points. Moxa can be added when appropriate. Some practitioners do not feel that treating the heart directly through heart channel points is correct treatment. Instead, pericardium channel points are used. Using CV 17, P 6, and the four gates may be inappropriate in advanced heart disease, because these points are dispersing and CHF indicates an advanced deficiency condition in which dispersing *Qi* may be contraindicated.

Auricular points: *heart, small intestine, liver, chest, brain, infra-antihelix crus end, shenmen.* Choose three or four points each time and retain for 20 min.

Nutritional:

- Steam 30 g *huang qi* in 200 ml of water for 2 h. Drink the fluid and eat the root with rice.

- Peel 30 g of garlic and boil it in water for 1 min; then place nonglutinous rice into the garlic water to cook as in congee. Add the garlic again to finish cooking the rice. Take warm in the morning and the evening.
- Steam Chinese white ginseng (*bai ren shen*) at low heat in a double boiler for 6–10 h. Drink ½-to-1 cup three times daily.
- *Gui jiang ren shen zhou* — *gui zhi* 6 g, *Sheng jiang* 6 g, *Bai ren shen* 3 g, *gou qi zi* 8 pieces, rice 100 g, Brown sugar to taste. Decoct the first four ingredients together until somewhat thicker in consistency. Cook the rice in the decoction with the brown sugar until a thick rice gruel or congee has formed. Take twice daily, in the morning and the evening. This congee is good for patients with *heart Qi* and *Yang deficiency*.

For deficient *Yin* patients, use *Yu zhu su rong yin* — *yu zhu* 250 g, white sugar 300 g. First, soak the *yu zhu* in cold water until it is soft and plump; add more water to the *yu zhu* and decoct three times, for 20 min each time. Mix the three cooks and decoct until almost boiled away; then add 300 g of white sugar, and dry and store. Infuse 10 g in boiling water three times per day and drink.

Sheng mai san has been researched and found to reduce the heart rate, improve left-ventricular performance, reduce camp levels in plasma after a myocardial infarction, and improve the overall function of the heart in acute myocardial ischemia. Thrombus formation time, prothrombin time, and prothrombin consumption time were all prolonged, and the plasma fibrinogen levels decreased, in patients given *Sheng mai san*.

Conclusions

The cultural expectations placed on males are often damaging to the spirit. As boys grow up and become men, they embody and incorporate these expectations into their very being. This way of being lays tracks of injury that are manifested in men's ability or inability to form relationships, nurture themselves and others both physically and emotionally, succeed without harming others, engage in war, express anger and frustration, and view the world as both interior and exterior, human and nature, male and female, without making distinctions or judgments based on hierarchy.

These are not gender problems. They are issues of learning and are cultural norms that have been handed down for generations. The world has reached a crisis point where changing this understanding of life and people's role in it must occur because we all may die as the injury increases exponentially. Cancer is emblematic of this injury. Prostate cancer is a metaphor for the lives that men must live in order to survive. It is an external manifestation of a life lived in a context where, starting in early childhood, men must not feel the tremendous pain of their loss — the loss of a connection to their interior self, their feelings of self, their relational self, and the child-hood spirit of love and devotion. This is an immense injury. This split allows them to live outside their bodies in ways that foster cruelty to the Earth, to animals, to women, to children and, most importantly, to themselves.

Men who survive as whole human beings in this world are bless-ings to the world. We so very much need them, want them, hope for them, and bless them. Healing the split between mind and *heart* is the primary way to enable men to grow and become whole. First, they must be willing to grieve for themselves. We must hold them through this.

References

1. www.unesco.org/opp/uk/declarations/seville.pdf
2. Earley J. (1997) *Transforming Human Culture: Social Evolution and the Planetary Crisis.* SUNY Press.
3. Eisler R. (1987) *The Chalice and the Blade.* Harper and Row, San Francisco.
4. Higgins R. (1973) *An Archaeology of the Minoan Crete.* The Bodley Head, London.
5. Hawkes J. (1968) *Dawn of the Gods: Minoan and Mycenaean Origins of Greece.* Random House, New York.
6. Echhart M. *Meister Eckhart: Selections from His Essential Writings.* HarperCollins (2005).

7. Thich Nhat Hanh *et al.* (1995) *Living Buddha, Living Christ.* Riverhead.
8. Goldstein J, Kornfield J. (1987) *Seeking the Heart of Wisdom.* Shambhala.
9. Eisler R. (2003) *The Power of Partnership: Seven Relationships That Will Change Your Life.* New World Library.
10. Hesse M. (1975) Criteria of truth in science and theology. *Relig Stud* **11(4)**: 385–400.
11. *Ibid.*
12. Peace, war and conflict. www.worldrevolution.org/projects/globalis-suesoverview/overview2/peacenew
13. Cancer facts and figures. 2012. www.cancer.org/acs/groups/content/@epidemiologysurveillance/documents/doc
14. Rocaht E. (2012) *Rhythm at the heart of the world.* Monkey.
15. Kramer H, Sprenger J. (2010) *Malleus Maleficarum.* Digireads.com
16. Zapotoczny W. German laws discriminating against Jews. www.wzaponline.com/germanlawsdiscriminatingagainstjews.pdf
17. The critiques. United Nations University website. www.archive.unu.edu/unupress/unupbooks/aa09ue/uv09ue0g.htm
18. Kauffman S. Breaking the Galilean spell. Edge. The Third Culture. www.edge.org/3rd_culture/kauffman08/kauffman08_index.html
19. Freud S. (1930) *Civilization and Its Discontents.* W.W. Norton (1989).
20. Schatzman M. (1973) *Soul Murder: Persecution in the Family.* Random House.
21. Barland JA. (1994) Splitting as a consequence of severe abuse in childhood. *Psychiatr Clin North Am* **17(4)**: 731–742.
22. National Council on Child Abuse and Family Violence. www.nccafv.org/child.htm
23. Miller A. (1984) *For Your Own Good.* Farrar, Straus and Giroux.
24. Romans 2:1. The Bible.
25. Gruen A. (2007) *The Betrayal of Self: The Fear of Autonomy in Men and Women.* Human Development.
26. Fromm E. (1992) *The Anatomy of Human Destructiveness.* Macmillan.
27. Jetzinger F. (1958) *Hitler's Youth.* Wilson, London.
28. Helfer R. (1999) Kempe C. (eds.). (1980) *The Battered Child.* University of Chicago Press.
29. Sattaur J. Perceptions of childhood in the Victorian *fin-de-siecle.* www.c-s-p.org/flyers/978-1-4438-2688-4-sample.pdf

30. de Mause L (ed.). (1974) *The History of Childhood.* Jason Aronson, New York.

31. Ehrenreich B. English D. (2010) *Witches, Midwives, and Nurses: A History of Women Healers,* The Feminist Press at CUNY.

32. Cohen J. Study suggests Adolf Hitler had Jewish and African ancestors. www.history.com/study-suggests-adolf-hitler-had-jewish-and-african-ancestors

33. *Op. cit.,* No. 23.

34. Fischer K. In the beginning was murder: destruction of nature and inter-human violence. www.jcrt.org/archives/06.2/fischer.pdf

35. Astati R *et al.* (eds.). (2007) *Questions of Anthropology.* Chap. 10 (Stewart M): How does genocide happen? Berg.

36. Pollack W. (1999) *Real Boys: Rescuing Our Sons from the Myths of Boyhood.* Owl.

37. Miller A. (1997) *The Drama of the Gifted Child.* Basic.

38. *Op. cit.,* No. 23.

39. Doran C, Parsons W. (1980) War and the cycle of relative power. *Am Pol Sci Rev.* **74(4)**: 947–965.

40. Goldstein J. (2001) *War and Gender: How Gender Shapes the War System and Vice Versa.* Cambridge University Press.

41. Men in families and family policy in a changing world. United Nations Publication Sales No. E, 11.IV.1 (2011).

42. Preparata G. (2007) *The Ideology of Tyranny.* Palgrave Macmillan.

43. Race and ethnicity in America: turning a blind eye to injustice. ACLU CERD Report. www.aclu.org/human-rights/aace-ethnicity-turning-blind-eye-injustice (2007).

44. Colloqium 2012: Extreme poverty is violence. www.atd-fourthworld.org/-colloqium-2012-extreme-poverty-is-violence.html

45. Bhutto B. Male domination of women. Beijing, Sep. 1995. www.famous-speeches-and-speech-topics.info/famous-speeches/benazir-bhutto

46. Hegstrom P. (2007) *Angry Men and the Women Who Love Them: Breaking the Cycle of Physical and Emotional Abuse.* Beacon Hill.

47. Adams D. (2004) *Why Do They Kill? Men Who Murder Their Intimate Partners.* Vanderbilt University Press.

48. Vitz P. (1997) Kleinian psychodynamics and religious aspects of hatred as a defense mechanism. *J Psychol Theo.* **25(1)**: 64–71.

49. Macioccia G. (2009) *Psyche in Chinese Medicine*. Churchill Livingstone.
50. Larre C, Rochat E. (1990) *Rooted in Spirit: The Heart of Chinese Medicine*. Barrytown/Station Hill.
51. Prostate cancer overview. Causes, risk factors, and prevention topics. American Cancer Society. www.cancer.org/cancer/prostatecancer/ overviewguide/prostate-cancer-overview
52. Ross R *et al.* (1985) Serum testosterone levels in healthy young black and white men. *J Nat Canc Inst* **76(1)**: 45–48.
53. Cao Y, Ma J. (2011) Body mass index, prostate cancer–specific mortality, and biochemical recurrence: a systematic review and meta-analysis. *Can Prev Res* **4**: 486–501.
54. Damone R. (2008) *Principles of Chinese Medicine Andrology*. Blue Poppy.
55. 2012 Science and Global Prostate Cancer Disparities conference. UF Shands Cancer Center. www.cancer.ufl.edu/research/symposia-and-conferences-2/symposia-and-conferences.
56. 1993 Causes of racial differences in testosterone levels of men. *J Natl Canc Inst* **85(6)**: 506–507.
57. Stress hormone blocks testosterone's effects, study shows. Available from Hormones and Behavior (*J Neurobiol*). www.utexas.edu/ news/2010/09/27/stress-hormone
58. Jeffries WM. (1991) Cortisol and immunity. *Med Hypotheses* **34(3)**: 198–208.
59. Ritchey J *et al.* (2012) A cross-sectional study of age, race and ethnicity, and body mass index with sex steroid hormone marker profiles among men in the National Health and nutrition Examination Survey (NHANES III). *BMJ open*, 2e001315.doi:101136/bmjopen-2012-001315.
60. Peterson C K *et al.* (2012) Anger and testosterone: evidence that situationally-induced anger relates to situationally-induced testosterone. *Emotion* **12(5)**: 899–902.
61. Male obesity linked to low testosterone level. *Diabetes Care.* May 2010.
62. Thomas J *et al.* (2012) Heart disease may be a risk factor for prostate cancer. *Cancer Epidemiol, Biomarkers Prev*, Feb. 8. As seen in dukehealth.org
63. *Prostate Cancer Prevention: Ways to Reduce Your Risk.* Mayo Clinic.
64. Ribeiro R. (2012) Overweight men more likely to develop prostate cancer. *J BMC Medicine. Sep.*

65. Friedland S. *et al.* (2012) Heart disease may be a risk factor for prostate cancer. *J Canc* Epidemiol. Biomarkers Prev, Feb.

66. Margel D *et al.* (2011) Correlation between female use of oral contraceptives and new cases of prostate cancer and mortality from prostate cancer. *BMJ* open, 67.

67. Cockburn M *et al.* Prostate cancer and ambient pesticide exposure in agriculturally intensive areas of California. *Am J Epidemiol.* dx.doi.org/10.1093/aje/kwr003.

68. Bertazzi PA *et al.* Environmental exposures and prostate cancer. *Am J Epidemiol* **129(6)**: 1187–1200.

69. Hajjar I *et al.* (2006) Hypertension: trends in prevalence, incidence, and control. *Annu Rev Publ Health* **27**: 465–490.

70. Cardiovascular disease. WHO/ISH hypertension guidelines. www.who.int/cardiovascular_diseases/guidelines/hypertension/en

71. Hypertension. Hormone Health Network. www.hormone.org/cardio-vascular/hypertension.cfm

72. Centers for Disease Control and Prevention. (2010) *A Closer Look at African American Men and High Blood Pressure Control: A Review of Psychosocial Factors and Systems-Level Interventions.* US Department of Health and Human Services, Atlanta.

73. High blood pressure: long-term effects and complications. www.servier.co.uk/disease-information/blood-pressure/long-term-effects-and-complications

74. Johnston S. Neurological complications of hypertension. www.expert-consultbook.com/expertconsult/ob/book-do?method=display&type

75. *Op. cit.* No. 72.

76. Lama G *et al.* (2006) American family physician. Hypertension in children and adolescents. *Am Fam Physician* **73(9)**: 1558–1568.

77. Centers for Disease Control and Prevention. Diabetes Public Health Resources. Children and Diabetes — More Information. www.cdc.gov/diabetes/projects/cda2.htm

78. Becker S *et al.* (2010) *Treatment of Cardiovascular Diseases with Chinese Medicine.* Blue Poppy.

79. Ma. Lecture notes.

80. Kuihara K. Lecture notes and class demonstration.

81. *Ibid.*

82. Gotto A. (1997) The Multiple Risk Factor Intervention Trial (MRFIT). *JAMA* **277(7)**: 595–597.
83. Fogyros R. All about hypertension treatment. www.heartdisease.about. com/od/highbloodpressure/a/all-about-hypertension-treatment
84. Web MD. Heart disease and beta-blocker therapy. www.webmd.com/ heart-disease/beta-blocker-therapy
85. *Ibid.* Heart disease and calcium channel blockers.
86. *Ibid.* Heart disease and ACE inhibitors.
87. Tomlinson C. Side effects of ACE inhibitors and beta-blockers. Liverstrong.com. www.livestrong.com/article/58961-side-effects-ace-inhibitors-beta-blockers
88. www.cancerres.aacrjournals.org/content/early/2010/07/16/0008-5472. can-09
89. Zhang H *et al.* (2010) Inhibition of cancer cell proliferation and metastasis by insulin receptor down–regulation. *Oncogene* **29(17)**: 2517–2527
90. National Heart Lung and Blood Institute. What is coronary heart disease? www.nhlbi.nih.gov/health/health-topics/cad
91. Hou JL *et al.* (1995) *Traditional Chinese Treatment for Cardiovascular Diseases.* Academy Press, Beijing.
92. Maciejko J. Management of hyperlipidemia. www.maofp.org/pdf/ cme%20lectures/aug2010/maciejko.pdf
93. Mayo Clinic. Erectile dysfunction: a sign of heart disease? www.mayo-clinic.com/health/erectile-dysfunction/HB00074
94. Yan DX. (1999) *Aging and Blood Stasis.* Blue Poppy.
95. National Research Center for Women and Families. A guide to cholesterol medication. www.center4research.org/2011/08/a-guide-to-cholesterol-medication
96. PubMed Health. Heart failure — overview. www.ncbi.nih.gov/pubmed-health/PMH0002211

CHAPTER 6

Fire — Chronic Viral Infection and Cancer

What would ancient Greece's Asklepio have thought of America's great bastions of health in 2000 ACE, her prestigious teaching hospitals? Strolling along hallways resonating with the sounds of beeping heart monitors and emergency audio pages, Asklepio might turn to daughters Panakeia and Hygeia.

Where is the solution to this mess? Asklepio might ask.

Panakeia would cast her eyes upon the plethora of high technology devices to which patients were attached and the long lists of drugs they were receiving. She would note the spread of diseases inside the hallowed chambers of panacea.

Sister, Panakeia would say in desperation, have you an answer?

And Hygeia would shake her head sadly, whispering, Most of these suffering souls should never have been here in the first place.

— from Betrayal of Trust: The Collapse
of Global Public Health, *by Laurie Garrett*

The Public Health Crisis

In 1996, Canadian scientist Joseph Decosas spoke of the crisis in underdevelopment of a global and local public infrastructure of public health at a gathering of AIDS researchers in Vancouver, Canada.

He held up a glass of water and said, "If the solution for AIDS would be to bring a glass of clean water to everyone in the world, we would not be able to bring it. We have not been able to stop children from dying from simple diarrhea by providing clean drinking water." A global initiative to address loss of life from completely preventable diseases, let alone AIDS, eludes us. It is only in very recent years that vaccination has been implemented in Africa against a resurgence of polio. The monies to fund these public health initiatives have come from private philanthropic foundations and not from a worldwide effort to organize an action against local endemic health hazards. Certainly, the epidemic of HIV infection is a global crisis, as is the resurgence of the poliovirus in Africa. But there are other chronic viral infections, including HPV, EBV, HSV, HBV, and HCV, that claim more lives every year than HIV.[1,2] These epidemics are silent killers.

One of the greater problems existing in global health from nation to nation is the lack of a well-organized global public health policy and infrastructure.[3–6] In a world where people are traveling to almost every corner of the globe, where food from other countries is being imported to the developed world and vice versa, where climate change is driven primarily by the actions of people in Western countries (the North) but currently primarily impacts people in the developing or undeveloped world (the South), where the public health components in even developed countries have become somewhat dilapidated, the spread of chronic viral diseases is becoming a major global concern.[7] Add to this the spread of Western diseases like heart disease, diabetes, and cancer into the developing world as a result of the dissemination of the Western lifestyle and diet via globalization, and the need is obvious for expanding the definition of public health to include these chronic noncommunicable diseases (NCDs), most of which are preventable.

Public health policy and implementation is not sexy. When people remain well, no plaques are handed out for a job well done. And as the United States becomes more and more of a class society, the decision-makers are insulated from danger since they are typically far more wealthy than those citizens in the line of fire of an emerging public health problem. They have elite health coverage on which to fall back. The scramble to gain meager support in the form of government allocations often forces public health agencies to bend to political and other whims just to survive and continue offering the most basic of care for the "underserved" and for the monitoring of those populations and for overall environmental quality.[8] When one looks at the state of international public health policy, the implications are far worse.[9]

The mission of public health no longer has a coherent definition. Medicine and public health have come to be indistinguishable. Public health is not curative medicine but rather is preventive medicine combined with public policy. For example, more than 44 million people in the US are uninsured, and there really is no coherent health care system or public health system that has been defined to begin to solve this major public health problem. Globally, the World Health Organization, once the conscience of global health, lost its way in the 1990s. Corruption, lack of leadership, and demoralization led the WHO away from its stated mission, and other international agencies took its place. Unicef, the World Bank, the International Monetary Fund (IMF), and the Gates Foundation began to be the biggest public health funders in the world. But a global public health policy cannot rely upon the generosity of philanthropy or major financial institutions to drive universal goals and the interpretation and implementation of those goals.[10–13]

Medicine has not been responsible for the vast improvements in public health. Even vaccines and antibiotics — tools of public health — have contributed comparatively little to population-based improvements in life expectancy, infant mortality, and infectious disease deaths.[13A] The bulk of the decline in infectious disease deaths has occurred prior to the age of antibiotics. There is some debate as to what contributed to the spectacular improvements seen in life expectancy and infant mortality in the US and Western Europe between 1700 and 1900. Nutrition, better housing, urban sewage and water systems, government epidemic control measures, road construction and paving, public education and literacy, access to prenatal and maternity care, smaller families, and overall improvements in standards of living and working were all key to these changes.

All of these same tools could be engaged to prevent many cancers. However, the established health care system does not view cancers as a realm of public health because, due to a semantic twist, the word "prevention," is not to be used when it comes to cancers. And the elephant in the room — contamination of the environment — is rarely scrutinized, unless it becomes clearly apparent that a specific contamination is responsible for human disease. Food quality and lifestyle issues, poverty, modern industrialized agriculture, the prepared food industry which uses primarily wheat, corn, sugar, and soy to produce pseudofoods, and industrial contaminants all remain outside of the purview of conventional medicine and public health to date. Even cigarettes, known for years to cause heart disease and almost every form of cancer, are still legal for sale in the US. Public health has always been thought of in terms of protection from biological contaminants, not NCDs. The chemical contaminants that are identified or probable causative factors for many cancers are under the surveillance of the EPA, an agency not specifically set up to protect public health. The EPA, as its name implies, was set up to protect the environment. This separation of human health from environmental health is emblematic of the struggle and confusion in which we now find ourselves.

In the 21st century, the dilemma of global public health seems embedded in the disparity between the rich and the poor, both within and between nations.[14] The alleged pharmacopeia of future disease prevention through biotechnology and protein-based public health does not exist for everyone even within the US. In much of the world, the core advances in public health pioneered between 1890 and 1920 have yet to take hold.[15] It sometimes even appears that the disparities of access to basic food and shelter are consciously engineered or held in place in order to ensure a cheap labor force for the developed world.[16] In the Third World, precious antibiotics are sold on the black market. Water, clean or otherwise, is a precious commodity. Public health infrastructures are left to local governing bodies, even in India — a rich and well-educated democracy. A few good people scramble to organize against epidemic diseases like malaria, diarrheal diseases, and HIV, HBV, and HCV infection. When it comes to cancers, only private and/or nonprofit organizations research environmental causative factors and prevention.

Public health has traditionally been rooted in two basic tenets: the germ theory of disease and the understanding that preventing disease in the weakest elements of society ensures protection for the strongest and the richest in the larger community.[17] Infectious diseases are less of a concern in the wealthy world. In the 21st century, the modern epidemics of cancer and heart disease in the developed world are for the most part nonmicrobial NCDs. And it has become a struggle to apply the basic tenets of public health policy to these collective health issues, because they are often caused by combinations of contaminants, and modern science has yet to develop a good strategy and understanding of how to research their combined impacts. There is a lack of will to interrupt the chemical soup in which we try to live, because these problems mirror the reality of life — they are interconnected in terms of biology and are interconnected between politics, economics, the theory of capitalism, and social and cultural understandings of who matters the most. The gross disparities of wealth and poverty, coupled with the lifestyles of the rich and famous, the capacity to fly almost anywhere, and the influx into the wealthy world of refugees from poverty and resource conflicts have changed the scene for public health not only in the poor countries but also in the wealthy nations. The global movement of refugees has never been as great as it is now.[18] The problems of poverty have been imported into the West, and there is no plan in place to manage the resulting issues that have come home to roost.

The challenges for public health have never been greater, either in the large metropolitan counties of the US or in Russia or in India, Southeast Asia, South America, and China. Although scientific and medical tools invented in the 20th and 21th centuries will help in the global public health efforts, the basic factors essential to a population's health are ancient, unchanging, and nontechnological: clean water; nutritious and uncontaminated food; decent housing for everyone; proper water and waste disposal; social and medical control of epidemics. They also include universal access to maternal and child health care, clean air, knowledge of self-care, and a health care system that follows the maxim of medicine — "First, do no harm." This maxim also means equal access for everyone. These are all essential components of a working public health system.

The Privatization of Public Health Services

The World Health Organization Commission on the Social Determinants of Health stated in 2008 that health inequalities were to be found all over the world — not just in the poorest countries, but even in wealthy countries. "The greater the social disadvantage, the worse the health."[19] There are many reasons for this.

Structural Adjustment Programs (SAPs), enforced by the IMF and World Bank for decades on poor countries, have had a disastrous effect on health. With the economic and Third World debt crisis in the 1970s and 1980s, developing countries were pressured to ensure debt repayment to the rich countries. This meant reducing the standard of living for most of their people. As a consequence of these actions by the IMF and World Bank, there was a drive toward privatization at all costs, the liberalization of capital markets, market-based pricing, and free trade. This meant that poor countries were driven further into poverty, while the costs of food and health services went up as important subsidies were removed, and social unrest came about as the cost of living became unbearable. As barriers to trade were removed the World Trade Organization (WTO) stepped in and the rich countries were favored.[20] It is almost as though the colonization of Third World countries by the West contributed to overall poverty in those countries; this poverty was then addressed by the West; and then the bill was given to the Third World to pay — all of which have contributed to an ongoing cycle of poverty as the Third World struggles to heal.

Despite all of these issues, the IMF recommended privatization of the health systems — a completely inappropriate solution for many poor countries. Studies of postcommunist Eastern European countries and former Soviet countries demonstrated that these IMF economic reform programs resulted in significantly worsened tuberculosis incidence, prevalence, and mortality rate. What had become an almost nonexistent disease found resurgence under the privatization of health systems fostered by the IMF in these countries.

Health is accepted as a fundamental human right, and not a privilege, in the UN Declaration of Human Rights (Article 25, paragraph 1). Therefore, in many of the world's richest countries a solely market-based system for health services is resisted. But, as of 2003, in the US 45 million people were without health insurance. Therefore, if even the richest country in the world continues to struggle with this issue, it is obvious that in poorer countries the struggle is even harder. The privatization of health care creates a two-tier system that reinforces economic and social inequalities across the world. And all of this is based on the World Bank and the IMF continuing even today to push for the privatization of public health services.[21]

As the world becomes in many ways one community, there is no longer "over there." Public health is now a matter of global prevention. And we must have the will to work with other nations to form a global infrastructure of public health networks that serves the here and now of everyone with the understanding that what benefits one will benefit us all. The organization and oversight of global public health must be taken out of the hands of financial institutions and the megawealthy. In the developed world, a world that is seeping and scraping across the globe, the issue of a global public health infrastructure must also include surveillance against industrial and other strategies that destroy and contaminate the land, air, water, and the right to live of all peoples and all species and ecosystems now and into the future.

Intellectual Property Rights and Corporate Profits

Multinational pharmaceutical companies neglect the diseases of the Southern Hemisphere, not because the science is impossible but because there is no profitable market. The market is there in terms of need, as evidenced by the HIV epidemic, which began in Africa — an epidemic that has killed over 50% of people in some African countries. But the market is not there in the sense that, unlike Viagra, an affluent drug for affluent people, the medicines needed in the Southern Hemisphere are needed by poor people in poor countries, where profit would be minuscule or nonexistent. The obligation of pharmaceutical companies to their shareholders demands that, they say, they put their effort into trying to find cures for the diseases of the affluent. Of the thousands of drugs that have been brought to the market in recent years, fewer than 1% are for diseases of poor people.[35] It was only in 2004 that HAART became available in South Africa for treatment of HIV/AIDS.

The issues of patents, access to essential drugs, and allowance for generics in life-threatening situations all go to the heart of the WTO and the global rules made at this organization to accommodate world trade. TRIPS (Trade-Related Aspects of Intellectual Property) is one of the main areas in the WTO agreements. Medicines were included in its patent rules, and some of these rules have come under severe criticism from many developing countries. Concerns have included the monopolization of life-saving drugs for 20 years, risking price increases, and even stifling innovation. Poor countries cannot wait 20 years to enjoy the benefits of important drugs.

The WTO imposed US-style intellectual property rights around the world. These rights were intended to reduce access to generic medicines, and they succeeded. Developing countries paid a high price for this agreement. The poor countries have received nothing in return.[36]

When it comes to the main institutions for cancer eradication and patient advocacy in the US, the CEOs of these organizations appear to play musical chairs between the cancer research industry, the pesticide industry, the chemical industry, the petroleum industry, the cancer drug industry, and patient advocacy organizations.[37,37B] Perhaps this explains how Nixon's war on cancer begun in 1972 has achieved such limited results.

Chronic Viral Infection

EBV and HPV[22]

There are several cancers that are caused by chronic viral infection. EBV (Epstein–Barr virus) is considered responsible for B-cell Burkitt's lymphoma. This cancer is found primarily in children with chronic malarial disease in sub-Saharan Africa and also in some advanced AIDS patients. Chronic malaria depletes the immune system in children to the extent that a ubiquitous virus, EBV, overwhelms the lymph system and causes low-level and persistent inflammation, which in turn causes cancer in the lymph system. In HIV infections, the immune deficiency caused by the virus and opportunistic infections is responsible for this type of lymphoma. EBV has also been found to be causative of several nasopharyngeal cancers (NPCs), cervical cancers, and prostate cancers. Oral cancers are becoming more common in the US. It is assumed that oral sex is the most common means by which EBV is transmitted. HPV (human papilloma virus) is also a main culprit, now found in oral cancers; it is considered a primary causative factor for many oral cancers. We know from HIV/AIDS that chronic viral infections potentiate each other and often become coinfections, each making the impacts of the others worse. Therefore, herpes simplex viruses couple with HPV and EBV especially in patients who are immune-compromised or HIV-positive.[23,24]

HPV has many strains. HPV 16 and 18 are responsible for high-risk cervical intraepithelial neoplasia (CIN), which leads to cervical cancer in women.[25] But there are other strains of HPV — HPV 31, 33, 35, 39, 45, 51, 66 — that are all implicated in cervical cancer. In the world at large, cervical cancer is one of the main killing diseases of women.[26] The rates of cervical cancer have gone down in the developed world, because of highly active health delivery systems making available the PAP smear, the main early screening tool for cervical dysplasia and other abnormalities. But, in the Third World, where health delivery systems are not available or funded or convenient, women do not have early screening as a tool for cervical cancer prevention. It is for these women that Gardisil, a vaccine against the several strains of HPV infection, is intended.

Since HPV is also responsible for anal condylomas which occur as a result of anal sex in both men and women, and for more and more oral cancers, it would seem reasonable and responsible to offer Gardisil[27] to both boys and girls who are not yet infected and to men and women who are not yet infected. The primary vector for spreading HPV is men. Inoculating men and boys against HPV should be a national health mandate. And offering Gardisil to Third World people, men and women, should be a global mandate.

HCV and HBV[28]

Today there are 400 million people worldwide who are living with chronic HBV infection. And 200 million people are living with chronic HCV infection. Together these two forms of chronic hepatitis are responsible for almost all hepatocellular cancers (HCCs) — liver cancers. Worldwide, HCC is the third-largest cause of cancer death.[29] HBV is the most important chronic viral infection in India despite effective vaccine. In that country there are 30 million carriers of HBV. In Brazil, in the state of Amazonas, 60% of the children are infected with HBV by the age of 10. In Brazil, 7.4% of all deaths are due to HBV infection. In the US, 4 million people are infected with HCV that we know of. Today HCV is the main cause of cirrhosis, and liver cancer, and the main reason for liver transplantation. In 1997 alone, 5.8 million people globally were newly infected with HCV. And 590,000 were children under the age of 15. In 2000, 200 million people worldwide were infected with HCV. In Egypt, 20% of the population is HCV+.[30]

Of those infected worldwide, 85% of HCV+ individuals who are initially infected will progress to being chronically infected and 15% of cases will spontaneously resolve over several weeks. HCV can avoid destruction by the body's own immune defenses, and when the infection does not resolve and becomes chronic it leads to inflammation, then to chronic hepatitis and to scarring in the form of liver fibrosis, and then to cirrhosis, and finally to liver failure and/or cancer.[31]

HCV belongs to the *Flaviviridae* family of viruses. It contains RNA genetic material and about 10,000 units of nucleotides organized to serve as a genetic blueprint for the structure and coat or envelope of the virus. There are six major genetic types of HCV that are often geographically distributed. In the US, genotypes 1a and 1b account for 80% of HCV found here. Genotypes 2 or 3 are generally found in people who have come into the US from other parts of the world. Identifying the type of HCV is important, because genotypes 2 or 3 have a better response to treatment with interferon. Genotype 1 does not have as good a response to interferon treatment.[32]

The damage done as a result of HCV infection may not be so much from the virus itself but from injury caused by the interplay between the virus and cytotoxic lymphocytes and specific inflammatory messengers called cytokines. Spread occurs as a result of infected blood or blood products, contaminated needles, and infected organ transplants including infected organs other than livers.[33] In the US, the most common cause of HCV infection is through intravenous drug use, although in the 1980s and 1990s it was mainly through contaminated blood products that went unscreened. Snorting cocaine also carries an increased risk of HCV infection. In new IV drug abusers, 50%–60% are infected in the first six months of drug use, and after one year 90% of IV drug users are positive for HCV. In the developed world, it is the abuse of drugs that is the primary public health issue regarding HCV infection.

HCV can be sexually transmitted but not very efficiently. It has been isolated in semen, vaginal fluids, and saliva. Therefore, it is important not to share razors, toothbrushes, and other hygiene implements because of blood transmission. Only about 1%–4% of HCV infections are transmitted via unprotected sex. Kissing is considered a risk only when there is an open oral wound. And 2%–5% of HCV infection is transmitted in health care workers through needle sticks.[34]

Unfortunately, only about 25% of newly infected people will exhibit any acute symptoms. There may be fatigue, muscle aches, low appetite,[35] and a low-grade fever. There is rarely jaundice. Most HCV+ individuals will remain asymptomatic.[35] As the cytokine injury to the parenchymal tissue of the liver progresses, fibrosis due to inflammation leads to cirrhosis, or scarring, and this results in muscle wasting, general weakness, bruising, fluid retention, lower extremity edema, ascites, internal bleeding due to varices, mental confusion, hepatic encephalopathy, and liver cancer, more or less in that order.[36] B-cell non-Hodgkin's lymphoma is also associated with HCV

Geology of Modern Cancer Epidemic

infection; the B-lymphocytes appear to be excessively stimulated by the virus.

Treatment for HCV infection[37]

There are three pattern responses to treatment for HCV:

- Sustained response — the absence of detectable HCV RNA using RT-PCR or TMA assay for at least six months;
- Relapse — an initial response to treatment but with a detectable level of RNA shortly after treatment ends; this is frequently called a breakthrough;
- Nonresponse — no response to treatment.

The goals of treatment for HCV infection are to:

- Eliminate the viral infection;
- Improve and normalize liver function tests and histology;
- Prevent progression to cirrhosis and liver cancer;
- Prolong survival;
- Improve the quality of life.

Therapy options are somewhat limited: interferon with ribavirin (Rebetol), pegylated interferon, and pegylated interferon with ribavirin. Pegylated interferon is a form of interferon designed to slow the clearance of interferon from the body. This allows the pegylated form to remain in the body longer, working against the virus. Polyethylene glycol (PEG) molecules are attached to interferon, allowing it to remain in the blood for seven days.

In all patients with any of the three types of HCV who were treated with ribavirin and interferon for 48 weeks, there was a 40% reduction in PCR assays of the HCV RNA. In patients undergoing the same regimen who had type 2 or 3 HCV, there was a 60% reduction in PCR levels of the virus.[38]

For nonresponse/relapsers, retreatment and no treatment are currently the only options. In those patients who present with acute

HCV infection, 85% will progress to acute liver disease. In patients who have a liver transplant, there is a universal HCV recurrence in the blood.

HBV[39]

HBV is transmitted blood to blood, through unprotected sex, from nonsterile needles, and from an infected woman to her newborn during delivery. This means that a great many people are at risk — Health workers, IV drug users, people with multiple sex partners, people who adopt a child from a country where HBV infection is high, and even people who share a toothbrush with an infected individual. Fortunately, there is a vaccine available to protect against infection,[40] but much of the Third World does not have access to this vaccine. This makes HBV infection very much an infection related to poverty.[41] And poverty is emblematic of a lack of will for international infrastructures to move toward the equitable distribution of resources, knowledge, and power that would enable an end to this form of human suffering.

Hepatitis B viral infection has a somewhat different course from HCV infection. It can progress from an immune-tolerant phase, in which the immune system ignores the virus, through an immune clearance phase, in which the immune system tries to eliminate the virus, to a quiescent phase, in which the virus is inactive. The course of chronic hepatitis B, however, is variable and relates to several factors, including the patient's age when they are infected. The course of HBV in people who are infected at a young age is quite different from those who are infected as adults. Ultimately, the course, in either case, depends on the balance between the immune system and the virus.

The immune-tolerant phase[42] is especially applicable to individuals infected at a young age. Children born in Southeast Asia, Brazil, and sub-Saharan Africa, for example, are more likely to become HBV-infected as children. The immature immune system of children initially does not recognize or react to HBV. The immune-tolerant phase is due to immaturity of the immune system itself. It may also be due to the virus expressing itself in liver cells during the early years of infection differently than in later years of infection.

During the immune-tolerant phase, little or no damage is done to the liver despite high levels of measurable virus in the body. Liver function tests remain normal and the infected individual remains asymptomatic. This phase can last up to two or three decades. Blood tests during this time reveal HBsAG positivity, HBeAG negativity, and HBV DNA positivity. This phase is generally not seen in individuals who become infected during adulthood, as usually occurs in North America and Western Europe.

The immune clearance phase[43] begins during the third to fourth decade of an infection that started during childhood. The immune system no longer ignores the infection. When an adult acquires an HBV infection, the immune clearance phase begins at the time of infection. In this phase, the immune system attacks and injures the HBV-infected liver cells. The immune system is attempting to clear and/or eliminate the virus. The paradoxical liver injury that results from this attempt leads to elevated liver transaminase levels, especially the ALT and the AST. Liver biopsy may show significant liver injury and inflammation, and the formation of scar tissue — fibrosis and cirrhosis. The severity of liver cell destruction and the duration of this phase determine whether the individual develops significant liver disease or cirrhosis — severe scarring. The more severe the destruction and the longer the phase, the more likely there will be cirrhosis.

The quiescent phase is a dormant phase during which the HBV levels become very low, the blood tests are near-normal, and biopsy reveals few inflamed or injured liver cells. The advanced fibrosis or cirrhosis that developed earlier remains. The individual will almost always remain HBsAG-positive but the markers of viral replication — HbeAB and HBV DNA — become negative and anti-HBe, denoting an inactive state of HBV and a smaller risk of spread.

Occasionally during the quiescent phase, there may be a flare or reactivation of the virus with associated symptoms, abnormal blood tests, and injury to the liver.[44] Disturbance in the balance between the immune system and the virus is the cause. A flare can be severe and result in more damage to the liver. Asian men over the age of 40 are at particular risk for flares. In many of these individuals the disease will progress and result in advanced or end-stage cirrhosis with the complication of liver cancer.

Most people with HBV infection have an insidious progression to cirrhosis. Many do not even know that this is occurring. Once cirrhosis is present, the risk of developing the primary complications of portal hypertension, fluid retention, hepatic encephalopathy, or bleeding is about 20%–25% over five years. The risk of developing primary liver cancer is about 200–300 times higher than in healthy individuals who have no HBV infection.[45]

HBV-infected people who have a brief and mild immune clearance phase before moving into the quiescent phase tend to do very well. They have normal liver function tests and are asymptomatic. These people are called healthy carriers of HBV.[46] Healthy carriers can transmit HBV to other people. The risk of HBV carriers developing cirrhosis and HCC is very small, although slightly higher than in people without HBV infection. In some healthy carriers who were infected as adults, there may be a seroconversion with no signs of HBV infection.

Chinese Medicine[47]

HBV and HCV infections enter the body differently than does HAV, which enters orally. Entry via the *Ying* and *blood levels* is a slightly different phenomenon and by its very nature eliminates the pathway through the outer defensive layers. The early symptomatic presentation, when observed, indicates, that there may be for some an entry through the *Qi level*. HCV does not manifest like a *warm disease*. Common presentations of a person with *heat in the exterior and interior* would include:

- Sweating;
- The body feels heavy;
- Very sleepy;
- Dry nasal passages;
- A dry throat with difficulty in vocalizing;
- Possibly delirium.

In the case of chronic hepatitis, these symptoms will present much later, even decades later, and are a result of the damage done by the *latent pathogenic factor* (LPF) and the body's response to it. When one is treating *warm diseases*, great care needs to be taken not to damage the *Yin*, because this will result in serious complications. In chronic hepatitis, when it becomes symptomatic, the apparent *Yin* deficiency is not due to an internal deficiency but to a *latent pathogen smoldering* in the *Ying* and *blood levels*. This smoldering may cause *Yin deficiency* or the patient may have a *Yin-deficient* constitution that acts like a magnet for the LPF. However, the *Yin deficiency* is not the primary issue in terms of treatment. Although the pathogen eventually enters the blood, there are no rashes, bleeding, or other signs of *heat* (including a red tongue). HBV and HCV infections are "*Yin* diseases" and are caused by LPFs. A *damp toxin* causes *damp* stasis and the formation of *phlegm* with *toxin* accumulation and the obstruction of *Yang*. Or a *heat* toxin enters the *Ying* or blood level with a similar affect. The *damp toxin* that enters in HBV or HCV infection is not the same *damp toxin* that enters in HAV infection; and this *damp toxin* acts differently. The *heat toxin* that enters is not well treated with *Yin*-nourishing herbs.

Latent pathogenic factors

The *Shang Han Lun* first mentioned the concept of latent pathogens when discussing the six stages.[48] The *Wen Bing Tiao Ben* evolved the concept into a more formalized discussion within the theory of *warm diseases* and the four levels.[49] *San Jiao* theory also speaks about latent pathogens and how to release them from the interior.

There are several terms that are used to describe stuck pathogens[50]:

- *Fu* refers to a latent, dormant, deep-lying pathogen that is barely perceptible. It is also used to describe abdominal masses and normal lymph nodes.
- *Fu Qi* refers to a *latent pathogen* that can emerge later, long after exposure to the pathogen.

- *Fu Qi Wen Bing* refers to interior latent diseases caused by a pathogen that obstructs the *Qi* mechanism: The pathogen sits until a later season, when it emerges or when another pathogenic event causes it to emerge to the surface.

Latent pathogens can be *heat, cold,* or *damp–heat pathogens. Heat,* as a pathogenic influence (EPI), elicits a fever caused by the *Wei Qi* battling with the pathogen. A sore throat in the *taiyang layer* manifests when there is an attack by *heat* in the superficial level; chills due to obstruction, a rapid and floating pulse, and a tongue that is normal are all signs and symptoms of a *heat pathogen.* However, a trapped *warm pathogen* elicits a low-grade fever with low-grade *heat* signs or none at all. The tongue will be red, with no coating or a thick, dry, sticky, and yellow coating. There may be thirst due to lingering *heat* and scorching of fluids. In fact, it may look like *Yin deficiency* but is not.

Etiology[51]

There are two routes of manifestation:

- A pathogen can enter the body, manifest a few brief signs, and move into the interior, where it may lie dormant; or it may emerge due to proper treatment or the body's own immune response;
- A *wind invasion* with an acute pathogen enters the body and is not expelled and sinks to the *Ying* or a deeper level.

Some people are predisposed to susceptibility to a *latent pathogen:*

- A weak constitution predisposes and may be at the level of the *jing* or via acquired constitutional injuries;
- Related to the above — poor self-care leads to a weak constitution or a moment of indisposition;
- An individual does not rest when sick but pushes through the illness, limiting the body's ability to heal itself;

- Increased use or overuse or improper use of herbs/supplements/ pharmaceuticals like antibiotics allows a portion of the pathogen to remain without being expelled.

Early-stage pathogens enter the *exterior* and are dispersed through the *exterior*. If the wrong treatment is utilized, especially treatment that cools the *interior*, then the intervention itself drags the pathogen inward. The treatment may have cleared the exterior symptoms but the pathogen remains. For example, antibiotics (*cold* in nature) have side effects that include gastrointestinal dysfunction, dizziness due to *cold–damp–phlegm*, and other *damp–phlegm* accumulations like candidiasis. Many of these antibiotics are contraindicated when kidney disease is present. Given their purpose and nature, Chinese medical theory considers antibiotics to be generally bitter and *cold*. Their side effects injure the *Qi* mechanism of the *lung, spleen, stomach, bladder,* and *kidney*. The *Qi* and *Yang* of the *spleen* and *kidney* is impaired. The patient appears to recover because the *heat* is cleared, but the *cold* nature of the drugs causes the original pathogen to smolder internally, thus injuring the *Yin*. This is why *LPFs* often look like deficiency *heat*. However, although the *Yin* is scorched, it is not the key. The root is a *heat* pathogen and the scorched *Yin* is the branch.

The pathogen can emerge symptomatically more easily when the resistance is low or when another pathogen enters to exacerbate the deeper level of injury. This mechanism of action may explain why HBV and HCV have periods of quiescence with flares and an ongoing progression that can remain asymptomatic for even decades. Combined HBV and HCV is called HEV, and viral cofactors in some patients make for an exceedingly complex treatment terrain, mainly because these patients are being treated with so many different antiviral drugs for each infection. The side effect picture becomes very complicated.

Predisposing factors

Why are some individuals able to resolve their infection without treatment? Given that many people may not know that they were ever exposed to and infected with HCV or HBV, if they do resolve these infections spontaneously, we may never be aware of their history to share and allow analysis. But the following predispositions may help in this quandary within the context of Chinese medicine:

- A Yin-*deficient* constitution tends toward *empty heat* which attracts inwardly unresolved pathogens.
- *Spleen deficiency* leads to a propensity for damp accumulations, and dampness can attract or transform external pathogens to *wind–dampness*, which in turn can lead to *damp–heat* in the interior.
- *Qi* stasis also generates *heat* and stasis, and can initiate a vicious circle.
- Diet can lead to *phlegm–heat, dampness,* and *damp–heat.* Alcohol, spicy foods, too much sugar and refined foods which raise blood glucose levels and increase insulin spikes all lead to internal conditions that act like glue for latent pathogens.

Diagnostic guidelines

LPFs are interior and, therefore, have no *exterior* signs or symptoms. Their direction is interior and as they resolve they move to *the exterior.* The symptoms are those of internal *heat* and steaming of the *yin* with damage leading to *dryness.* The *interior* refers to the *Qi, Ying,* or *blood levels.* At the *Qi* level we are looking at symptoms or signs that reside in the *lung, stomach, gallbladder, urinary bladder,* or intestines. At the *Ying* or *blood level* we are looking at signs and symptoms that reside in the *kidney, heart,* or *liver.*

Heat or *lingering heat* combines easily with *damp–heat.* Watching for this is essential and can become a clue for treatment. If the *kidney Yin* is nourished, the pathogen will be tonified. Therefore, nourishing *Yin* is the wrong treatment for *LPFs.* Determination of what *Yin deficiency* is and what an *LPF* is can be done through taking a very careful history of the patient. An example is "This all started when I went on a trip to Barbados, or "when I started using heroin," or "when I started that relationship with so-and-so." If such a clear historical demarcation is not available, treatment can either confirm or deny your diagnosis. *Yin*-nourishing techniques that do not resolve the condition confirm that *Yin deficiency* is not the root. Compliant treatment for two weeks without a 30% improvement implies that you are treating the patient incorrectly. If treatment is stopped and all previous symptoms return, the diagnosis and treatment are wrong.

Treating chronic hepatitis infection that is asymptomatic may require the use of conventional medical measurements of the viral load. Also, liver function tests (LFTs) will be essential in understanding the efficacy of your treatment. If you are treating alongside conventional agents, like interferon and ribavirin, then the side effects of those drugs must be taken into account. Enabling a patient to continue to undergo antiviral treatment with these drugs may enable them to live longer and with better health. Chinese herbal medicine may potentiate the treatment with these agents by allowing the patient to remain on them longer, by increasing the antiviral effect of the agents, and by protecting normal liver cells.

Laboratory tests for monitoring

Prodromal phase

- Aminotransferase elevations are the hallmark of HCV infection.[52] The AST and the ALT are high in the prodromal phase, peak before maximum jaundice, and then fall slowly in the recovery phase. They are typically 500–2000 IU/L and the ALT is usually less than the AST (normal values rarely exceed 300 IU/L). High levels of either enzyme show activity of HCV and not the amount of disease damage.[53]
- Urinary bile usually precedes jaundice. The WBCs will be in the low range and a smear test will show atypical lymphocytes. Anti-HCV serum antibodies will appear several weeks after infection and after this phase.
- Albumin under 3.5 shows liver inflammation, cirrhosis, and edema.
- The alkaline phosphatase level, called ALP or alk phos, is in the normal range when between 50 and 135. If high it indicates a bile duct problem or obstruction. The GGT is normal when between 15 and 85. If high it indicates a bile duct problem also.

- The alpha feto protein (AFP) is normal when under 25. If it is over 20, however, there is a high risk of liver cancer.
- Ammonia is in the normal range when between 11 and 35. When high and combined with a presentation of mental confusion, it indicates hepatic encephalopathy.
- Bilirubin is within normal limits when under 1.0. Higher levels will usually accompany jaundice. Bilirubin is measured in a conjugated and an unconjugated form. High unconjugated levels of it probably indicate fibrosis and cirrhosis.
- The BUN refers to kidney function and has a normal range of 7–18. It is possibly low in cirrhosis and liver failure.
- Total cholesterol within normal limits is below 200. Low cholesterol, for example 130, indicates cirrhosis. High cholesterol may indicate bile duct blockage.
- Creatinine levels also refer to kidney function. The normal range is between .6 and 1.3. The later stage of liver disease will manifest higher creatinine levels.
- The normal limit for ferritin, which indicates iron storage levels in the body, is between 15 and 200. This can be high in HCV infection.
- INR has a normal range of 0.9–1.1. High levels indicate prolonged coagulation time.
- Platelets range between 140,000 and 440,000 when normal. Low platelets indicate cirrhosis.
- The WBCs are normal between 4 and 10, and can be low in the presence of portal HTN.

Using these guidelines for normal blood values, the practitioner can evaluate the status and treatment efficacy in an asymptomatic HCV+ patient. All of these study guidelines can be found at the Hopkin website on HCV infection.[54]

Treatment guidelines for LPFs

Identifying the *level* where the *latent pathogen* is residing is very important. The possibilities include the *Qi level*, and the *Ying* and *blood levels.* There are many herbs that are used to vent the *pathogenic Qi* to the *exterior.* They include:

* *Bo he,*
* *Lian Qiao,*
* *Sang ye,*
* *Dan dou chi,*
* *Jin Yin hua,*
* *Ge gen.*

Eliminate the pathogenic *heat* to the *Qi level* — this means *heat* in the *lungs, spleen, gallbladder, urinary bladder,* or intestines. Choose herbs or techniques that address the correct organ. Measure the *zheng Qi* versus the *pathogenic Qi.* Generally, the *zheng Qi* is weakened before exposure, then weakened again by pharmaceutical drug therapies, and then again by the *lingering pathogen.* Therefore, it is important to nourish and strengthen the *zheng Qi.* This makes the *heat-clearing* treatment different from that to which we are accustomed when treating an EPI. Herbs like *huang Qi, xi yang shen,* and *dang shen* can be used. No *Yin*-nourishing herbs should be used. But herbs that clear deficiency *heat* are not contraindicated. Neutral temperature *Qi* tonic herbs are also used, including *tai zi shen.* *Deficiency-heat-clearing herbs* include *sheng di, xuan shen,* and *zhi mu.* If the pathogenic *Qi* is resolved, then and only then is it all right to go back and nourish the *Yin.* However, if the pathogen is cleared on its own in a relatively short period of time, then the Yin should recover on its own. This is unlikely in a chronic hepatitis patient at the present time. And it indicates that the sooner we treat patients who are newly infected, the better the outcomes. The outcome will depend on how long the *LPF* has been present and how much organ damage has been done.

Qi-level treatment

An acute pathogen that goes to the *Qi level* will manifest as a vigorous fever. Locating the organ affected, usually the *lung* or *large Intestine,* leads us to proper treatment strategies. When a patient does not rest to recover from the pathogen, it becomes a *lingering patho-gen* that is not entirely expelled from the body. When lingering, a pathogen will elicit symptoms that include a low-grade fever, chest constraint, a sore throat that comes and goes, thirst, dry mouth and lips, and insomnia. This can look like chronic fatigue syndrome. It can also appear to be deficiency *heat* but is not; this is evidenced by a pulse that is rapid but deficient.

The *wen bing* school uses phrases like "out-thrusting" of *internal lingering heat*. Special herbs are used to accomplish this. They include *dan dou chi, ge gen, bo he, xuan shen*, and *bai shao*. A formula used to clear lingering *heat* from the *Qi level* is *huang qing tang*.[55] This *lingering heat* is sometimes called "spring warmth." It is a pathogen that comes in the spring, when the patient's *zheng Qi* is weak because they did not replenish the root in the winter. The pathogen gets trapped in the *Qi level*, and the manifestation is mild rather than vigorous. This kind of presentation can happen in modern times as a result of travel from a *cold* climate to a warm climate and then a return to the *cold* climate. The adjustment in a weak constitution contributes to a mild *lingering heat pathogen* in the *Qi level*.

Damp–heat in the *Qi level* is also a common presentation. The body feels heavy and there is body aching, chest oppression, and afternoon feverishness. Damp obstructs the clear *Yang* and this causes a disturbance in the ascending and descending functions. The tongue is sticky, with a thin white or yellow coating. The pulse is thin because of fluid damage but also soggy due to *dampness*. There is aversion to cold due to *Yang* obstruction by *dampness*. Antibiotics injure the *Yin–Yang* balance. There is *spleen* damage due to cold. So here the *damp–heat* issues from the treatment with antibiotics. What was once a climatic event has become an iatrogenic event. The cold damage leads to *spleen* injury, which in turn leads to damp and then to *damp–heat*. This occurs especially in a person with a *spleen-deficient* constitution. *San ren tang*[56] is the formula of choice, because it resolves *damp–heat* and leads the *heat* to the *exterior*. It is important to add herbs that tonify the *zheng qi*. In this case, the sweetness of *huang qi* contributes to *dampness*, and so *dang shen* is a better choice.

Another example: *Yin Qiao San*[57] is the typical formula to clear *wind–heat* from the *wei level*. This formula can be modified to treat *lung heat* or *heat* in the *Qi level*. It is specific to the respiratory system. Herbs can be added to modify: *jie geng* opens the *Qi* mechanism of the lung; *sheng di, mud an pi,* and *xuan shen* clear *deficiency heat*. To clear *Qi level heat*, one can add *shi gao, dan zhu ye,* and *zhi mu*. If a patient is being treated for chronic sinusitis that has been treated with multiple courses of antibiotics over a longer period of time, then *cang er zi san*[58] can added to the above formula. To this formula herbs that tonify the *zheng qi* can be added: *huang qi* or *xi yang shen*. Another approach to the same problem could be to use *cang er zi san* and add *yu ping feng san*.[59] This combination treats the overall *LPF* and the presentation.

Shaoyang damp–heat

Damp–heat becomes obstructed in the *shaoyang* and manifests symptomatically as fever, chills, a smoldering sensation in the late afternoon (not a deficiency type of malar flush), sweating as the sun rises but which stops later in the early morning hours, sweating which is in only a small amount because *dampness* obstructs (the sun rising is *Yang* and empowers that *heat* aspect of the *damp–heat*), agitation, and thirst. Earaches may also be present. When treated with antibiotics these earaches may appear to resolve but the patient will retain a kind of dizziness. This is due to the *LPF* remaining because the pathogen was not released outward but became obstructed in the *shaoyang level*. This is not uncommon in childhood chronic earaches where antibiotic therapies have exacerbated the condition, creating an *LPF* stuck in the *shaoyang*.

Qing hao is a special herb for *LPFs*, because it vents *heat* outward, clears deficiency fevers, and acts like a damp curtain for the wind to waft through, thus clearing the *heat* in a very mild way. It is the chief herb in the formula *hao qin qing long tang*.[60] In the theory of the six stages we would use *xiao chai hu tang* but this formula is not very cooling. *Hao qin qing long tang* contains:

- *Qing hao* — vents *heat* outward;
- *Huang qin* — clears *shaoyang heat;*

- *Zhu ru*;
- *Ban xia*;
- *Zhi ke* — transforms damp–*heat* in the *shaoyang level*;
- *Chen pi*;
- *Fu shen* — calms;
- *Gan cao*;
- *Hua shi* — clears *heat* from the *Qi level* via the *bladder*;
- *Qing dai*.

Ying-level LPFs

The construction aspect (*Ying level*) helps form blood, which then circulates in the vessels to the organs, especially the deeper viscera. *Ying-level LPFs* are generally not differentiated from blood-level LPFs. They are taken as a unit. The injury is to the *heart, kidney*, and *liver*. Trapped *heat* in this layer can manifest as mental disturbance, night sweats, agitation, restlessness, a red tongue with no coating, and a fine and rapid pulse that may be deep. This presentation is easily confused with *Yin deficiency*. If the *Yin* is nourished, there will be no change. A good history will help determine whether or not an *LPF* is present. In the case of HBV and HCV infection that has been identified via blood chemistries and PCR *assay*, one cannot assume that this *Ying-level* presentation will be identifiable until later in the infection, when the infection is advanced and more *liver* damage has occurred. However, similar treatment strategies are used even when patients are asymptomatic.

In this level of trapped *heat, or LPF*, there will be no *Qi-level* symptoms. Treatment involves the use of a combination of formulas. A base formula is *Qing hao bie jia tang*[61]:

- *Qing hao*;
- *Bie jia* — goes with *Qing hao* to deeper levels and moves or vents outward;
- *Sheng di*;
- *Zhi mu*;
- *Mu dan pi*.

The above formula tonifies and clears deficiency *heat*. Add it to the following formula of *Qing wen bai du yin*[62]:

- *Shi gao* — the following three herbs clear *heat* from the *Qi level*:
- *Zhi mu*;
- *Dan zhu ye*;
- *Xi jiao* — substitute *shui niu jiao* times 10; it clears *blood heat*;
- *Sheng di*;
- *Dan pi*;
- *Chi shao*;
- *Xuan shen* — this and the above three herbs clear *Ying-level heat*;
- *Huang lian*;
- *Huang qin* — these two herbs clear *Qi-level heat*;
- *Lian qiao* — vents *heat* to the exterior.

The combination of these two formulas clears *heat*, clears *deficiency heat*, and clears deeper level *heat pathogens* that are difficult to clear. This is done by clearing the *heat pathogen* at the trapped level and by clearing the *heat pathogen* by lifting it to a ventable level.

In addition, there are possibly wind issues that arise from trapped *heat*. When these *LPFs* obstruct heat in the *Ying* or *blood levels*, the injury is primarily to the *liver* and *kidney*. *Kidney* injury can result in the *kidney water* failing to nourish the *liver wood*, and this can evolve into wind. This kind of wind is called *wind stirring*. It is not due to extreme *heat* but rather an emptiness pattern. It may manifest as twitching and low-grade tremors or fasciculations rather than convulsions or stroke or more severe symptoms of internal wind. Mineral herbs are commonly added in this presentation of wind stirring, because they nourish the *kidney* and *liver* and help anchor the *Yang*.

The main principles in treating all *LPFs* are to:

(1) Dispel the *heat toxin* pathogen;
(2) Tonify the *zheng qi*.

HBV and HCV infection

The mechanism begins primarily in the spleen and progresses to liver and kidney failure. Following is a schematic for the progression of chronic hepatitis:

Acute →	Chronic →	Fibrosis and cirrhosis →	HCC →	Encephalitis
=	=	=	=	=
Damp–heat	Sp/Lv Yin and blood	Blood stasis due to damp–heat in blood level	Blood stasis with toxin	Lv/K failure

Comparison of HBV and HCV by Chinese medicine diagnosis

	HBV	HCV
Damp–heat LPF	41%	26%
Blood stasis	1%	12%
Liver and kidney Yin deficiency	15%	8%
Liver Qi stasis with Sp Qi deficiency	42%	54%
Sp and K Yang deficiency	1%	1%

Strategies for treatment

Strategies for treatment depend on the type of virus and the stage of the infection, and therefore the presentation of the patient. Treating an asymptomatic patient who has yet to develop symptoms or who is in the quiescent phase is highly valuable but also difficult. Conventional treatments are toxic and carry many side effects. Some patients cannot manage these side effects and opt out of treatment with ribavirin and interferon. Others may chose to do combined care using Chinese medicine to treat the side effects of conventional agents and also enhance that treatment by utilizing Chinese herbs that have antiviral effects. How these two systems combine to improve outcomes will depend on the ability of the practitioner to read the diagnostic pattern in the patient. The following are possible diagnostic patterns for chronic hepatitis:

(1) *Damp–heat in the stomach–spleen axis*
	Rx: *Bu huang jing zheng qi san*,[63] *yin chen hao tang*[64]

(2) *Damp–heat in the liver/gallbladder*
	Rx: *Long dan xie gan*[65] *wan* or *qing gan cao*

(3) *Qi stasis in the spleen and liver*
	Rx: *Chai hu shu gan san*[66] with *liver*-predominant symptoms,
		Xiang sha zhi zhu[67] *wan* with *spleen*-predominant symptoms,
		Xiao yao san

(4) *St/Sp deficiency*
	Rx: *Gui shao liu jun zi tang*

(5) *Liver Yin deficiency*
	Rx: *Yi guan jian*[68]

(6) *Blood stasis in the liver/spleen*
	Rx: *Dang gui huo xue san* or *xue fu zhu yu tang*,[69]
	Tao hong si wu tang jia jian[70]

(7) *Spleen and kidney Yang deficiency*
	Rx: *Wen zhong jian pi zhi gu tang*

There are some herbs that are contraindicated for use with interferon. They are primarily *chai hu* and milk thistle. Since *chai hu* is ·contained in some of the above formulas, substitutes need to be used. A good substitute for *chai hu* is *gotu kola*. *Chai hu* and milk thistle can be used at other times in treatment for chronic hepatitis when interferon is not being used.

The following herbs are *liver*-protective, because they either nourish *liver Yin*, clear *liver heat*, or regulate the *liver blood*:

- *Chai hu,*
- *Milk thistle,*
- *Han lian cao,*
- *Haung qin,*

- *Zhi zi,*
- *Yin chen hao,*
- *Gou qi Zi,*
- *Yu jin.*

The following herbs are antiviral for HBV or HCV:

- *Da qing ye,*
- *Pu gong ying,*
- *Ban lan gen,*
- *Zi cao,*
- *Di er cao,*
- *Hu zhong,*
- *Ban zhi lian.*

The following herbs vitalize the *liver blood*:

- *Dan shen,*
- *Ji xue teng,*
- *Ba yue zha.*

Patterns, symptoms, treatment principles

(1) *Liver/gallbladder damp–heat*

- Sx — bright-yellow face and sclera, fever, costal pain, jaundice, bitter taste;
- Pulse — wiry or wiry and sliipery;
- Tongue — red body with a yellow greasy coating;
- Treatment principle — clear *damp–heat*, and regulate the *liver* and *gallbladder;*
- Points — Lv 14, Gb 24, Du 9, *da nang xue,* Lv 3, Bl 18, Bl 19.

(2) *Spleen damp–heat*

- Sx — jaundice, abdominal pain, nausea, loose foul-smelling stools, fever, anorexia;
- Pulse — slippery and fast;

- Tongue — a red body with a greasy coating;
- Treatment principle: — clear *damp–heat* and tonify the *spleen*;
- Points — Lv 13, Sp 9, St 36, Bl 20, Bl 21, St 44, Gb 34.

(3) *Spleen damp–cold*

- Sx — a sallow face, abdominal pain, nausea, undigested food in stools, feels cold even with fever, anorexia;
- Pulse — slippery and tight;
- Tongue — a pale body with scallops and a white greasy coating;
- Treatment principle — clear *dampness*, and warm and tonify the *spleen*;

- Points — Needle — Sp 3, Bl 20, Bl 21; moxa — Sp 6, Sp 9, CV 12, CV 4, St 36, Du 4.

(4) *Liver Qi stasis — excess type*

- Sx — PMTS, fatigue, hypochondrium pain, abdominal fullness, nausea, gas with bloating, elevated liver enzymes, hepatomegaly, splenomegaly;
- Pulse — wiry and forceful;
- Tongue — a purple body with a thin white coating;
- Treatment principle — move and regulate *liver Qi*, and tonify the *spleen*;
- Points — Lv 14, CV 12, CV 13, Bl 18, Bl 19, four gates.

(5) *Spleen Qi deficiency*

- Sx — fatigue, abdominal tenderness, nausea, anorexia, muscle weakness, loose stools;
- Pulse — soft, soggy, moderate, weak, or slippery;
- Tongue — pale and swollen, with tooth marks; a wet thick coating;
- Treatment principle — tonify the *spleen* and transform *dampness*;
- Points — needle — Sp 3, Sp 6, Bl 20, Bl 21, Sp 9; moxa — CV 12, CV 4, St 36.

(6) *Liver Yin deficiency*

- Sx — dry eyes, dry throat, brittle nails with lines, fatigue, blurred vision, dizziness, muscle spasms, numbness on some extremity channels, red cheeks and eyes, irritability;
- Pulse — thready and rapid;
- Tongue — redder edges;
- Treatment principle — nourish *liver* and *kidney Yin* if the *LPF* and resulting hepatitis is at a stage where it makes sense to nourish Yin;
- Points — Lv 2, Ht 8, K 7, Gb 40, Bl 18, Bl 23, Sp 6, Lv 3, Lv 8, K 10.

(7) *Overall systemic Qi deficiency*

- Sx — fatigue, bruising, bleeding, leg edema, ascites;
- Pulse — soft, soggy, weak, or slippery;
- Tongue — pale, with a swollen body;
- Treatment principle — nourish blood, and tonify the *spleen* and *kidney*;
- Points — Bl 20, Bl 23, Sp 10, Lv 14, Lv 13, Gb 24.

(8) *Blood stasis*

- Sx — signs and symptoms of liver cancer, stabbing pain, abdominal pain with movement, symptoms that are worse in the night, a dark face, cyanosis of the lips, spider veins;
- Pulse — choppy and wiry;
- Tongue — a purple body with ecchymosis;
- Treatment principle — move blood and regulate *liver Qi*;
- Points — Bl 17, 18, 19, Lv 13, Lv 14, SJ 6.

The side effects of interferon and ribavirin treatment can be quite severe. Liver and kidney function tests (LKFTs) can be abnormal as a result of treatment. They need to be monitored and evaluated within the context of Chinese medicine. Treating those side effects can allow a patient to remain on primary cytotoxic treatment. Other side effects include unclear thinking and depression. These can be easily treated with Chinese medicine. Fibrosis is also a result of treatment and not only of the infection. The signs of fibrosis are:

- High bilirubin levels — these are indicative of *damp–heat* in the *liver*, *damp–heat* in the *spleen*, and *damp–cold* in the *spleen*;
- Low blood glucose — indicative of *spleen Qi deficiency* and/or *blood deficiency*;
- Low albumin — indicates *San Jiao* disharmony and *kidney/spleen deficiency*;
- High ammonia — can indicate a *shen* disturbance;
- Low cholesterol — indicates *kidney deficiency*;
- An abnormal INR — indicates that the *spleen* is not holding the blood in the vessels, and/or sinking *spleen Qi*.

Ascites is another result of HCV or HBV infection that is advanced. It is secondary to portal HTN and may also be caused by interferon. In Chinese medicine this is due to *spleen Qi deficiency*, *spleen Yang deficiency*, or *San Jiao* disharmony. Moxa on CV 9 will help resolve or stabilize ascites. Ascites can lead to other conditions:

- Bacterial peritonitis — caused by *toxic heat* or *damp–heat*;
- Gastrointestinal bleeding — due to varices from the *spleen* not holding the blood in the vessels this may cause *blood stasis*;
- High estrogen levels — due to *liver Qi stasis* and *kidney deficiency*;
- Spider veins — from *Yin deficiency* and/or the *spleen* failing to hold in the blood.

Encephalopathy is caused by *heart blood deficiency*, *heart fire*, or *spleen* and *kidney deficiency*. Muscle wasting or cachexia is due to *spleen Qi* deficiency or *spleen Yin deficiency* (a precursor of *spleen Yang deficiency*). Finally, *liver* cancer is caused by *blood deficiency* leading to *blood stasis*.

Jaundice is rarely seen in chronic liver infection with these viruses.

Liver cirrhosis

(1) *Qi stasis from damp accumulation*

- Sx — distension in the abdomen, tympanites, subcostal distension, anorexia, better after belching or passing gas;
- Pulse — bowstring;
- Tongue — white greasy fur;
- Treatment principle — regulate *Qi*, relieve distension, and transform *damp*;
- Rx — Li *qi chu zhang zhi gu tang*.

(2) *Entanglement of Qi and fluid*

- Sx — marked abdominal distension and fullness but flaccid, decreased urination, a bitter taste, a dry mouth;
- Pulse — sinking and bowstring;
- Tongue — a dark body with thin yellow fur;
- Treatment principle — regulate *Qi*, vitalize blood, clear *heat*, and drain fluid;
- Rx — *li qi tong luo li shui tang*.

(3) *Retention of fluid/damp*

- Sx — a distended abdomen with a firm tympanic surface, *restless heat* symptoms, a bitter taste, decreased urinary output, hard and marble stools;
- Pulse — wiry and rapid;
- Tongue — thick yellow greasy fur;
- Treatment principle — promote urination and expel fluid, vitalize blood, and circulate *Qi*;
- Rx — *Huo xue xing qi zhu shui tang*.

(4) *Confined entanglement of damp–heat*

- Sx — restless *heat*, a bitter taste, thirsty but cannot drink, jaundice, concentrated dark urine, constipation with dry stools;

- Pulse — wiry and rapid;
- Tongue — a yellow greasy coating;
- Treatment principle — attack and expel evil fluid;
- Rx — *Da jig an sui qian hua san.*

(5) *Hepatosplenomegaly with retention of fluid*

- Sx — a distended and enlarged abdomen with ascites that is hard and firm, intolerable urgency of urine, venous (*luo*) dilation, a dull black facial complexion, cyanotic lips;
- Pulse — thready;
- Tongue — purple, with dark spots;
- Treatment principle — crack the blood, open the *luo* vessels, and drain fluid;
- Rx — *Huo xue tong luo li shui tang.*

Supplement therapies for HCV

- Magnesium,
- Zinc picolinate,
- Vitamin A,
- Vitamin E succunate,
- Vitamin buffer,
- B12 and folic acid,
- Aqueous liver extract,
- Lecithin,
- Flax oil,
- CoQ10,
- Evening primrose oil.

Diet

The general caloric needs of an HCV-positive patient are higher than normal. Whatever the caloric intake should be for the individual's body weight should be multiplied by about 1.4. The protein intake should also increase by 0.5–0.7. With encephalopathy the protein intake should decrease to 0.5 g/kg. Soy protein should be decreased and instead the following should increase: rice, whey, vegetables, legumes, and whole grains.

Iron increases oxidative damage and this is true of cancer as well. Therefore, reduced intake of iron is appropriate with HCV and should be eliminated in all cancer patients. In HCV infection, eliminate red meat and the patient should take no vitamin C with iron. The body stores iron as the liver moves toward cirrhosis.

Bile salts decrease in concentration and this leads to fat malabsorption. This means that fat-soluble vitamins are also malabsorbed.

Insulin resistance increases in HCV infection before the onset of cirrhosis and fatty liver. Vitamin E 1200 IU daily, Betine 20 mg daily from beets, and magnesium 500 mg daily will help prevent insulin resistance in an HCV-positive patient.

Vitamin A storage is altered and over 10,000 IU daily may be toxic. Use beta-carotene 150,000 IU daily instead, or use mixed carotenoids.

Fats should be decreased. Trans fats should be completely eliminated for everyone, regardless of health status. Omega-3 fatty acids should be 20%–30% of fat intake. More than 2 g daily may be difficult to assimilate if there are digestive difficulties.

Ascites is a condition where lymph fluid leaks into the abdominal cavity. Salt should be reduced when this condition is present. Also, processed foods that are commonly high in salt, fats, and sugar should be eliminated.

Encephalopathy occurs in 50%–70% of cirrhosis patients and is caused by elevated ammonia levels in the brain from bacterial fermentation of proteins in the gut with liver cirrhosis. The cirrhotic liver cannot metabolize ammonia, and this circulates to the brain, where it causes swelling. The symptoms of encephalopathy include sleep disturbance, personality changes, speech disturbances, poor muscular coordination, tremors, muscle rigidity, and postural changes.

Treatment for this condition in HCV infection is reduction in protein intake — the body weight times 0.23–0.34. Reduction in lactolose is also important, otherwise it will cause diarrhea. L-ornithine/L-asparate at 6 g twice daily, *Enterococcus faecium* 6 g thrice daily, and lactobacillus acid at ¼–½ teaspoonfuls between meals three times daily will help in managing encephalopathy.

Antioxidants:

- Glutathione — to aid in detoxification lost when HCV+ = 10 g daily;
- Silymarin — 2 g twice daily at 80% standard extract when not on interferon;
- Alpha-lipoic acid (ALA) — improves glutathione levels 450–1200 mg daily;
- Selenium — levels are reduced by up to 40% in HCV; 200 mcg yeast-based Se;
- Zinc — reduced levels in HCV+; helps to transform ammonia 200–400 mg daily between meals (citrated not chelated);
- Vitamin E — 400–1200 IU daily (gamma-tocopherol only, and not with coumadin and not with a vitamin K deficiency);
- SAMe — normalizes bile secretions; 800–1000 mg daily.

Conclusions

The worldwide epidemic of chronic viral infection has been happening primarily in the developing world. However, the modern movement of people across the globe, if for no other reason, demands that a global public health system be instituted. In the developed world, and especially in the US, the problem of drug addiction is also a major public health problem, not only for the US but also for all of those countries that are part of the supply end of this epidemic. The result of illegal drug abuse is not only loss of health from addiction and spread of viral disease but also loss of life due to violence. The disruption of normal life due to the drug trade is an epidemic in and of itself. All of these issues intersect and are driven by poverty. Poverty is the No. 1 issue of life on the Earth, and until it is addressed these issues of chronic disease will persist even in the midst of plenty.

Cancer has many causes, including chronic viral infection, immune deficiency, other chronic diseases, and exposures to environmental contaminants. Ultimately, all of these causes, infectious and otherwise, fall into the sphere of public health and global health. In the developed world, cancer is primarily caused by lifestyle, poor dietary habits, and environmental contamination. In the developing and underdeveloped world, the causes of cancer are primarily chronic viral infection, tobacco smoking, food contamination, and contamination of the environment, all linked by poverty. All of these causes are converging. And until we have viable local, regional, and international public health systems in place, they will continue to converge and overlap. The main driving force is poverty — material poverty and the poverty of the spirit known as apathy.

The genocides that have occurred in the 20th century and continue today are also caused by these two kinds of poverty. It is impossible to know how many people would have been spared if the rest of the world had become involved in WWII sooner than it had. At Nuremburg some of the living perpetrators of that war were brought to justice. Today, even as this writing is taking place, 1.5 million people are at risk in Darfur, and no one is acting. The International Criminal Court (ICC) has moved to apply for a warrant for the arrest of the president of Sudan for crimes against humanity. He laughs, because he knows that no one will enforce this warrant against him. The US, Russia, and China are not members of the ICC. In the rest of the world, 92 nations are members. It may be that these three countries do not join in because they engage in activities that would themselves be called crimes against humanity.

As has been stated many times here, many of the actions of the Western world have contributed to the demise and breakdown of the developing or "undeveloped" world. Global climate change is very much a product of the West and yet the countries most harmed to date are in Africa and South Asia. This diminishment of quality of life in Africa is primarily the responsibility of the US and Europe. This is only one reason why the US does not join the ICC. In Russia today the replacement of a semidemocratic society postcommunism with a dictatorship that is immensely corrupt is the main reason why it does not join the ICC. These two countries would be found guilty of crimes against humanity.

There are an overwhelming number of examples that can be shared about how various countries have contributed to human societal damage, death, and the destruction of the environment. In China, the death toll from the Tiananmen Square massacre was reported by the Red Cross in Beijing as 1650 the day after the massacre. The injury toll was given as 7000. These numbers stood for one day and then were pulled from history as though they had never existed. To this day, no numbers are available about the death and injury tolls from that time, and the children of the people involved do not know of the events that occurred in 1989. Their parents do not talk go out those events, and the Internet access to anything about Tiananmen during that time is blocked in China. If China were to be held accountable for these actions, the ICC would be called in and reparations demanded and paid to the Chinese people. This is one reason why China does not belong to the ICC.

Those events are blatant examples of the cruelty of humanity when power and resource ownership is at stake. The ownership of the modern cancer epidemic by the medical industry is also an example of a form of genocide by greed. The medical, pharmaceutical, and research industries all own cancer by defining what it is and, therefore, how it can be treated. There is no definition of health, only a definition of disease. The NCI and ACS have for many decades said that cancer is not preventable, that it is only treatable. If cancer went away or diminished in incidence, these institutions and all of the money that they generate would be unnecessary. In 1974, the NCI was mandated by the Congress to spend at least 10% of their research dollars on prevention. In all of the years since that time, they have never spent more than 4% of their research dollars on prevention. They have even defined prevention — it is early detection through screening. The long latency period of cancers, they say, makes it impossible to ever track back to an original causative factor unless it is a biological hazard. This means that chemical carcinogens are discovered only after the fact and not because anyone is actually looking. The only researchers looking at environmental contamination are those in private nongovernmental institutions funded by private citizens who also pay for the research at the NCI through their tax dollars.

The truth is that modern research has the capacity to develop new chemicals and uses for these new chemicals, including medical uses. But it does not have the know-how to understand how these new chemicals interact with the human body, with each other, and over time. Because this is true, the European Union has developed a new oversight agency that demands that any new chemicals be tested *before* use in any product. This is called the precautionary principle. Here in the US the precautionary principle is applied to medical drugs used in cancer and treatment for other diseases, but not to the very chemicals that may have caused those diseases in the first place. The human body has become the test tube for the largest uncontrolled study ever conducted. The amount of profits made from this study by the chemical industry is the largest of any industry in the world. The amount of apathy it takes to let this happen is equally astounding and is emblematic of a heart–mind split.

It has taken decades for states to develop public health offices that track the incidence of all types of cancer by county and by state. Some states still do not have any public tracking system in place. Devra Davis has written about this in *The Secret History of the War on Cancer.* As one of those researchers in the cancer industry, she has stepped into the shadows of the truth about the tobacco industry and many other industries that have contaminated life and covered that up for many decades. And she did this at the risk of her own professional career. All researchers who do so risk their reputations as "real" seekers of the scientific truth.

The environment is the Commons and, as such, is part of public health. The Commons are the terrain of public health. This automatically makes cancer a public health issue. With one in two men and one in three women being diagnosed with cancer in their lifetime in the US, it is obvious that we are in the midst of an uncontrolled and unacknowledged epidemic. Public health agencies have traditionally been involved only with infectious and biological causes of disease. However, even within the context of virally caused cancers, there is no will to monitor, prevent, inform, and

save the many millions of people on the face of the Earth who struggle with chronic viral infection. Now, we need to extend the realm
of public health agencies, reinvigorate their mandate, and engage
with the burgeoning problem of the cancer epidemic and all that it
means.

References

1. Powles J, Comim F. World Health Organization. Trade, foreign policy,
   diplomacy and health. 6. Public health infrastructure and knowledge.
   www.who.net/trade/distance_learning/gpgh6/en/index1.html
2. For the United States Senate Appropriations Committee. Public health
   infrastructure: a status report. CDC. www.uic.edu/sph/prepare/courses/
   ph410/resources/phinfrastructure.pdf
3. Global health overview. www.globalissues.org/print/article/588
4. Cohen M. Herpes virus remains a global cancer. UNC Institute for
   Global Health and Infectious Diseases. globalhealth.unc.edu/2010/03/
   herpes-virus-remains-a-anational-concern
5. www.worldhepatitisalliance.org/libraries/English_fact_sheets/
   WHD_2012_media
6. Fuster V *et al.* (2007) Low priority of cardiovascular and chronic diseases on the global health agenda. *Circulation.* www.circ.ahajournals.
   org/content/116/17/1966.full
7. Commission on Social Determinants of Health, World Health
   Organization. Closing the gap in a generation: health equity through
   action on the social determinants of health. *WHO,* Aug. 28, 2008,
   p. 60.
8. www.kaiseredu.org. The state of public health preparedness. www.kai-
   seredu.org/issue-modules/the-state-of-public-health-preparedness
9. Stiglitz J. (2002) *Globalization and Its Discontents.* AllenLane Books/
   PenguinBooks, London
10. Colgan A. (2002) Hazardous to health: the World Bank and IMF in
    Africa. *Africa Action,* Apr. 18.
11. Bretton Woods Project. (2009) World Bank health work flawed; still
    pushing privatization of services. July 10.

12. Khor M. (2002) *Intellectual property, biodiversity, and sustainable development; resolving the difficult issues.* United Nations Environment Program, pp. 27–28.

13. Dasgupta R. (2001) Patents, private charity and public health. *Himal Asian,* Mar.

13A. Schlipkpter U, Flahault A. (2010) Communicable diseases: achievements and challenges for public health. *Health Rev* **32**: 90–119.

14. Alwan A, Assistant Director-General, Noncommunicable Diseases and Mental Health. (2011) Global Status Report on Noncommunicable Diseases. 2010. World Health Organization. Apr., pp. vii, 2, 3, and Chap. 2.

15. How NCDs contribute to poverty and how poverty contributes to NCDs. Global Status Report on NCDs 2010. *WHO,* Apr. 2011, p. 35.

16. Chassudovsky M. (2003) *The Globalization of Poverty and the New World Order. Global Research,* 2nd ed.

17. Teutsch S, Churchill R (eds.). (2000) *Principles and Practice of Public Health Surveillance,* 2nd ed. Oxford University Press, New York.

18. UNHCR. Asylum and migration. www.unhcr.org/pages/4ald406060.html

19. WHO. (2008) Closing the gap in a generation: health equity through action on the social determinants of health. Commission on Social Determinants of Health. *WHO,* Aug. 2008, p. 31.

20. Stiglitz J. (2003) *The Roaring Nineties: Seeds of Destruction.* AllenLaneBooks/PenguinBooks, London.

21. Bretton Woods Project. World Bank/IMF governance. www.brettonwoodsproject.org/topic/governance/index.shtml

22. Talbot S *et al.* (2005) Viruses and cancer. *Medicine* 39–42.

23. Balfour H. (2004) Herpes group viruses and HIV infection. *PRN Notebook,* Dec. Vol. 9.

24. Cuadros D, Garcia-Ramos G. (2012) Variable effect of coinfection on the HIV infectivity: within-host dynamics and epidemiological significances. *Theor Biol Med Model* **9**: 9.

25. HPV and cancer. NCI. www.cancer.gov/cancertopics/factsheet/risk/hpv

26. Cervical cancer statistics. www.Cervicalcancer.org

27. Rabin R. A vaccine may shield boys too. www.nytimes.com/2011/07/19/health/19garda.html?_r=0

28. WHO. Global Alert and Response (GAR). Hepatitis.

29. Altekrause S *et al*. (2009) Hepatocellular carcinoma incidence, mortality, and survival trends in the United States from 1975 to 2005. *J Clin Oncol* **27(9)**:1485–1491.

30. CDC. Data and statistics by date. www.cdc.gov/features/dshepatitis-awareness

31. NIH News. NIH scientists identify likely predictor for hepatitis C severity. www.nih.gov/news.health/jul2012/niaid-23a.htm

32. WHO. Global Alert and Response. Hepatitis C. www.who.int/csr/disease/hepatitis/whocdscrlyo2003/en/index2.html

33. CDC. Hepatitis C. www.cdc.gov/hepatitis/hcv/pdfs/hepclivingwith-chronic.pdf

34. WHO. Medical Centre. Hepatitis C. www.who.int/mediacentre/factsheet/fs164/index.html

35. Hilton I. (2000) A bitter pill for the world's poor. *Guardian*, Jan. 5.

36. Stiglitz J. (2006) Scrooge and intellectual property rights. *Br Med J* **333**: 1279–1280.

37. Hepatitis Help Center. WebMD. Treatment overview. www.webmd.com/hepatitis/hepc-guide/hepatitis-c-treatment-overview

37B. Epstein S. (1998) *The Politics of Cancer Revisited*. East Ridge.

38. Arora S *et al.* (2011) Outcomes for treatment for hepatitis C virus infection by primary care providers. *NEJM* **364: 2**199–2207.

39. CDC. Hepatitis B information for health professionals. www.cdc.gov/hepatitis/hbv

40. CDC. Hepatitis B vaccine. www.cdc.gov/vaccines/pubs/downloads/vis-hep-b.pdf

41. Leroux-Roels G *et al.* (2001) Prevention of hepatitis B infections: vaccination and its limitations. *Acta Clin Belg* **56(4)**:209–19.

42. Tran T. (2011) Immune tolerant hepatits B. *Gastroenterol Heptol (NY)* **7(8)**: 511–516.

43. Elgouhari H. Hepatitis B infection: understanding its epidemiology, course, and diagnosis. *Cleveland Clin J Med.* www.cejm.org/content/75/12/881.full

44. Perillo R P. (2001) Acute flares in chronic hepatitis B: the natural and unnatural history of an immunologically medicated liver disease. *Gastroenterology* **120(4)**: 1009–1022.

45. *Ibid.*

46. Hoofnagle J *et al.* (1987) Chronic type B hepatitis and the "healthy" Hbsag carrier state. *Hepatology* **7(4)**: 758–763.
47. Cohen M. (2000) *The Hepatitis C Help Book: A Groundbreaking Treatment Program Combining Western and Eastern Medicine for Maximum Wellness and Healing.* St. Martin's Press.
48. Zhang ZJ. (1999) *Shang Han Za Bing Lun (On Cold Damage), Translation and Commentaries.* Paradigm.
49. Guo HL. (2005) *Warm Pathogen Diuseases: A Clinical Guide.* Eastland.
50. Ma SC Lecture notes.
51. *Ibid.*
52. Digestice Disorders Health Center. WebMD. Aspartate amino transferase (AST) and ALT. www.webmd.com/digestive-disorders/aspartate-amino-transferase-ast
53. Viral hepatitis C. Johns Hopkins Medicine. Gastroenterology and Hepatology. www.hepatitis-gi.org/GDL_disease_aspx?currentudv=31&GDL_disease_ID
54. *Ibid.*
55. Bensky D, Barolet R. (1990) *Formulas and Strategies.* Eastland, p. 195.
56. *Ibid.*, p. 186.
57. *Ibid.*, p. 44.
58. *Ibid.*, p. 51.
59. *Ibid.*, p. 352.
60. *Ibid.*, p. 141.
61. *Ibid.*, p. 101.
62. *Ibid.*, p. 81.
63. *Ibid.*, p. 182.
64. *Ibid.*, p. 189.
65. *Ibid.*, p. 96.
67. *Ibid.*, p. 146.
67. *Ibid.*, p. 460.
68. *Ibid.*, p. 271.
69. *Ibid.*, p. 314.
70. *Ibid.*, p. 250.

CHAPTER 7

Epigenetics, the *Source*, and the Precautionary Principle

> When we were given these instructions, among many of them, one was that when you sit in council for the welfare of the people, you counsel for the welfare of the seventh generation to come. They should be foremost in your mind — not even your generation, not even yourself, but those that are unborn so that when their time comes here, they may enjoy the same thing that you are enjoying now.
>
> — *Chief Oren Lyons*, Faithkeeper of the Turtle Clan of the Onandoga Nation

The Ages of Civilization — The Macrocosm

Life on the Earth has been evolving since its beginning in time. This evolution has involved every species and has been impacted by the myriad of things. Weather, meteors, bacteria, viruses, yeasts, plants, and all of the communities of life that have existed and now exist have acted on others and been acted on by others and by themselves. From the eons before us we have been able to gain information and utilized the knowledge of chemistry and biochemistry, geology, archeology, and so on to construct what is meant to be a best guess of how all of this evolution took place.[1] In what would be modern times in the history of the Earth, i.e. from about 500,000 years ago to the present, we have looked at the eras of time in the context of hominid and human development and called them ages or epochs.[2] And studying the last 50,000 years is valuable in terms of understanding

401

life on the Earth as an evolutionary process that involves the physical, mental, emotional, and spiritual aspects of life.

Astronomically speaking, the day marks the period of the Earth's rotation on its axis. The year marks the revolution around the sun. The Great Year equals a period of approximately 25,000 years during which the poles of the Earth's axis trace an imaginary circle in the sky. It is divided into 12 time periods of approximately 2500 years. These periods are called the Great Months. The Great Months have traditionally been named after the zodiacal constellations, even though they are actually eras of time and not areas of space.[3] According to some, they are phases of evolutionary life and growth for everything that is influenced by cosmic, and possibly, sacred activity.[4]

The constellations cannot be permanently associated with a place in the sky, because everything in the universe is in movement. This means that every place must eventually become the focal point for the operation of all conceivable cosmic activities. And this in turn implies that the cosmic organism itself is developing by passing through successive phases of experience.[5]

The vital process of the movement of the universe, its galaxies and constellations, refers mainly to dynamic relationships rather than to static objects. This truth remains a part of all perennial philosophies.[6] Although modern astronomy and physics are bonded in their search for the makeup of these objects in space and how they act, modern science is not interested in how the dynamism of celestial bodies might affect life on the Earth. Nevertheless, the philosophy of ancient and modern astrology/astronomy has persisted, and utilizing the knowledge of the Great Months coupled with archeological history and anthropology has led to the concept of processional epochs to track and understand the collective evolution of the human race and all life on the Earth.[7]

Hominids have been on the Earth for about four million years, evolving toward a modern human form for several hundred thousand years. The last 50,000 years have been very active for all of those hominids we have called "*Homo* _____ " and there have been many close calls for us when it comes to outright extinction. For example, one recent near-extinction event, a megadrought across the Earth, lowered the numbers of humans, *Homo sapiens*, on the Earth to about 600 individuals in Africa about 76,000 years ago. It is from those individuals that all the rest of us *Homo sapiens* have come.[8]

Homo sapiens evolved from *Homo heidelburgensis* in Africa. Those *Homo heidelburgensis* members who moved out of Africa and into Europe became Neanderthals. Those who stayed in Africa became *Homo sapiens*, or modern humans. *Homo sapiens* also moved through time and into all of the rest of the world. As they moved into Europe, Neanderthals, who were also a form of humans, were pushed out. Their last stronghold was on the Rock of Gibraltar, about 28,000 years ago.[9] And as modern humans moved across the Earth, their movement could be charted by the fall of all of the large animals on each continent as they were hunted into extinction.

One of the major differences between Neanderthals and *Homo sapiens* was the ability of the later to adapt versus the inability of the former to *flex* with changes in the environment. Although Neanderthals lived and flourished for 300,000 years in Eurasia, much longer than *Homo sapiens* have now lived, they were unable to adapt to the different hunting techniques forced on them by a highly adaptable hunting style utilized by modern humans. Neanderthals stuck to the use of heavy jabbing spears that forced them to get very close to their prey. *Homo sapiens* utilized much smaller, shorter, and lighter spears with bone points that could be thrown, giving them distance and safety from their prey. The elimination of large prey in Europe by modern humans pushed Neanderthals to extinction. They were able to survive alone in the harsh and cold environment of Europe longer than any other human species across the entire world. But once modern humans were in Europe, they could not compete for food.[10]

Modern humans have been shaping the environment ever since they came into being in Africa. The ability to use the environment in such a successful way is one of the hallmarks of *Homo sapiens*. The ability to more successfully bear and raise young is another. These two characteristics are part of the reason why we find ourselves in the modern world predicament. Can we use the understandings we have gleaned from our superior minds and the study of humanity through time to once again adapt and help ourselves find a path on the Earth today that preserves the Earth and its environment and communities and, therefore, save ourselves? This is the quandary we must learn about in the modern epoch — the Aquarian Age.

Most of human history for which we have some form of records includes archeological, anthropological, written, and other forms of evidence, and begins around 50,000 years ago.[11] This changes almost annually as a result of new finds and research methods that become available. But, beginning in 11,000 BCE, when there were a substantial number of human beings and the beginnings of written historical documents, the epoch and the cosmic mandate for the Earth, cosmologically speaking, was called the Golden Age, when humankind worshipped the sun. Many have interpreted this time as a cosmic assignment to the task of searching for the light of the sacred, or consciousness, within rather than without. As part of this subjective influence, a flowering of scientific discovery took place during this time. The Atlantean culture that many have deemed to be a part of Minoan culture occurred during this time and may have annihilated itself as a result of early failures of scientific efforts.[12]

The next age or epoch occurred during the times between 8850 and 6700 BCE. The orientation was towards understanding the Earth as Mother and away from the sun as God. This time may have been a reaction to the exploitation of the Atlanteans which nearly destroyed the Earth, especially around the Mediterranean. There are other explanations for the destruction of that time, including volcanoes and tidal waves. Whatever the truth, the result was an effort on the part of humankind in the cradle of civilization to gestate the seeds of an entirely new civilization. Housing was improved, and basic skills and techniques were learned anew during a time of great austerity.[13]

The next Great Month brought forward writing as a form of communication. Logic and reasoning, the growth of commerce, vast migrations of people, and the exchange of ideas ushered in the seeds of science and philosophy. Concepts of good and evil were incorporated into religious doctrine.[14]

The temples of Latin America and the pyramids of Egypt exemplify the aspirations of the people of the next epoch — the evolution of concrete structures and security based on possessions. The expression of ideas was inspired by their preservation. The agrarian time and animal husbandry were essential to the economy. Copper was discovered. Metal money came into use. Competition, jealousy, and greed were expressed on the side of evil, solidifying the concepts of good and evil and perhaps a societal class system.[15]

From 2400 to 250 BCE, the growth of city states and outright greed led to organized warfare, which made the next epoch a time of incessant strife. Ramparts and fortresses were constructed to preserve resources and war plunder. Land was fought over. And iron replaced copper, allowing more effective war machines. On the opposite side, principles of law and order were introduced. Weights and measures were standardized. Hammurabi, Moses, and Solon played roles in regulating human conduct, and a series of great religious teachers, including the Old Testament prophets and the authors of the Upanishads and Vedas, instructed humanity in the spiritual laws.

This time was also a time of heroes. The divine right to rule was supplanted by the right of superior mortals who achieved glory to rule through physical prowess, leadership, and courage. Women suffered greatly during this time and were seen more as objects of plunder than as heroines. This may have been the initial time when the original separation of male and female, humans from nature, and nature from mind took place.[16]

From 250 BCE to 1900 CE, emotionalism and fanatic devotion spread throughout the world, laying the foundations for Christianity and the mystical sects of all the great faiths. After the brutal wars of the previous epoch, compassion became a tide of healing that flooded the world. Asoka founded the first animal hospital in India in *c.* 250 BCE. Buddhists in China founded hospitals for the sick and dying at about the same time. Charity became a socially sanctioned ideal. Ocean voyages and circumnavigation of the globe occurred during this time. Hygiene and the healing arts made great progress. And, in fact, modern medical advisers believe that it has been public health works more than medicine that have contributed to longevity.[17]

The first half of the last epoch featured the growth of religious and monastic orders, and ended in the Age of Reason, which led to the scientific materialism of the 18th–20th centuries. The current epoch will end in 4050 CE. We are now in the major transition of the Piscean Epoch to the Aquarian Epoch.

On a cosmic and macrocosmic level, these collective changes in human understanding and culture form an evolutionary mechanism of large-scale change on the Earth. At the same time, and unbeknownst to us, another change, on the microcosmic level, was driving changes in the very fiber of humans, and these cellular changes in turn have affected the external world in which we all live. The world has changed immensely since the Neanderthals struggled to survive in Europe. And the human body, mind, and spirit are also changing the world and being again changed by it, in a circle of evolving manifestation.

Introduction — The Microcosm

The human genome has recently supplied us with a map of where the human physical expression is at this time.[18] It has helped us to understand that the concept of race occupies less than 1% of the human genome and that the racial differences occupy only the super-ficial aspects of the human body. Chimpanzees differ from us only in a very small percentage of the genome we share. The truth is that humans and all other life forms on the Earth are constructed from the same Earth materials and in the same architectural format. It is an immensely beautiful home we make up.

And it turns out that what happens to us on a daily basis, as opposed to over a millennium, also affects who we are and who we become. Although changes in the human genome take literally thousands of years,[19] the way in which that individual genome is expressed is flexible and constantly changing. These more subtle expressions change who we are and how we handle all of what life brings to us.

There are hundreds of different kinds of cells in the human body. Although each one derives from the same starting point, the features of each type are different. Over 30,000 genes make up the human genome, and as cells develop, their development is governed by the selective use and silencing of genes. It appears that the way our genes perform can change dramatically between generations without any alteration in the DNA sequence. The field of epigenetics seeks to determine how genome function is affected by mechanisms that regulate the way genes are processed.[20]

DNA methylation is the primary mechanism by which epigenetics takes place; DNA methylation patterns play a role in all sorts of phenomena, from the color of a rose to the growth of a cancerous tumor, where genes are switched on or off. Failure to silence genes can be as problematic as failure to turn one on. Too little DNA methylation can alter which genes are silenced after cell division. Too much DNA methylation can interfere with the protective work of tumor suppressor genes and DNA repair genes.[21] Epimutations have been observed in a wide range of cancers.[22]

Epigenetics also provides knowledge about the means by which genetic material responds to changing environmental conditions. For example, although plants do not have a nervous system or brain, their cells have the ability to memorize seasonal changes. In some biennial species, this ability is linked to their capacity to flower in the spring, when warmer ambient temperatures are detected. Exposure to cold during winter triggers structural changes in chromatin that silence the flowering genes. These genes are reactivated in spring, when the longer days and warmth are more conducive to reproduction.

The environment can also prompt epigenetic changes that affect future generations. Inbred mice have demonstrated how changes to their diet might influence their offspring. These methylation changes to a particular gene during embryonic growth can trigger brown, yellow, or mottled color fur. Foxes raised in the wild demonstrate what we would call typical fox coloration. But those that are raised in captivity demonstrate how changes in coloration occur that are very similar to those of many modern *Lupus* species away from the typical coloration of their predecessor, the wolf.

Epigenetic factors govern the interpretation of DNA within each living cell. Understanding them could revolutionize evolutionary and developmental biology, and affect practices from medicine to agriculture.

The Dynamic Epigenome and Its Implications in Disease

The epigenome serves as an interface between the dynamic, ever-changing environment and the static, inherited genome. It is sculpted during development to shape the diversity of gene expression programs in the different cell types of an organism. Epigenetic aberrations have similar consequences to genetic polymorphisms resulting in variations in gene function.

Recent data suggest that the epigenome is dynamic and is therefore responsive to environmental signals not only during development but also during later life. Some of the exposures that have been understood so far to affect changes in the genome include not only chemical exposures but also social behavior, including abuse and maternal care.[23] Exposures to different environmental agents could lead to interindividual phenotypic diversity as well as differential susceptibility to disease and behavioral pathologies.[24] Interindividual differences in the epigenetic state could also affect susceptibility to xenobiotics.

Epidemiological evidence increasingly suggests that environmental exposures early in development have a role in susceptibility to disease in later life.[25] Some of these environmental effects seem to be passed on through subsequent generations. Recent studies have demonstrated for the first time that heritable, environmentally induced epigenetic modifications underlie reversible transgenerational alterations in the phenotype.[26]

Cancer is a disease that results from both genetic and epigenetic changes.[27,28] Differences in environmental exposures have long been attributed to cancers in identical twins. However, disparities in gene expression resulting from variable modifications in DNA methylation and chromatin structure in response to the environment also play a role in differential susceptibility to disease. The environmental agents most strongly affecting the epigenome and the critical windows of vulnerability to alterations from these exposures are not, as yet, fully defined. This incomplete knowledge should drive the precautionary principle, especially when it comes to new exposures never before seen, like modern chemicals both as single entities and in combinations.

The developing fetus is especially sensitive to maternal nutrition, exposure to environmental toxins, and psychological stress.[29] Social behavior, including maternal care, can affect the epigenome. There is a link between the social environment early in life and long-term epigenetic programming of behavior and responsiveness to stress and health status in later life.[30] Epigenetic equilibrium remains responsive throughout life. Therefore, environmental triggers could play a role in generating interindividual differences in human behavior later in life.[31] It is speculated that exposure to different environmental toxins alters long-established epigenetic programs in the brain as well as in other tissues, leading to late-onset disease.

Previous studies on rats have shown that parenting has a measurable physical impact on behavioral responses to stress. The way in which a mother treats her offspring determines the extent to which certain proteins get made from DNA. In particular, the expression of glucocorticoid receptors associated with mood disorders in the brains of abused humans who committed suicide had different epigenetic marks than in people who were not abused. The results of several research findings suggest that childhood experiences can lower the expression of glucocorticoid receptors. This has a knock-on effect on the HPA (hypothalamic–pituitary–adrenal) function. The overactivation of the HPA axis affects our ability to cope with stress, leaving individuals at risk for suicide.[32]

The biological implications of psychological abuse, whether its source be from maternal, familial, or sociocultural exposures, are deeply meaningful. The forms that shame binds take and the physical and emotional abuse of young children are all linked to future behavior in ways that we have not imagined.

Environmental cues trigger changes to epigenetic tags on our genome. These tags on the genome can be carried through from cell to cell as we replace damaged body tissue. When such changes occur inside egg or sperm cells, they can pass through to the next generation. Based on recent research, which indicates that low birth weight is associated with increased risk of obesity and diabetes and cardiovascular disease during adult life, it was found that these effects occurred in the next generation as well.[33] Males from the first-generation crosses were found to be glucose-intolerant and this increased with age. It was found that diabetes can pass through more than a single generation via the maternal line.[34]

We now have explanations from many angles of conventional science, including the fields of psychoneuroimmunology, neurotransmitter science, and epigenetics, for the so-called mind–body connection. What we have traditionally thought of as mind and emotion residing in the brain, or from the neck up, we now must understand as being ubiquitous in the human body. And we must understand that the continuum of life reaches forward and backward through our bodies and our psyches, changing who we are, who we are to become, and the world in which we live.

Endocrine-Disrupting Chemicals

Endocrine-disrupting chemicals (EDCs) are of increasing concern, because of their potential impacts on the environment, wildlife, and human health. Pesticides and some pesticide metabolites are an important group of EDCs, and exposure to them is obviously damaging but poorly quantified. Many ED pesticides are harmful at very low doses, especially if exposure occurs during sensitive stages of development, producing effects that may not manifest for many years or that affect descendants via epigenetic changes.[35]

For example, the effects of cigarette smoke exposure on early immune development and respiratory disease include data indicating that second-hand smoke affects the developing fetus *in utero* as well as *ex utero*. This exposure impacts the individual's risk of asthma and other respiratory disease, and it also impacts immunity through immunoglobulins in all tissues that are mucus-producing ones.[36]

Another example is the effect of vinclozolin, an antifungal chemical, on the prostate transcriptome initiating adult-onset disease of the prostate. Vinclozolin is a pseudoestrogenic chemical that mimics human estrogen and fills estrogen receptors in the human body. Early estrogenic exposure increases the risk of prostate cancer.[37,38] The fungicide vinclozolin acts as an antiandrogenic, and also acts transiently at the time of embryonic sex determination to promote in the F1 generation a spermatogenic cell defect and subfertility in the male. The animal lines in the laboratory in one study that were allowed to develop up to one year were found to develop a number of other diseases. This phenotype was transferred through the male germ line to all subsequent generations analyzed. These lines went out four generations. It is not only habitat loss that is responsible for some species' extinction; it is also the loss of male fertility and the inability to carry on the line.[39]

The ability of an environmental factor like an endocrine disruptor to promote an epigenetic transgenerational phenotype spotlights the potential hazards of environmental toxins. There is a distinct pattern of gene expression throughout mammalian development that is heritable from parents to offspring. This lineage-specific pattern establishes DNA methylation for somatic cell development after fertilization. Epigenetic reprogramming is based on the genetic material transferred from egg and sperm. Alterations in the lineage-specific epigenetic reprogramming result in developmental defects or embryonic death. The germ line DNA methylation pattern is established during gonadal development and is gender-specific. Epigenetic reprogramming of the germ line is critical for imprinting. Unlike the lineage-specific reprogramming, the alterations in the germ line epigenetic reprogramming can alter the heritable epigenetic information, resulting in a transgenerational phenotype. The embryonic period is the most sensitive for chemical and environmental effects on the epigenetics of the male germ line.[40]

This epigenetic effect on the germ line could reprogram the germ cell through an event such as altered DNA imprinting. It could then have a transgenerational effect on subsequent generations through the germ line. Epigenetic alterations that lead to transgenerational transmission of specific genetic traits or molecular events like imprinting have recently been identified. The impact this has on human health and evolutionary biology is significant.

Environmental effects of irradiation, chemical treatments like chemotherapy, and environmental toxins such as endocrine disruptors have been observed over the past decade.[41] The majority of the observations are of the effects of the agent on the gestating mother

(F0) and subsequent actions on the offspring associated with the F1 generation. Examples of the environmental factors during environmental development that influence the F1 generations are the effects of heavy metals causing cancer, abnormal nutrition that causes diabetic and uterine defects, chemical exposure having brain and endocrine effects, and endocrine disruptors like DES and phthalates causing reproductive tract and endocrine defects.

These effects are on the F1 generation *in utero*. To be transgenerational it is required that minimally these effects be reflected on the F3 generation. This is because the F3 generation is the first generation not directly exposed to the original environmental factor. Transgenerational effect has been shown to occur. Irradiation exposure was one of the first transgenerational impacts observed to be transmitted through the germ line to multiple generations, often associated with mutagenesis and tumor formation. The chemotherapeutic treatment of cancers has been shown to cause F1 generation effects, but the transmission to multiple generations has not yet been thoroughly investigated.

Environmental factors do appear to promote transgenerational susceptibility to cancer.[42,43] Gestating nutritional deficiency effects on the F1 generation have been observed, and recently these nutritional effects on a diabetic condition and growth defects have been shown to be transgenerational to the F2 generation. Several environmental chemical exposures have also been shown to transgenerationally affect the F2 generation; they include benzpyrene, orthoaminoasotoluol, and dioxin. Environmental toxins such as endocrine disruptors have also been shown to influence the F1 generation after parental exposure.

Many reports have suggested that environmental endocrine disruptors, which act to mimic estrogens or act as antiestrogens or antiandrogens, are detrimental to reproduction and may promote abnormalities such as a decrease in the sperm count, an increase in testicular cancer, and an increase in abnormalities in sex determination for many species. These chemicals include pesticides like DDT and methoxychlor, fungicides, insecticides like trichorfon, herbicides like atrazine, plastics, phthalates, and a wide range of xenoestrogens.[44] Most of them are ubiquitous in the environment, resulting in daily exposure for humans and other animals. Many of these compounds can be metabolized into both estrogenic and antiandrogenic activities. Methoxychlor and vinclozolin have been used as model endocrine disruptors that have estrogenic, antiestrogenic, and antiandrogenic metabolites.

A large number of environmental EDs are weakly estrogenic and elicit their actions through estrogen receptors.[45] Mammalian estrogen receptors are widely distributed throughout the reproductive tract, and are made up of ER-alpha and ER-beta receptors. ER-beta is present in higher concentrations in the testes and ovaries of the fetus. ER-alpha is present mainly in the uterus. Neonatal exposure to estrogen alters the ER-alpha and ER-beta expression during postnatal testis and hypothalamic/pituitary development.

Antiandrogenic EDs can also influence fetal gonadal development.[46] Androgen receptor (AR) expression is very similar to ER-beta expression in the developing testis. AR is detected in Sertoli, myoid, and prespermatogonial cells just after cord formation. It is proposed that AR is present in cells that migrate from the mesonephros and enables cord formation to occur. Flutamide administered to pregnant rats at different ages of gestation impairs fertility in the male offspring, because this drug blocks the ability of androgens and epidermal growth factor to stabilize the Wolfffian duct in the male reproductive system. A commonly used antiandrogenic ED is vinclozolin, which is employed in the wine industry as a fungicide.

Transgenerational actions of EDs have also been found to affect future generations. Endocrine disruptors appear to induce an epigenetic transgenerational disease condition for four generations through the male germ line. Although most genes get reset in early embryonic development, a subset of genes called imprinted genes maintain their DNA methylation pattern. In contrast to all somatic cells, the primordial germ cells undergo a demethylation during migration and early colonization of the embryonic gonad, followed by a remethylation starting at the time of sex determination in a sex-specific way. The exposure of the pregnant mother at the time of sex determination appears to have altered the remethylation of the germ line and permanently reprogrammed the imprinted pattern of the DNA methylation.[47]

If the exposure of your grandmother at midgestation to environmental toxins can cause a disease state in you with no exposure, and you will pass it on to your grandchildren, it becomes obvious that the potential hazards of environmental toxins need to be rigorously assessed. Equally important, the epigenetic component of disease now needs to be seriously considered.

Epigenetics has shown that cancer cells are originally normal cells that have been injured in some way. These cells proliferate partly because they are unrecognized by the immune system. The immune system sees foreign antigens as they sit in our cells alongside the same identity tag borne by the immune system itself. This tag allows the immune system to recognize what is us and what is outside of us. This is called antigen processing, and in the earlier phases of cancer the damaged cells still look enough like us that they are not screened.[48]

A second way that cancer cells develop is through the loss of tumor suppressor genes. The knocking-out of these genes, which are part of the immune system, will allow mutated cells to continue and grow. The loss of genes that tell cells where they can and cannot go in the body can lead to metastasis. The loss of genes involved in the MHC and antigen processing is another common finding. By not displaying the right identity tag, cancer cells can go unrecognized by the immune system.[49]

An organized workforce of proteins ensures that the correct ID (MHC) is properly assembled on the surface of our cells. Proteins are encoded by distinct genes and each gene is potentially affected in cancer. The best-understood is a protein called TAP (transporter associated with antigen processing). It has been observed that in many different types of cancer the amount of TAP is reduced or even absent, prompting a reduction or loss of MHC and therefore a fraudulent ID. This defect can be used to predict cancer progression and survival rates in humans. Faulty TAP protein results from changes in the epigenome of cancer cells.[50] Thus, an epigenetic way for cancers to dodge the immune system has been identified.

The modern science of genetics and epigenetics is laying a foundational language for concepts within many perennial forms of medicine that have to do with the paradigm of a source for all of life. Ayurvedic and Chinese medicine, in particular, have very sophisticated explanations of how life comes about and is changed by the act of living itself. But because these perennial systems never had to analyze the effects of environmental and sociocultural contamination, they do not have the modern tools for understanding the specifics of that contamination. Combining bioscience with perennial sciences to understand our pathway in this morass is essential. On one side, we have the biochemical and genetic/epigenetic understanding of how these things work. On the other side, we have the prelinear understanding of how nature works and how to protect and rehabilitate life. Each perspective is equally valuable. They are the *Yang* and the *Yin* of understanding.

Chinese Medicine

The discussion of water as a primary necessity for life on the Earth is descriptive of how water is perhaps an analog for the esoteric and material concept of the *San Jiao* and more particularly the *Source* from Chinese medicine. It makes its origin in the moving *Qi* between the *kidneys*. This place and its opening complexity into all of the communications that run a living being is like the river source in the high mountains, gathering momentum as it moves down toward the ocean. It is difficult to locate the exact spot where it all begins. Just like the source of the Nile is somehow Lake Victoria, the truth is that it is a phenomenon of weather systems, rainfalls, streams, rivers, and springs that ultimately include and feed into one another in the vast system we call East Africa. This phenomenon is not unlike the flows of the meridians, fascia, *Luo* Vessels, *Ying* and *Wei*, connective tissues and membranes of Chinese medicine and its concepts from the *San Jiao* and the *Source*.

Source theory is the *Yin* and *Yang* of Chinese medicine. As such it is perhaps the genome and the epigenome according to Chinese medical theory, if such an analog can be constructed between the two systems — one ancient and one modern. If in modern theory genetics loads the gun for human injury, then the environment pulls the trigger. The *Source* and *San Jiao* theory exemplify this statement.

Source theory finds that human beings have a compound beginning that includes a sacred or cosmological continuum between Heaven (*Tao and Yang*), the Earth (*Yin*), and the individual (both *Yin* and *Yang*). It begins as a concept in the ling shu[51] and is taken up subsequently in the *Nan Jing*[52] and later commentaries. *Nan Jing Source* theory revolves around the functions of the *San Jiao* and the master of the *heart. Jing* (essence) and *shen* (spirit) are received from the *Tao*, and the form and the body are received from the Earth. This statement implies that we are at once cosmic and material. The theory states that there is an energetic center of the body that has a physically central location and is the root of the body energetically. It is an underlying energetic substratum called the *Source*, the place where energy, or enlivening force, meets matter. As the root of all the organs and meridians, it is located in the abdomen below the umbilicus at the gravitational center of the body. This energetic center of the body is the fulcrum for balance between the sacred and the mundane, now and the future, the material and the nonmaterial, the inheritance of our life and what we do with that inheritance.

The *Source* has certain qualities. It is the *Source* of all movement and is itself described as a moving *Qi*. Most frequently it is known as the moving *Qi* between the kidneys. This is thought to be a manifestation of an even more profound energy in the universe. It is constant and, when it ends, the person, i.e. the body, dies. It regulates and is interdependent with other energetic properties, the *jing, shen*, and *Qi*. If the *Source* is strong and healthy, then a person with a disease can recover from that disease. If it is weak and poorly nourished, or is itself diseased, no matter how strong the energetics in the other strata of the body, it will be very difficult for the person to recover.[53]

The *Source* is the "gate of breathing." This refers to physical breathing and also to taking in sacred *Qi* or enlightenment. Poor breathing habits can weaken the *Source* both physically and spiritually. *Mingmen*, as a part of the *Source*, is the actual gate; the word means literally "bright gate." It links the gate at *mingmen* to the lungs and to Heaven. It is a profound physical place within the human body. Although this was not an issue when the *Ling Shu* or *Nan Jing* was written, in modern times the quality of the air we breathe, whether we breathe it in poorly or not, must certainly contribute to a draining of the *Source Qi*. Since the *Source* is at the physical center of the body, i.e. the fulcrum, physical imbalances can also affect its energetics. When I use the term "energetics," I mean the place and the process whereby the spirit meets matter. I also mean the enlivening force for all of life that Chinese medicine calls *Qi*. Emotions affect energetics and, therefore, affect the correct functioning of the *Source*. That the world has seen 250 wars in the 20th century underscores the fact that the human psyche has been suffering under the weight of unresolved tensions. This affects us physically and spiritually.

Not only do air and water quality affect the *Source*. Diet can also affect it. What is referred to is not only the diet of highly refined foods from the center aisles of grocery stores but also the modern monocultural industrial agricultural system that is harming the human body with poor-quality foods and degrading the Earth on which we live with environmentally destructive agricultural practices.

Injuries to the *Source* can go unnoticed until it is too late.[54] The *Source* is the "*shen* that protects against evil." If the root is dying, the stems and branches (the organs and meridians) will dry out but appear normal at the pulse. The *Source*, the root, is dying in the interior but is still there in the exterior. This is one of the early questions asked of the Yellow Emperor by *Qi Bo*. He asks how the pulse can feel normal but the patient dies soon after the taking of the pulse. The 21st century may be the century during which we find out exactly what has been done to our bodies and our world; you cannot change what you do not see or acknowledge. The modern cancer epidemic is but one manifestation of the injury. Cancer is not just a disease of aging. It is a disease of living poorly. It is a disease of living off the land but not as part of the land. It is occurring in younger and younger people, perhaps partly as a result of epigenetic changes to the *Source* from present and earlier generational impacts.

The *Source* is also connected via the *shen* to the *heart*. The attraction of "*heaven Qi* " into a person and the resulting creation of *shen* that protects the body is part of breathing. This is why cultivating the breath is part of so many meditation techniques. Air is as important to life as is water. As stated earlier, the moving *Qi* is also the origin of the

San Jiao. The *San Jiao* transports the *Source Qi* from its origin to the *Source* points of each of the 12 meridians. In this way, it maintains the basic energetic connection of the 12 meridians to the *Source.* The *San Jiao* also unites *Qi* at the *kidneys,* the *Source* of *Yuan Qi,* or ancestral *Qi. Yuan,* the *Source,* refers to a spring of water that flows from behind the rocks of a ravine. "*Yuan* is the root origin of water." The meridian point *taiyuan* is the *Source* point of the *lung* meridian and is an immensely important point clinically. It is the place where the underground source of water reaches the surface. So *Source Qi* is the spring of *Qi* that rises from a deeper level, especially at Lu 9 — *taiyuan.* The *yuan, basic Qi,* the original or *fundamental Qi, prenatal Qi,* is the surfacing of an underground river — the aquifer of material and spiritual DNA, if you will. And the *yuan Qi* is the enfolded or implicate order; the *Source Qi* is the first unfolding of the *yuan Qi.* The *yuan Qi* is the *prenatal Qi,* and the *Source Qi* is the root of the *postnatal Qi.* The *Source Qi* is formed when the breath comes to the moving *Qi* between the *Kidneys,* the gate of breathing.[55] This is the cosmology of Chinese medicine.

If it is possible to compare this understanding of *Source* theory — an ancient theoretical concept from a culture and time where the knowledge of genetics did not exist — to modern genetic theory, then it is here at these early junctures with the *Source* and the *San Jiao* that injury to the DNA, and injury that causes a mishap in the expression and interpretation of DNA, first happens. The *Source* and the *San Jiao* are the primal and foundational expressions most vulnerable to the exposures we have constructed in modern life. Perhaps we could say that inherited predispositions to cancers come from injuries to the *Source,* and that in many solid tumors and cancers where there is no predisposition it is injury to the *San Jiao* and the weakest organ/meridian that manifests as a cancer of that organ. The hematopoietic cancers in young children who have not yet established a mature presence of the *San Jiao* throughout the body are caused by a direct hit to the *Source* from their environment.

When we were very young, we reveled in learning about the new world we had been born into. Then we became a part of it. And finally we acted on it and made that world for our own children.

When we were young, we were part of the world in which we lived. But over time we became separate from it and learned to make it our own rather than to understand it and make our self a viable part of it. The modern constructed and "civilized" world seems to require that we learn how to stand outside of nature. Science is emblematic of this split. But what we are splitting from is our *Source*, in the microcosm of our bodies and in the macrocosm of our industrialized world and in the cosmos. The slow progression of this split has taken place over millennia of evolution but truly the most destructive actions of the split have occurred in the last 200 years and in the West. This has deconstructed our own DNA, both material and spiritual, and the expressions and interpretations of that DNA. DNA could be thought of as the *water–fire* duality of life — the receptive and the initiatory, the *Yin* and the *Yang*, the science of meaning in material life.

Wang Shu He's commentary on the *Nan Jing* discusses the *San Jiao* in relation to the water–fire duality expressed by the *kidney* and *mingmen* interaction. "The *kidney* belongs to *water*; *mingmen* (the gate of breath) belongs to *fire*. The *Qi* comes out from inside of the *water–fire*. The *Qi* of the *San Jiao* starts there. Therefore, the *Source* of the *San Jiao* is the *shen* which protects against evil." This is one reason why the *San Jiao* has a connection to immunity in modern parlance. But perhaps the reference can also be construed as saying that protection against evil equals the material and spiritual wisdom to know what evil is and that knowledge is the protection. It is a knowledge that all healthy beings are born with. This is one reason why *mingmen* is often called the small *heart* (*su wen* 52:275). The *heart* is the void in which the *shen* or universal *spirit* (*Tao*) resides. *Mingmen* is the *Source* for the *shen* at the *heart*. This relates, in my mind, to having access to and knowing the truth. When we breathe and cultivate the breath, we are cultivating the *shen* and improving our capacity to know the truth. It quiets the mind and connects it to the *shen*, the spiritual truth, of the *heart*. When there is injury to this very early spring of knowledge and truth, we become lost.

Zhang Jie Bin says of *mingmen*: "*mingmen* totally controls the *kidneys* and both *kidneys* belong to *mingmen*. Therefore, *mingmen* is the *fu* of *water* and *fire*. It is the home of *Yin* and *Yang*. It is the ocean of the *jing Qi*. It is the passageway of life and death. If *mingmen* is depleted, the five *Yin* and six *Yang* organs all lose some of their function; *Yin* and *Yang* are diseased and changed. Therefore, there is no place unaffected."[56]

This apparently esoteric iteration of the anatomical and energetic mechanisms of Chinese medicine describes from a perennial point of view how the emotions and all of their ramifications, including cultural decisions, diet, and how food and the agricultural system to grow food, and environmental destruction and contamination, can cause injury at the very basic DNA and pre-DNA levels of all life on the Earth. It describes how the seventh generation can become affected by the injuries and actions from previous times, whether those actions or injuries involve the *shen* (*spirit*), the *jing* (essence or DNA stream/pool), the *Yuan Qi*, the *San Jiao*, or even the *Source*.

Certainly, these changes have been seen throughout the existence of humankind. And the very world in which we live has been constructed by the choices and the damage humans and other forms of life and even the weather and geological changes have inflicted upon this world. However, in modern life, especially during the past 200 years, the damage to the very fabric (*Source*) and essence (*jing*) of our world, and therefore to ourselves and to other life forms, has taken on a new potency, level, and catastrophic quality that impacts the future of all life on the Earth and has done so in a very short period of time. The essence of the injury began many millennia ago, when humankind started to separate itself from nature, and the *shen* or *spirit* of life was changed. As this separation has unfolded it has changed the world in which we live to the extent that we may no longer be able to survive. Our journey now is to take the understandings we have gleaned from living in all of these millennia and to reconstruct and rehabilitate them in ways that allow all life to survive and flourish. The Aquarian Epoch has the capacity to rebuild and reinvent our world as one where meaning and knowledge are one. This rehabilitation will involve physical, mental, emotional, and spiritual actions.

Thoughts

At the material and philosophical levels, the interlocking economic structures that bind the direction of medicine and science to the interests of industry have been developing since the Age of Enlightenment. And the arrival of the atomic, nuclear, and chemical age that followed WWII has produced on a large scale carcinogenic[57] and other chemicals that contribute to the modern cancer epidemic. These carcinogens, chemicals, endocrine disruptors, and so on are manufactured in such a diverse array and in such large quantities that they are no longer confined to the workplace where they were conceived or manufactured or utilized. They have seeped into the general environment, where we all come into intimate and daily contact with them. And the lives that many humans are forced to live in the modern world contribute to culturally imposed emotional and psychic injuries that are unbearable. Making visible the links between cancer, environmental contamination, poverty, violence, loss of hope, and the current economic structure of a globalizing world is a difficult task.

In fact, the human environment has become a massive uncontrolled experiment when it comes to exposure to new chemicals and ways of being never before seen on the Earth. There remains no unexposed control population to whom the cancer rates of exposed people can be compared. Each of us is exposed repeatedly to minute amounts of many different chemicals, carcinogens, and amoralities through many different routes as the injured ecology and spirit of the Earth struggles to continue to function. We are forced to live without connection to the natural world, to the production of our food, to the *Source.* The ever-present trauma of this way of living is causing us all to live in deep grief without even knowing it. Science loves order, simplicity, and the manipulation of a single variable against a background of constancy. When everything is changing all at once, the tools of science do not work well. The science of how these cumulative and combined chemical exposures and emotional injuries in modern life affect the human and animal body over time is almost nonexistent. Epigenetics is beginning to give us some idea of how these issues impact not only us but future generations as well.

Modern capitalism is the operating system of the world economy. Private employers hire workers to produce products and services, which the employers own and then sell for profit. Competitive markets, the price mechanism, the modern corporation as the principal institution, the consumer society and materialistic values that sustain it, and an administrative state actively promoting economic strength and growth make up a capitalistic society.

These features as constituted today work together to produce an economic and political reality that is highly destructive to both the physical and the spiritual environment. It is difficult to understand that this destruction is intended in any cosmic mandate for the evolution of our species or our world.

What Is Needed

The Earth is a community. *Homo sapiens*, as one form of animal within that community, has the cosmic mandate of the Aquarian Epoch to learn how to protect the rights and welfare of all species and all people. Part of what this means is that cruelty and violence must be eliminated. Freud was wrong; cruelty and violence are not part of the human genomic manifestation. Cruelty and violence are reactions, just as cancer is a reaction to injury. These injuries do not just happen; they are caused, and the causes must be identified and eliminated.

All species and cultures have intrinsic worth. They are intrinsic beings and not objects for manipulation or ownership. No humans have the right to own other species, other people, or the knowledge of other cultures, or the knowledge of life as a capitalistic forum for profit. Defending biological and cultural diversity is a duty of all people, because diversity is an end in itself, and a value and source of richness in life. Defending diversity equals defending the source and the universal Chain of Being.

All members of the Earth community have the right to sustenance — to food and water, to safe and clean habitat, to security of ecological space. These rights are natural rights and birthrights given by the fact of existence on the Earth. They are best protected through community rights and the rights of the Commons. These rights are not given by states or corporations, nor can they be extinguished by state or corporate action. They are part of the higher order of creation. No state or corporation has the right to erode or undermine these natural rights or to enclose the Commons which sustain all, through privatization or monopoly controls.

Earth democracy[58] is a philosophy of the Commons and is based on economic democracy. Economic systems in Earth democracy protect ecosystems and their integrity. They protect people's livelihoods and provide basic needs to all. There are no disposable or dispensable species or people. The Earth economy is a living economy based on sustainable, diverse, and pluralistic systems that protect nature and people, all of whom are a part of nature.

Conservation of the Earth's resources and creation of sustainable and satisfying livelihoods is most caringly, creatively, and equitably achieved at the local level. Localization of economics is a social and ecological imperative. The global economy should not crush and destroy local economies. Local economies support national and global economies. This is welling-up economics as opposed to trickle-down economics.

Earth democracy is based on local living democracy with local communities, organized on principles of inclusion and diversity and with ecological and social responsibility having the highest authority on decisions related to the environment and natural resources.

Earth-centered and community-centered knowledge systems are what form the foundation of Earth democracy. Living knowledge is knowledge that maintains and renews living processes, and contributes to the health of the planet and people. It is knowledge that is embedded in nature and society, and is not abstract, reductionist, linear, or antilife. Living knowledge is a Commons. All humans have a duty to share knowledge. No person or corporation has a right to enclose or monopolize or patent or exclusively own as intellectual property living knowledge.

Rights are derived from and balanced with responsibility. People can be connected in circles of care, cooperation, and compassion instead of being divided through competition and conflict. Earth democracy globalizes compassion, not greed, and peace, not war.

The Precautionary Principle

"First, do no harm" is a profoundly emblematic statement of the precautionary principle.[58,59] It is based on the Great Chain of Being, which is so elegantly expressed in the Chinese medicine concept of the *Source* or in the concept of the seventh generation of Native American beliefs. Unfortunately, in the cancer epidemic, modern medicine is one of the first sciences to give up the precautionary principle. In Chinese medicine, chemotherapy and radiation are attack arrays utilizing poison to treat poison. And, in the Eight Methods, or *ba zheng*,[60] it is the last technique to be used and then only in certain circumstances. When poison is used to treat an illness in Chinese medicine, it is always balanced with the simultaneous use of techniques for protection and rehabilitation. In truth, this is one of the major reasons why Chinese medicine is so good at supportive care in standard oncology treatment. It has a long history of working alongside drastic purging and draining techniques, the modern analogs of which are chemotherapy and radiation.

When it comes to extracting resources from the natural environment, these techniques of rehabilitative medicine are not utilized although the environment in many circumstances is grossly undermined and damaged by injuries similar to cancer. The modern solutions for the provision of food, manufacturing, energy production, mining, logging, shelter, and even medicine itself are all based on attack arrays that are not balanced by rehabilitation and are grossly inappropriate techniques in and of themselves. In cancer treatment, for example, modern conventional medicine leaves patients to their own devices to recover from the cytotoxic and damaging therapies to which they are exposed. They are left to recover and rebuild an immune system, blood, organ function, and so on, all of which function to protect them from the occurrence of the same or another cancer, often caused by the therapies used to treat their original cancer. These same techniques are used in agriculture and resource mining with no thought of the damage done to the soil, the Earth geology, water, or the *Source*. What we are doing to the environment we are also doing to ourselves. The same linear thinking is constantly repeating the same injuries over and over again.

The science and way of thinking and knowing that drives modern industrial agriculture, chemistry, manufacturing, medicine in all of its specialties, and war, is one of attack — that is, poison to treat poison. Much of the writing in this book is an attempt to show how this is true and to begin to build a bridge of understanding about how we got here, especially in the context of cancer.

Principles of the Precautionary Principle — the Wingspread Conference[61]

"The release and use of toxic substances, the exploitation of resources, and the physical alterations of the environment have had substantial unintended consequences affecting human health and the environment. Some of these consequences include high rates of learning deficiencies, asthma, cancer, birth defects and species extinctions, along with global climate change, stratospheric ozone depletion and worldwide contamination with toxic substances and nuclear materials.

"We believe existing environmental regulations and other decisions, particularly those based on risk assessment, have failed to protect adequately human health and the environment — the larger system of which humans are but a part.

"We believe there is compelling evidence that damage to humans and the worldwide environment is of such magnitude and seriousness that new principles for conducting human activities are necessary.

"While we realize that human activities may involve hazards, people must proceed more carefully than has been the case in recent history. Corporations, government entities, organizations, communities, scientists and other individuals must adopt a precautionary approach to all human endeavors.

"Therefore, it is necessary to implement the Precautionary Principle: When an activity raises threats of harm to human health or the environment, precautionary measures should be taken even if some cause and effect relationships are not fully established scientifically.

"In the context the proponent of an activity, rather than the public, should bear the burden of proof.

"The process of appling the Precautionary Principle must be open, informed and democratic and must include potentially affected parties. It must also involve an examination of the full range of alternatives, including no action."

These words are from the Wingspread Conference on the Precautionary Principle, which was convened by the Science and Environmental Health Network in 1998.[62]

The European Commission established the EC Treaty in February 2000.[63] This treaty tries to establish common guidelines on the application of the precautionary principle, partly in the hope that it will have positive repercussions at the international level. The principle has been recognized in various international agreements, notably the Sanitary and Phytosanitary Agreement (SPS) included in the framework of the World Trade Organization.[64]

According to the Commission, the precautionary principle may be invoked when the potentially dangerous effects of a phenomenon, product, or process have been identified by a scientific and objective evaluation, and this evaluation does not allow the risk to be determined with sufficient certainty. Hence, the use of the precautionary principle belongs in the general framework of risk analysis which, besides risk evaluation, includes risk management and risk communication, and more particularly includes the context of risk management corresponding to decision-making.

The Commission stresses that the precautionary principle may only be invoked in the event of a potential risk and that it cannot be used to justify arbitrary decisions. Therefore, it can only be invoked when the three preliminary conditions are met:

- Identification of potentially adverse effects;
- Evaluation of the scientific data available;
- The extent of the scientific uncertainty.

It goes on to state that measures from the use of the precautionary principle may take the form of a decision to act or not to act depending on a political decision, and are a function of the level of risk considered acceptable by the society on which the risk is imposed. This determination is made according to certain legal tools and is subject to review by the courts. The outcomes that are possible from this legal review include funding a research program and informing the public as to the adverse effects.

Guidelines on the use of the principle should be informed by three specific principles:

• Implementation of the principle should be based on the fullest possible scientific evaluation. As far as possible, this evaluation should determine the degree of scientific uncertainty at each stage.
• Any decision to act or not act pursuant to the precautionary principle must be preceded by a risk evaluation and an evaluation of the potential consequences of inaction.
• Once the results of the scientific evaluation and/or risk evaluation are available, all of the interested parties must be given the opportunity to study the various options available, ensuring the greatest possible transparency.

According to the Commission, an action taken under the precautionary principle may in certain cases include a clause shifting the burden of proof to the producer, manufacturer, or importer. This possibility should be examined on a case-by-case basis. Products for which the burden of proof already rests with the manufacturer include products such as drugs, pesticides, and food additives.

A related act from the European Parliament laid down general principles and requirements of food law, establishing the European Food Safety Authority,[65] which laid down procedures in matters of food safety. These principles also include the precautionary principle, which may be invoked where a food might have harmful effects on health.

At this time, the US, Canada, and the Communication of the Commission of 2000 (E.U.) have all drafted similar papers on the precautionary principle. The EC has been in existence longer than any other commissions or public agencies that have been gathered for this purpose, and has rejected some unauthorized use of the precautionary principle. For example, the Upper Austria provincial government notified Brussels that it proposed a ban on genetically modified seeds. This rejection was based on the fact that the requirement for a scientific evaluation had not been met by Upper Austria. At the same time, Italy, France, Germany, Luxembourg, and the UK have banned GMOs from their territories, even if these have been approved at the EU level. The Commission took the scientific evidence provided by these member states as justification for the bans and submitted it to the European Scientific Committee for an opinion. The Committee deemed that there was no new evidence that would justify overturning the original authorization for the use of genetically modified seeds.[66,67]

The National Foreign Trade Council[68] states that the EU is using the precautionary principle to create obstacles to trade. The NFTC has been portrayed as imagining that European officials work day and night to develop schemes to make life difficult for US industries. But, as the second-largest exporter in the world, the EU has much to lose if the precautionary principle is abused.

When evaluating the case of hormones, Directive 2003/74 from the EC concluded that:[69]

- Risk to the consumer has been identified with different levels of conclusive evidence for the six growth hormones — endocrine, developmental, immunotoxic, genotoxic, and carcinogenic effects could be envisaged with prepubertal children among the most vulnerable.
- Estradiol 17 beta has to be considered a complete carcinogen.
- As for the other five, risk has been identified, but no acceptable daily intake can be established. The new Directive keeps a permanent ban on estradiol 17 beta and places a provisional ban on the other five, pending further scientific information. Three therapeutic uses of estradiol will still be allowed under tight conditions, to be phased out in the future.

Conventional wisdom tells us that the US is far behind the EU when it comes to use of the precautionary principle. However, when compared piece by piece, Europe appears to be more precautionary than the US about such risks as GMOs, hormones in beef, toxic substances, phthalates, and climate change. The US appears to be more precautionary than Europe about such risks as new drug approval, mad cow disease in beef, nuclear energy, diesel, lead in gasoline, and the phaseout of CFCs. When compared to most of the rest of the world, the US and the EU are probably both at the high precautionary end of the spectrum of risk management actions. However, it is obvious that the precautionary principle is an element in the culture war, one part of which is the disagreement between corporate business practices and the beliefs of much of the consumer public.

The precautionary principle (PP) has taken center stage in a number of recent international discussions on trade, the environment, and human health. As a result, there are criticisms and qualifications that have been repeated with some frequency. The Science and Environmental Health Network has offered responses to these criticisms. Following are the main criticisms and the Network's responses.

The precautionary principle has been worded differently each time it has been articulated. The criticism that it is vague and has conflicting definitions is not uncommon in international customary law. The statements of the precautionary principle, however, contain no major conflicts among them. At the core of each statement is the idea that action should be taken to prevent harm to the environment and human health, even if scientific evidence is inconclusive. As the principle has been elaborated recently, it nearly always implies three additional concepts beyond harm reduction and current scientific uncertainty. They are:

• The idea of seeking alternatives to harmful technologies;
• The idea of shifting to proponents of technology the responsibility for demonstrating its safety;
• The goal of transparency and democracy in making decisions about technologies.

Taken together, these concepts provide what is believed to be a sound overarching approach to assessing and making decisions on products and technologies and other human activities that may impact health or the environment.

Another concern has been that if precaution is applied to everything, then all technology would be stopped in its tracks. But this criticism confuses the broad, common sense precautionary approach to decision-making with specific precautionary action. Precautionary action does not always mean calling a halt or implementing a ban. It can also mean imposing a moratorium while further research is conducted, or calling for monitoring of technologies and products already in use, adopting safer alternatives, and so on. A broad precautionary approach will encourage the development of better technologies. Making uncertainty explicit, considering alternatives, and increasing transparency and the responsibility of proponents and manufacturers to demonstrate safety should lead to cleaner products and production methods.

The concern that zero risk is an impossibility is pointless. The real goal must be to impose far less risk and harm on the environment and human health than we have in the past. The idea is not to harness human ingenuity but to reduce the harmful effects of our activities. The same ingenuity can be applied to safer products and activities. The precautionary principle is based on the assumption that people have a right to know as much as possible about the risks they are taking, in exchange for what benefits, and to make choices accordingly. With food and other products, the choices are often played out in the marketplace. A major factor in the controversy over genetically engineered food is the consumer understanding that benefits of these products (which accrue more to producers than to consumers) do not outweigh the risk of harm to themselves or the environment. In the current climate, manufacturers are choosing to reduce risk themselves by substituting safer alternatives in response to consumer uneasiness, the threat of liability, and market pressures. A number of toy manufacturers, for example, have voluntarily stopped using phthalates in soft plastics. This is the spirit of the precautionary principle.

Risk assessment is the prevalent tool used to make decisions about technologies and products. Many say that these are sufficient. However, risk assessment is often used to delay precautionary action. It is not necessarily inconsistent with the precautionary principle. But because it omits certain basic requirements of the decision-making process, the current type of risk assessment is helpful only at a narrow stage of the process, when the product or technology and alternatives have been well developed and tested and a great deal of information has already been gathered about them. Standard risk assessment is useful only in conditions of relatively high certainty, and generally only to help evaluate alternatives to damaging technologies.

The precautionary principle not only applies to risk management. It is a comprehensive approach to preventing harm. Current and prospective alternatives to harmful technologies, like GMOs, must be scrutinized as carefully as the technologies they replace. Therefore, the idea that the precautionary principle will prevent us from adopting technologies that are actually safer is a consideration built into the precautionary principle.[70]

The precautionary principle is not antiscience. In fact, it calls for more and better science, especially investigations of complex interactions over longer periods of time. Taking action in advance of full scientific proof does not undermine science. Scientific standards of proof are high in experimental science, and they should be. Science should serve society and not vice versa. The decision is society's and science's.

The precautionary principle was created to protect public health and the environment, not to restrict valid trade. The idea that it is a cover for trade protectionism is not the real issue. The real issue is whether a nation has the sovereign right to impose standards that exceed the standards of international regimes. The recent European Commission statement on the precautionary principle and the Cartagena Biosafety Protocol[71] both assert that right.

Some Conclusions

Scientific uncertainty and ignorance about the effects of human-made stress on ecological systems are the underlying rationales behind a precautionary principle. It is necessary to define uncertainty in broader terms than we do now. There is uncertainty about the models used to relate exposure to disease. The exposures that are occurring now are much different than the exposures of our ancestors. The timing and dosage of the exposures is very important when one is weighing the impacts. Variability in humans poses another form of uncertainty. Politically imposed uncertainty requires that uncertainty be exposed as an unavoidable component of decisions involving environmental and public health harm. The uncertainty regarding the short- and long-term effects of a substance or intervention becomes the very reason for taking action to prevent harm and for shifting the benefit of the doubt to those beings and systems that might suffer harm. Currently, we are functioning within the framework that requires that harm be proven before a substance or action is terminated or stopped.

Precaution challenges science in fundamental ways. The traditional model of academic or laboratory science uses a high standard for establishing conclusive knowledge. For the problems relating to environmental hazards, the ideals of laboratory science often cannot be achieved or are achieved only at the expense of prevention-oriented actions. The traditional model of science also suppresses speculation and cross-discipline studies. Therefore, some fundamental changes in science will be needed if precaution is to be embedded in research design and public policy. These changes include a change in incentives given to scientists that allow them to examine problems and hypotheses outside the boundaries of normal science; and a need to encourage scientists to make policy conclusions on the basis of not only what they know statistically and scientifically, but also what they believe. Other types of legitimization other than pure science must be augmented and used. Science and meaning must be reunited.

We have not only inherited the Earth from our ancestors, we have also borrowed it from our children and great-grandchildren. The Great Chain of Being moves backward and forward. The *Source* is universal, ancient, present, and is the foundation for our seventh generation.

Precaution is an issue of ethics, morality, and truth. For those who are affected harmfully, it is an issue of right and wrong. Precaution is about protecting present and future generations, who have no power over the decisions made today. Decisions about a toxic chemical should ask the basic question of whether exposure is safe for a six-week-old embryo. Decisions about harm to human health are public decisions and require the maximum feasible participation of people affected by the decisions.

Precaution is also about human rights. There is a disconnect between those who benefit from harmful activities and those who are harmed. There is also a lack of consent among those who suffer the burden of "acceptable risks." Medical ethics requires informed consent. Exposures to harmful activities that also cause medical injury should require informed consent too. There is no difference between the types of experiments conducted to test drugs and the experimentation that occurs every day on humans and ecosystems from exposure to untested synthetic chemicals and technological innovations.

Given the uncertainty and ignorance of the vast complexity of ecological systems, it can no longer be asked what level of harm is safe. The world is all one. What is needed is to question basic human activities like consumption, materialism, and resource exploitation, and ask questions about how we can avoid harm and live in sync with our environment, learning from millions of years of ecological self-regulation.

Precaution must become a moral imperative, of equal or greater importance than economic growth or military security. The elevation of precaution can drive science toward solving problems for the public good. Our government agencies need to shift their focus from protector and mediator of interests to public and environmental trustee. In the long run, growth, sustainability, and prosperity will be a reflection of the extent to which we are creatively just.

References

1. Bada J. (2004) How life began on Earth: A status report. Science Direct. *Earth Planet Sci Lett* **226:** 1–15.
2. Geological time scale. www.hyperphysics.phy-astr.gsu.edu/hbase/geophys/geotime.html
3. Kragh H. (2007) *Conceptions of Cosmos: From Myths to the Accelerating Universe; A History of Cosmology.* Oxford University Press.
4. Margulis L. (2007) *Dazzle Gradually: Reflections on the Nature of Nature.* Sciencewriters.
5. Charisson E. (2012) Researching and teaching cosmic evolution. In Rodriguez *et al.* (eds.), *From Big Bang to Global Civilization: A Big History Anthology.* University of California Press, Berkeley 2012.
6. Huxley A. (2009) *The Perennial Philosophy: An Interpretation of the Great Mystics, East and West.* Harper Perennial Modern Classics.
7. Collective evolution: a documentary series. www.collective-evolution.com
8. Ancient timeline of concordances. www.well.com/mareev/portal/pre-history/ancient_prehistory_timeline2.html
9. Hall S. Last of the Neanderthals. National Geographic. www.ngm.nationalgeographic.com/2008/10/Neanderthals/hall-text
10. Hayes J. Humans and Neanderthals interbred. *Cosmos,* Nov. 2, 2006.
11. Wade N. Scientists rough out humanity's 50,000-year-old story. www.webfamilytree.com/50,000_year_human_history.htm
12. The ages of the world. About.com
13. *Ibid.*
14. *Ibid.*
15. *Ibid.*
16. *Ibid.*
17. *Ibid.*
18. Human Genome Project information. genomics.energy.gov www.ornl.gov/sci/techresources/human_genome/home.shtml
19. Sagan C. (1986) *The Dragons of Eden: Speculations on the Evolution of Human Intelligence.* Ballantine.
20. Church D. (2009) *The Genie in Your Genes: Epigenetic Medicine and the New Biology of Intention.* Elite.
21. *Ibid.*

22. Weidman J *et al.* (2007) Cancer susceptibility: epigenetic manifestation of environmental exposures. *Canc J* **13(1):** 9–16.
23. Szyf M *et al.* (2007) Maternal care, the epigenetic and phenotypic difference in behavior. *Reprod Toxicol* **24(1):** 9–19.
24. McGowan P *et al.* (2008) The social environment and the epigenome. *Environ Mol Mutagen* **49(1):** 46–60.
25. Doliney DC *et al.* (2007) Epigenetic gene regulation: Linking early developmental environment to adult disease. *Reprod Toxicol* **23(3):** 297–301.
26. Anway M, Skinner M. (2000) Epigenetic transgenerational actions of endocrine disruptors. *Endocrinology* **147(6):** 43–49.
27. Epigenetics? Catching the criminal. The enemy within. The Epigenome Network of Excellence. www.epigenome.eu/en/2,54,1051
28. Steingrabber S. (1998) *Living Downstream: An Ecologist's Personal Investigation of Cancer and the Environment.* Vintage.
29. Meaney MJ. (2005) Maternal care as a model for experience-dependent chromatin plasticity. *Trends Neurosci* **28(9):** 456–463.
30. Francis DD *et al.* (1999) Maternal care and the development of stress responses. *Curr Opin Neurobiol* **9(1):** 128–134.
31. Lederbogen F *et al.* (2011) City living and urban upbringing affect neural social stress processing in humans. *Nature* **474(7352):** 498–502.
32. Epigenetics? Abuse affects genes. The Epigenome Network of Excellence. www.epigenome.eu/en/1,65,0
33. Raloff J. (2012) Pollutants long gone, but disease carries on. *Science News,* Feb. 28. www.sciencenews.org/view/generic/id/338832
34. Zambrano E. (2009) The transgenerational mechanisms in developmental programming of metabolic diseases. *Rev Invest Clin* **61(1):** 41–52.
35. McKinaly R *et al.* (2008) Calculating human exposure to endocrine-disrupting pesticides via agricultural and non-agricultural exposure routes. *Sci Total Environ.*
36. Prescott SL. (2008) Effects of early cigarette smoke exposure on early immune development and respiratory disease. *Pediatric Respir Rev,* Mar.
37. Anway MD *et al.* (2008) Transgenerational effects of the endocrine disruptor vinclozolin on the prostate transcriptome and adult onset disease. *Prostate,* Apr.
38. Skinner M. (2012) Early estrogen exposure increases risk of prostate cancer. *Cancer,* June.

39. Vanishing species. *Endangered Species Handbook.* www.endangered specieshandbook.org

40. Merlet J *et al.* (2007) Development of fetal testicular cells in androgen receptor deficient mice. *Cell Cycle* **6(18):** 2258–2262.

41. Szyf M. (2007) The dynamic epigenome and its implications in toxicology. *Toxicol Sci* **100(1):** 7–23.

42. Weidman JR *et al.* (2007) Cancer susceptibility: epigenetic manifestation of environmental exposures. *Canc J* **13(1):** 4–16.

43. Jirtle RL, Skinner M. (2007) Environmental epigenomics and disease susceptibility. *Nat Rev Genet* **8(4):** 253–262.

44. Davis DL *et al.* (1993) Medical hypothesis: xenoestrogens as preventable causes of breast cancer. *Environ Health Perspect* **10(5):** 372–377.

45. Li Y *et al.* (2012) Differential estrogenic actions of endocrine-disrupting chemicals bisphenol A, bisphenol AF, and zearalenone through estrogen receptor alpha and beta *in vitro. Environ Health Perspect* **120(7):** 1029–1035.

46. Uzumcu M *et al.* (2004) Effect of the anti-androgenic endocrine disruptor vinclozolin on embryonic testis cord formation and post-natal testis development and function. *Reprod Toxicol* **18(6):** 765–774.

47. Skinner M. School of Biological Sciences. Research interests; brief analysis of mammalian reproduction and environmental epigenetics. www.sbs.wsu.edu/faculty/?faculty/155

48. Wesach P. Antigen processing and presentation. Nature Reviews Immunology. www.nature.com/nrl/posters/antigenprocessing/index.html

49. Sadikovic B *et al.* (2008) Cause and consequences of genetic and epigenetic alterations in human cancer. *Curr Genom* **9(6):** 394–408.

50. Kaklamanis A *et al.* (1994) Loss of major histocompatibility complex-encoded transporter associated with antigen-presentation (TAP) in colorectal cancer. *Am J Pathol* **145(3):** 505–509.

51. Wu JN. (2002) *Ling Shu, The Spiritual Pivot.* University of Hawaii Press.

52. Unschuld P. (1986) *Nan-Ching, The Classic of Difficult Issues.* University of California Press.

53. Birch S, Matsumoto K. (1988) *Hara Diagnosis: Reflections on the Sea.* Paradigm, pp. 109–110.

54. Unschuld P. (2003) *Huang Di Nei Jing Su Wen: Nature, Knowledge and Imagery in an Ancient Chinese Medical Text.* University of California Press.

55. Wang M. (2011) *Foundations of Internal Alchemy. The Taoist Practice of Neidan.* Golden Elixir.

56. Zhang JY. (1981) *Zhi Yi Lu (Record of Questions and Doubts).* 1687 C.E. Jiangsu Science and Technology.

57. Shiva V. (2005) *Earth Democracy: Justice, Sustainability, and Peace.* South End.

58. Science and Environmental Health Network. Precautionary principle. www.sehn.org/precaution.html

59. Europa. Summaries of EU legislation. The precautionary principle. www.europa.eu/legislation_summaries/consumers/consumer_safety/132042_en.htm

60. Zhang L. (1989) *WojiJing. Zhanongguo da baike quanshu, Junahi,* Vol. 2, p. 1067.

61. Science and Environmental Health Network. The precautionary principle. www.mindfully.org/precaution/precautionary-principle-common-sense.htm

62. www.sehn.org/precaution.html

63. *Op. cit.,* No. 59. Summaries of EU legislation.

64. WTO. The WTO Agreement on the Apllication of Sanitary and Phytosanitary Measures (SPS Agreement). www.wto.org/english/tratop_e/spsagr_e.htm

65. European Food Safety Authority. www.efsa.europa.eu

66. Health and consumers. EU Register of Authorized GMOs. www.ec.europa.eu/food/dyna/gm_register/index_en.cfm

67. GMO Free Europe 2012. www.gmo-free-regions.org/gmo-free-regions.html

68. National Foreign Trade Council. www.nftc.org/?id=1

69. Health and consumers. Hormones in meat — introduction. European Commission. www.ec.europa.eu/food/chemicalsafety/contaminants/hormones/index_eu.htm

70. Myers M. Debating the precautionary principle. www.environmentalcommons.org/precaution-debating.pdf

71. Convention on Biological Diversity. The Cartagena Protocol on Biosafety. www.bch.cbd.int/protocol

CHAPTER 8

The Geology of Hope

Visitor: Sir, what happens when the soul leaves the body?
Ramakrishna: To bother what happens after death!
How silly!
You are born as a human being only to experience
pure love.

— from *The Great Swan*:
Meetings with Ramakrishna

Introduction

In the United States as of 2010, one in every two men and one in every three women are diagnosed with cancer in their lifetime.[1] Since 1970, the incidence of testicular cancer has risen by 115%,[2] and that of non-Hodgkin's lymphoma by 67%.[3] Breast cancer occurred in 1 out of 22 women in 1940, and in 2000 it occurred in 1 out of 8 women.[4] Childhood leukemia has the greatest rate of increase of any cancer. This throws new light on the traditional view that cancer is a disease of aging and that the rise in rates is due to a growing aging population. When adjusted for an increased population with a longer lifespan, it remains true that the rates of almost all cancers are rising and are far above what is medically and scientifically expected. Something happened in the 20th century to drive this increase. What happened?

The geology of the modern cancer epidemic is lodged in the bedrock of a way of life that has evolved over many generations of humans. The institutions that have evolved alongside these generations are emblematic of a way of thinking that is linear, as opposed to the circular philosophies of almost all of the perennial

439

philosophies and their cultures. This linear way of thinking about and viewing the world has brought us to a place in time where human beings no longer see themselves as part of nature. We have become the manipulators of nature. We are no longer members of an Earth community made up of many beings, both fauna and flora. As we act on our Earth community, we act on ourselves unknowingly. This denial is a symptom of the split between heart and mind. The mind should act from knowledge gained from the heart, the residing place of the spirit or Tao — the whole truth. We must heal this split and ourselves. The Earth will follow. And the modern plague of cancer will once again become the disease of only a few.

Reconnecting Science and Religion

Although quantum uncertainty has to some extent surpassed general relativity and quantum mechanics, the most important part of reductionism remains: the world is still nothing but particles in motion. The reductionist view[5] is that, at bottom, there is nothing but whatever is the bottom line base of physics. The evolution of what is down there at the infinitesimal baseline or basis of mechanics has evolved and probably will continue to evolve. We have moved from electromagnetism to the atom, to the proton, the neutron, and the electron, to particle physics and string theory.

However, reductionism remains in place and everything points downward, from societies to people, to organs, to biochemistry, to genetics, to physics. Physicists have given up trying to reason "upward" from the apparently ultimate physical laws to larger-scale events in the universe. Most would say that the generation of explanations upward is ultimately an esthetic and not a scientific question. This scientific worldview of reductionism is immensely important, because it does not speak to or explain or involve itself with the evolution of the universe and all that is in it. Modern science does not say anything about values, doing, action, meaning, or history. And yet all of these things are part of the universe. The why of it all has been left to philosophy and religion. Modern science is linear thinking.

Some would say that we are not humans having a spiritual experience. Ramakrishna said that we are spiritual beings having a human experience. And the root of all faiths, paths of seeking, and religious philosophies is to make a better or more complete human being. To make spirit and humanity one and to grow the soul; to resolve the matter-versus-spirit dichotomy; to connect the mind with the heart and the spirit; to experience pure love — all seem to be the goal of most religious philosophies.

String theory has led some to the idea that there may be multiple universes, with some of them containing constants of nature that are somehow tuned to support life. Unfortunately, no one is able to write down the equations of explanation/proof for string theory as is required in physics. But it appears that we are reaching for a new scientific worldview that is moving forward to the concept of "emergence" and to vast unpredictability and unending, ever-new diversity and creativity which appear to be beyond natural law as we understand it. We are perhaps going back to circular thinking.

Evolution as an historical fact does not stand isolated from the rest of science but is an integral and interwoven part of the tapestry of our understanding of nature. Some of the religious people of the Abrahamic traditions still deny evolution, perhaps out of fear that the ethical foundations of Western civilization will crumble if evolution is factually true. At the same time, there is considerable doubt on the scientific side about the power and sufficiency of natural selection as the sole motivator of evolution. Natural selection has become a poster child for reductionist thinking. Evolutionary theory became united with genetics in such a way that we can now draw causal arrows from traits and behaviors to genes to molecules to chemistry and on down.

However, within the theory of natural selection[6] there do seem to be some features that cannot be reduced to physics: natural selection itself, and the attribution of functions to parts of organisms as being due to natural selection. The existence of the part of the organism being analyzed cannot be reduced to physics or chemistry. How did the organ or part come into existence in the universe in the first place in order to be selected for? Things that have causal consequences in their own right are real. The organ, the organism of which it is part, and the biosphere in which it lives are all real entities and not essentially and only reducible to particles or strings or atoms or whatever comes next in the linear "down-low" of physics.

The physicist cannot take the Newtonian scientific framework[7] where we can prestate the variables, the laws among the variables, and the initial and boundary conditions, and then compute the forward behavior of the system. Physics cannot help us predict future states of our world. Physics cannot tell us *why* anything exists. This is because the universe is partially lawless and ceaselessly creatively enfolding itself and unfolding new and changed expressions. The evolution of any biosphere or life system is firmly beyond reductionism. It is part of the Great Chain of Being, and to a large extent a mystery.

The implication is that life is almost certainly not constrained to the Earth. A general biology of life in the cosmos awaits our discovery. Although *Darwin's on the Origin of Species* has no equations in it, it still can be stated mathematically. Darwin's law did not need physics and uses the law of biology. The concept of natural selection was inferred and never inductively examined by Darwin. He was a stunning observer of the natural world, never reducing his idea to the list of possible organisms in possible universes. Natural selection was not reduced to physical laws, and it stands on its own and at its own level — biology.

The limitations on reductionism and linear thinking are important, because they imply that something else is possible and real. Biology is really not just physics. Organisms are really not just physics. Organisms are part of the universe and change the actual physical evolution of the universe in a ceaseless and ever-changing cycle. Life, agency, value, meaning, and consciousness have all emerged in the evolution of the Earth and perhaps elsewhere. They change the evolution of life and are changed by it.

The Earth, a biosphere, is indescribably creative. We may never know the history of the creation of life on the Earth. It takes DNA, RNA, and encoded proteins to carry out the process of translating genes into proteins — the stuff of which living cells are made.[8] In modern cells, the molecular mechanisms by which cells reproduce form a complex self-referential system that is highly evolved.

The central dogma of molecular biology[9] is that DNA structural genes are transcribed into RNA molecules, which are then translated into proteins via the genetic code. But self-reproduction of a cell is vastly more complex than the central dogma. There is a propagating organization of linked processes that complete a set of work-related construction tasks that closes on itself in such a way that the cell as an entire entity reproduces itself. In so doing, the cell replicates its DNA using protein enzymes, synthesizes its boundary membrane, and recreates a variety of intracellular organelles like the mitochondria. After 40 years of work, no one has been able to build DNA from even a modest number of nucleotides.

Experimental demonstrations have now proven that amino acid sequences can produce copies.[10] This has proven that molecular reproduction does not need to be based on DNA or RNA. All of these results open the way for us to consider that many different sets of molecules might form collectively autocatalytic sets and be the basis of life on the Earth and in the cosmos.

The creativity in the universe is tied to the explosions into what has been called the adjacent possible.[11] The more connections made, the more collectively autocatalytic sets occur as natural phenomena. The result of these connections is more diversity. And this diversity makes the universe a ceaselessly creative phenomenon — one in which heritable variations are probable and a top-down selection of whole systems would be allowed. These ideas are all beyond reductionism and none of them are reducible to any known theory in physics. They do not point downward but upward to the collective emergent properties of complex chemical reaction networks and the organizational mathematical law that may govern a spontaneous emergence of collectively autocatalytic sets. Therefore, it is scientifically plausible that life arose from nonlife, probably here on the Earth.

The original face of this world is one we can only imagine. The commonplace and uncommonplace activities of humans and of all other forms of life are literally altering the physical universe. Human agency in the earliest roots of life was action, meaning, doing, and value as emergent realities in the universe. The 600 *Homo sapiens* members living with their backs to the sea in a cave on the southern tip of Africa 76,000 years ago would attest to this. They were the agents of the survival of the human race as we know it. Agency is also present in animals and perhaps in all expressions of the physical world. All of life everywhere may be an expression of evolving consciousness. And consciousness may be the result of what many call the Sacred.

In physics there are only happenings, no doings. In biology there are functions. With agency values have emerged in the universe.[12] And with values comes meaning. The relevant features of actions, like biological functions arising due to evolution, cannot be discriminated by the physicist. Teleological language refers to conscious reasons, motives, intentions, purposes, and understanding. It is not considered scientific but it cannot be replaced by physical language. Teleological language is the language of agency. It is beyond reductionism. It is not linear.

The origin of agency is not reducible to physics. Is it possible to trace the origin of action, value, and meaning to the origin of life itself? Without a cyclic process and a self-resetting work cycle of purpose and function, the entity, the living organism, will not continue. Part of the propagating organization of process is continuity. When the possibilities are linked into a web of propagating work, there is enormous selective advantage. The emergence of agency via selection was of selective advantage. It is an expression of the evolution of consciousness. It is a circular process.

With agency meaning, values, doing, and purposes emerge in the universe. Once the value of something is true, meaning and "ought" enter the universe. Values, meaning, doing, action, and ought are all real parts of the structure of the universe.

The attempt to find the concepts needed for propagating organization is an example of the conundrum in which modern science finds itself and of the requirement for imagination and even wonder in science. The 20th century focused on information about how it all works through genetics. But the other properties of cells have been ignored. The one-way flow of information from DNA to RNA to proteins has remained molecular biology's central dogma. There are still many parts of molecules that are not understood. The web of propagating organization of processes that are part mechanical, chemical, electrochemical and other unknown processes are for the most part being ignored, perhaps because we remain locked into linear thinking, which possibly in this case at least is a form of denial. This is why the questions regarding certain concepts and realities of perennial forms are not understood or pursued. We are locked into a particular way of thinking and seeing. In Western science, these complex processes exist to perform a task — work. And yet the definition of work exists only within the field of physics.[13]

Cells have evolved to do work to construct constraints on the release of energy, which in turn does further work, including the construction of parts of the mechanistic action of their function, and also the construction of further constraints on the release of energy. A self-propagating organization of processes arises in cells, and they build their own boundary conditions. They build a richly interwoven web of boundary conditions that further constrains the release of energy so as to build yet more boundary conditions. We have as yet no theory for systems that do work and work cycles to build their own boundary conditions, which thereafter modify the work that is done, which in turn modifies the boundary conditions in the myriad ways that occur in a cell as it propagates organization of the process. The ancients called it the Great Chain of Being.[14] The Chinese called it many things in medicine but the theory of the *five phases* comes to mind initially.

The interwoven web of work and constraint construction, whether of a cell or life and its evolution on the Earth, has not been interwoven into our modern understanding. Perhaps the science of ecological systems comes the closest. A living cell is much more than molecular replication. It is a closure of work tasks that propagates its own organization of processes. It is awesome in its wonderful warp and woof of persistent becoming.

How matter, energy, and information may come together is unknown. But R. Ulanowitz, an ecologist, has introduced a measure for workflows in ecosystems.[15] The measure is the total energy flow in an ecosystem times the diversity of that energy flow. He has shown that mature ecosystems maximize this measure, while it drops to lower values for disturbed ecosystems. Diversity and organization are part of the essence, or *Jing*, of healthy life.

Since Descartes, Galileo, Newton, and La Place, all of reality has been understood in terms of particles in motion, or whatever physicists currently suppose is down there. From this point of view, all arrows point downward. What about the Sacred — agency, meaning, values, purpose, all of life, the planet? Is the concept of the Sacred a human illusion? Are we truly outside nature? And is not nature sacred?

The apparent schism between religion and science is ultimately a disagreement over the existence of meaning. The vast unrepeatability of the universe at all levels of complexity leaves room for creativity in the way the universe unfolds — a creativity that is unpredictable. The radical implication is that we live in an emergent universe in which ceaseless unforeseeable creativity arises and surrounds us. We cannot predict what will happen and, therefore, reason (linear thinking) alone is an insufficient guide to living our lives forward. The ceaseless creativity in this universe is the bedrock of the Sacred.

Many complex systems, including the Earth, share the property of an evolutionary process that is radically unpredictable and ceaselessly creative. This means that the universe is not governed only by natural laws. This idea means that we are entering new scientific and philosophic ground. A partially lawless universe cannot be proven. We cannot predict the past or the future, and we cannot even make probability statements. We are forced to get out of linear thinking.

The explanatory arrows point upward to the evolutionary emergence of preadaptations via natural selection for non-prestateable selective environments. The evolution of life violates no law of physics but cannot be reduced to physics. In this new scientific worldview, our place in the world is very different from that envisioned by pure reductionism.

Galileo believed that science, not revelation, was the only true path to knowledge. We have come to believe that we will understand everything, and that everything will be understandable by natural law. Based on this, spirituality seems pointless. If we were to reinvent the Sacred as the creativity of the universe, the Source of Chinese medicine, we could from there invent a global ethic to orient our lives, and our emerging global civilization — a global civilization that we will partially coconstruct. The Earth has been coconstructing itself for 3.8 billion years. How does the whole remain coherent so that species continue to be able to coexist, even as extinction events occur and new species evolve? This is the unknown mystery into which we must live our lives.

Reason is not a sufficient guide to living our lives forward. Reason is only a part of a still-mysterious entirety of our lives. We are in the process of reinventing ourselves. And, if we are to survive, we must reinvent ourselves as part of all that is sacred.

The Now

We face limited resources and a warming planet. The growth of the economic web is also emergent and may parallel the evolution of the biosphere. The unknown practical potential in understanding how the economic web drives its own advance with the persistent creation of ever-new economic niches may give us, on the positive side, the knowledge of these processes and how to harness them to lift the world out of poverty. Certainly, ending poverty would be a sacred action.

During the Upper Paleolithic, no one saw a machine tool industry known as the Stone Age. We constantly use our tools in new ways. The Industrial Revolution was a transition that expressed physically the ideas of reductionism. In the process of the Industrial Revolution, the horse-and-buggy culture was destroyed, along with the use of manure on agricultural fields. It was replaced by a new culture with new accoutrements like cars, roads, petroleum-based economies, suburbia, petroleum inputs in agriculture and chemistry, and so on. This creative destruction of a whole way of life forced us into the adjacent possible, where existing tools and goods were used for novel purposes. This then becomes an economic revolution and is part of the endless creativity in the universe. The question is how to use this creative expression in a positive way.

We are called upon to reintegrate our entire humanity in the living of our lives. Certainly, our modern time forces us to think locally and globally and act locally and globally. The human creativity of this process is sacred.

The mind connected to the void of the heart, in the Chinese philosophical sense, is what in the West we call sacred consciousness. Consciousness is incompatible with reductionism. Consciousness is a meaning and doing organic system. It is nonalgorithmic. It slips free of computation to go where it will. This freedom of consciousness is part of the creativity of the universe. Consciousness makes meanings and understandings. As such it is sacred.

Our entire historical development as a species, our diverse cultures have been self-consistent, coconstructing, evolving, emergent, and unpredictable. All of life is constantly evolving. To be part of it in time is amazing — and a gift. Ecosystems are the coevolution of organisms and their processes that coevolved together to mesh their functionalities into evolving physiologies that sustain life and also evolve over time. They are a self-consistent community assembly forming niches in which the species can exist and sustain mutual life, and yet evolve. Law as governance is partially beyond natural law. "God's laws" is our name for the creativity in the universe. The creativity in the universe is the Sacred.

Reason cannot be separated from all the rest of our sensibilities. Part of our evolution is to heal this fracture that influences the deepest parts of our humanity. Perhaps part of the evolution of the Aquarian Epoch is to heal this fracture. Re-examining ourselves as evolved living beings in nature is both a cultural task — with implications for the roles of the arts and humanities, legal reasoning, business, practical action — and part of reinventing sacredness, i.e. living with the creativity in the universe that we partially cocreate. We cannot know everything but must live anyway. We must live forward into mystery. So our deepest need is to better understand how we do so.

The discrimination of the Western way of life with the spirit of reason and the rest of human sensibilities driving the reductionist model is an opportunity for the West and the whole human house to reassemble the diverse parts of the human house on a single foundation without losing diversity. We are now at a juncture for the first time in human culture to understand and heal this split, to answer the need for the invention of a global ethic for a global ongoing civilization with faith and courage and with at least one view of "God" that is the sacred creativity of the universe. We can refashion how we use the symbol of God as the creativity of the universe to shape our own single and collective lives.

Science and the humanities must be brought back into the whole. Science has achieved a kind of unspoken hegemony with regard to access to "truth." The humanities are how we know ourselves. Science, as the highest form of reason, says that the pre-eminent goal of humanity is reason. However, it cannot begin to tell us about the self-consistent coconstruction and partially lawless evolution of the Earth, nor can it predict the evolution of technology or the coconstruction and coevolution of human cultures. Therefore, we need to re-examine and reintegrate the arts and humanities along with science, practical action, politics, ethics, and spirituality. Sublime poetry and literature is a lens through which to view our selves, our lives, our world. The Milky Way is truly a speck of foam on the ocean of ecstatic love. It also can show us the truth. Science is not the gold standard for truth. In this respect, science is a belief system. Being in the world is not merely cognitive; it is the full integration of all of our humanity, imagination, invention, thinking, feeling, intuition, sensation — our full emotional selves.

The old propensities for profit, power, and empire are no longer useful. We are still a diverse global community with the widest communication in the history of the Earth. We can no longer survive failure. We cannot survive culture wars. There is no longer "the other." We do not know the future but must act anyway. A wise coevolution of our traditions is humility, because humility invites tolerance. Humility and tolerance are creative. And creativity is sacred.

Natural Selection for Human Agency and the Sacred

Agency emerged in the universe and with it came values, doing, and meaning. Moral law is consequential — a form of evolutionary morality. Agency equals values, meaning, doing, action, and purpose. There is no single moral law from which all moral action can be derived. In the West, we use the utilitarian theory of the "greatest good for the greatest number" but this is not a universal principle. The union of our emotional and rational systems in moral reasoning seems to have evolved by natural selection and reason, emotions, and intuitive capacities that have come into play in our moral reasoning. The ancient moral policies under which we have been living must evolve; leaving out, leaving behind, destroying one group — these all lead to global grief and moral trauma, especially at the level of the receptive.

The virtues inherent in the evolution of law as a model have been accumulated wisdom, the capacity to change as society changes, and a tendency to reject totalitarian ethics. The virtues inherent in law point to a far greater depth than the simplicity that the Abrahamic God handed down in the Ten Commandments.

What is lacking is a global ethic. When formed it must embrace diverse cultures, civilizations, and traditions. The sacred in life pertains to all life and, as we unleash the vast extinction that accompanies our global ecological footprint, we are destroying the creativity in the biosphere that is the Sacred. We are one with all life, with all creativity, with a God that is creativity. And the whole liberating creativity of the universe that we share and partially cocreate invites us to take the next step in evolving an emerging global ethic that respects all of life and the planet.

Capitalism

Modern capitalism is the operating system of the world economy that has evolved out of the Industrial Revolution and reductionism, and the separation of science and religion, meaning and truth. Private employers hire workers to make products and services, which the employers own and then sell for profit. Competitive markets, the price mechanism, the modern corporation as the principal institution, a consumer society and the materialistic values that sustain it, and an administrative state actively promote economic strength and growth. This system has been very good at generating growth.[16]

At the same time, these features as constituted today work together to produce an economic and political reality that is highly destructive to the environment. The powerful drive to earn profits, invest them, innovate, and grow the economy has resulted in remarkable exponential expansion and growth of the world economy. Society-wide the commitment is to economic growth at almost any cost, plus an enormous investment in technologies designed with little regard for the environment, plus powerful corporate interests whose overriding objective is to grow by generating profits including the profit from avoiding the environmental costs they create, and markets that systematically fail to recognize environmental costs unless corrected by government.[17] Rampant consumerism is spurred by the worship of novelty and by sophisticated advertising; and economic activity is so large in scale that its impacts alter the fundamental biophysical operations of the planet and combine to deliver an ever-growing world economy that is undermining the planet's ability to sustain life.

Expansion of economic activity is the predominant cause of environmental decline. The world economy, increasingly integrated and global, is poised for unprecedented growth. A mutually reinforcing set of forces associated with today's capitalism combines to yield economic activity inimical to environmental sustainability. A political default perpetuates the world market environmental costs for which no one is paying, ending in and perpetuating widespread market failure due to deep and environmentally perverse subsidies.[18]

Societies face environmental threats of unprecedented scope and severity, especially as environmental issues link with social inequities and tensions, resource scarcity, and other issues. And mainstream environmentalism has proven insufficient to deal with these challenges as we run from one catastrophe to another but with no overriding approach. However, now these approaches remain essential to laying down the path to address problems with these tools. But it is still true that the momentum of the current system is so great that only very powerful forces will alter the trajectory.

Most environmental deterioration is a result of systemic failures of the capitalism we have today. This includes the internal human environment and human health. And the capitalism we have today is the product of a way of thinking driven by the separation of values and meaning from scientific truth and profit. The market must work for the environment, and therefore us — not the reverse. The field of ecological economics[19] is a critique of endless economic growth and explores the dimensions of a "postgrowth society" where neither nature nor community is sacrificed to the priority of economic growth. Economic growth in affluent societies is not materially improving human happiness. Economic growth is a poor way to generate solutions to pressing social needs and problems. Consumption is a term of affluenza and needs to be substituted for green consumption and living more simply.[20] Corporate dynamics need to be transformed and challenged. The dominance of the corporation and its profit motive are outdated. We need to move beyond capitalism and socialism.

How do We Harness Economic Forces for Sustainability and Sufficiency?

Creativity, innovation, and entrepreneurship of businesses operating within a vibrant private sector are essential to designing and building the future. Growth and investment are needed across a wide front:

- Growth in the developing world that is sustainable and springs from people-centered growth[21];
- Growth in the human incomes of those in America who have far too little; growth in human well-being along many dimensions;
- Growth in new solution-oriented industries, products, and processes;
- Growth in meaningful, well-paying jobs, including green collar jobs;
- Growth in natural resource and energy productivity and in investment in the regeneration of natural assets;
- Growth in social and public services and in investment in public infrastructures.

This is where growth should occur. Harness market forces to these ends.

Natural Capitalism

Natural capitalism redesigns industrial systems to mimic biological ones and progressively eliminate waste.[22] This is an economy based on provision of services rather than the purchase of goods. And it would reverse worldwide resource deterioration and generate natural capital. The market would be transformed into an instrument for environmental restoration and this, in turn, would equal human health restoration. Humanity's ecological footprint would be reduced to what can be sustained environmentally. Incentives that govern corporate behavior can be rewritten. Growth would be focused on things that truly need to grow, and consumption on having enough and then only on having what is healthy. Thus, the rights of future generations and all species would be respected.

Many worlds exist in today's world[23]:

- *The fortress world* is the one in which today's well-to-do escape to protected enclaves like gated communities with armed civilians and private security; mercenary armies are included here, like Black Water hired by the US military services in Iraq and Afghanistan; including prisons, which in the US hold the highest number of inmates of any prison system in the world; a society in which there is a rich minority and a poor majority.
- *The market world* is the world in which nature is considered boundless, where there are no constraints, and economic growth and innovation is key to environmental problems.
- *The policy reform world* is that part of the world where skillful policy guidance will recognize emerging scarcities and threats, and devise responses; economic growth can be consistent with environmental preservation.
- *The new sustainability world* protects and reclaims natural and human communities, and envisions major changes in values, lifestyle, and human behavior. Deep change in social values away from ever-increasing material consumption and toward close community and personal relationships, social solidarity, and a strong connection to nature all require a new consciousness essential to resolving today's social and environmental dilemmas.

- *The social greens world* states that dilemmas have to do with power within society and inequitable resource distribution and access. The focus is on redistributive policies including power redistribution to address environmental questions. Decentralization and protection of local economies and communities is essential. There is a basic question about the ability of government and political impartiality of expertise to guide behavior.

The market world has controlled the levers of power and decision via the market. Today's environmentalism operates in the policy reform world. Solutions of the new sustainability world and the social greens world both point positively beyond today's situation to a new vision and worldview. They relate the human venture to the larger destinies of the universe spoken of in the science and religion section. And they believe that now is the time to carry out the transition from a period of human devastation of the Earth to a period when humans would be present to and for the planet in a mutually beneficial manner (Thomas Berry).[24] The planet is partially us and vice versa. What we do or don't do now will determine our future health and that of our world. They are inexorably intertwined.

Modern Capitalism

Modern capitalism has become the secular religion of advancing secular societies. Anything that will hurt the economy is verboten. The ruthlessness of the marketplace has led to increased foreign competition, deregulation, weakened labor unions, the consumption of natural resources (both renewable and nonrenewable), and the release of pollutants on a scale never before known.[25] Paul Ekins says in *Economic Growth and Environmental Sustainability*, "The sacrifice of the environment to economic growth…has unquestionably been a feature of economic development since the birth of industrialism."[26] The sacrifice remains enormous.

- World economy = +14-fold;
- World population = +4-fold;

- Water use = +9-fold;
- Sulfur dioxide emissions = +13-fold;
- Energy use = +16-fold;
- CO_2 emissions = +17-fold;
- Marine fish catch = +35-fold.

The impacts are increasing, not decreasing. Many of our environmental resources are unprotected by appropriate prices that would constrain their use. The market system simply does not allocate the use of these resources properly. Economic and political interests stand to gain by not allowing connections in government policies that would enable a correction of the market's failure to work for the environment rather than against it. Water would be conserved and used more efficiently if it were sold at its full cost, including the environmental damage of overusing it. But politicians and farmers (especially agribusiness) have a stake in keeping water prices low.[27] Organic and sustainable farming uses less water but industrialized farming continually receives subsidization of its poor practices, with water being one resource lost in the process.[28] Polluters could be made to pay the full costs of their actions, in terms of both damage and cleanup, but typically do not. Natural ecosystems give societies economic services of tremendous value. A developer's actions can reduce these services to society, but rarely does the developer pay fully for those lost services.

Modern technologies are changing the economy of the future to one where opportunities to reduce materials consumed and wastes produced per unit of output are opening up new areas and new products that are lighter, smaller, and more efficient. But, right now, one can conclude that growth is the enemy of the environment, and the economy and the environment remain in collision. The environment includes the human body, which lives as part of it. Therefore, human health in the modern age is partly driven by the capitalist economy. It is partly this economy and the profit motive that drives environmental degradation which pollutes our water, air, and Earth and drives the manufacture of pseudofoods which fill our center aisles in grocery stores with food not worth eating. Food, air, and water contaminated with additives and contaminants that are known carcinogens; and foods grown under conditions that are not supportive of the rest of life surrounding the fields in which they were grown contribute to environmental and human degradation.

In a capitalist economy, survival requires growth, and growth requires profits. This exponential growth economy is a life-and-death matter for any firm. The profit motive powerfully affects the capitalist's behavior. Surplus products (profit) can be increased through environmentally perverse subsidies and other advantages. Today's corporations are committed to keeping the real costs of their activities off the books. They are committed to finding subsidies, tax breaks, and regulatory loopholes from the government. Modern capitalism demands and is allowed to be the sole director of the fate of human beings and the natural environment.[29] This is resulting in the demolition of society.

Fundamental biases in capitalism favor the present over the future and the private over the public. The essence of sustainable development is equity toward future generations. But future generations cannot participate nor are taken into account, in capitalism's markets. The future is part of the public now and greater emphasis on the public side would serve our environment better. Large public investments are overdue in land conservation, in environmental education, research and development, and in incentives to spur new ecologically sophisticated technologies. We have not inherited the Earth from our parents. We have borrowed it from our children.

Today there are more than 63,000 multinational corporations. In 1990 there were fewer than half that. ExxonMobil is larger than 180 nations. The corporate sector wields political and economic power, and has routinely used that power to restrain ameliorative government action. It has driven the rise of transnational capital as the basis for economic globalization.[30] We are becoming a single global economy. But, unfortunately, what we have today is the globalization of market failure. And, as the developing world catches up, it will also begin to suffer from the same diseases that the developed world now suffers from — cardiovascular disease, diabetes, and cancer. All of these diseases are preventable and are the result of a life lived within the constraints of modern capitalism and all that it means.

Globalization scholar Jan Scholte has put it this way: "Students of globalization must surely take seriously the possibility that the underlying structures of the modern (now globalized) world order — capitalism, the state, industrialism, nationality, rationalism — as well as the orthodox discourses that sustain them, may be in important aspects irreparably destructive."[31]

Perhaps part of what makes us human is the capacity to transcend the violence, poverty, ecological decay, oppression, injustice, and secularism of the world into which we were born and which we also continue to make. If it is true that there is selection for agency and the universe is an evolving process, then we can hope for this and see our way into a new and yet-to-be-predicted future. The transcendence and transition requires confidence in the future. And it requires a vision and willingness to risk a great deal to attain it. Sacrifice, commitment, and risk are essential for confronting successfully a well-entrenched system of beliefs, institutions, and practices that do not serve our world. We must transform the essential nature of the main pillars of modernism — the state as a focus for political loyalty, of nationalism as a mobilizing ideology, of the market as a basis for allocating resources, and war as the fulcrum of international stability.

In this age of plenty, there is a spiritual hunger that requires new words of action:

- Nonviolent practices,
- Participating organizations,
- Soft energy paths and gentle technology,
- Democratizing politics,
- Feminizing leadership and tactics,
- Spiritualized nature,
- Green consciousness.

We must replace the ideology of self-help, free enterprise, and competition, on which the United States was founded, with these new concepts. This ideology has coincided with the rise and spread of modern industrial capitalism. Material power and productivity can no longer be considered emblematic of flourishing success. Our society is not in good shape, nor is our mental/emotional/physical/ spiritual health. The modern cancer epidemic is emblematic of this failed lifestyle.

The Environment

Today's environmentalism:

- Believes today's problems can be solved within the system and with new policies;
- Is pragmatic and incremental, addressing the results versus the cause;
- Believes that problems can be solved at acceptable economic costs without significant lifestyle change;
- Sees solutions coming from within the environmental sector;
- Is not focused on political activity or organizing a grassroots movement, which are always second to lobbying, litigating, and working with government agencies;
- Entrusts major action to expert bureaucracies like the EPA and the Department of the Interior.

But the results over the past 25 years have been that trends of destruction have worsened.[32] International treaties are weak and non-bonding, with no clear requirements, targets, and timetables. And there is no enforcement. None of the climate conventions or any other conventions held on a global scale to protect biodiversity, reduce desertification, and protect the world fisheries have had any impact. The world forests have never had a convention. Although air and water pollution standards are vigorously made, air and water quality problems have persisted. In the early 1970s, laws set the goal of returning freshwater bodies to being fishable and swimmable by 1983. The EPA in 2002 reported that one-half of the lakes and one-third of the rivers in the US were still too polluted to fish or swim in.[33] In 2007, 37% of the nation's estuaries were in poor condition. In 2006, the EPA reported that the Great Lakes were again at a tipping point, beyond which their ecosystems could not recover. And in 2007, the EPA reported that one-third of all Americans lived in counties with air pollution levels that fall short of EPA standards. All of these standards were set to protect not only the environment but, in the process, also human health.

We need effective fundamental, nonincremental change in the American government. Exposure to chemical cocktails is a serious and ongoing concern after three decades of the Toxic Substances Control Act.[34] Pesticides, including insecticides, herbicides, fungicides, rodenticides, and other biocides, pour 5–6 billion pounds of toxics into the world's environment each year, with one-quarter released or sold in the US Less than 1% actually reach a pest. In 2005, the EPA's Toxics Release Inventory reported that 4.34 billion pounds of some 650 chemicals (for which reporting is mandated) were disposed of in the environment, as opposed to being treated or recycled. Of this amount, 40% was released to surrounding air or waterways.[35]

Why are We Losing?

- The media has lost interest. News outlets are all owned by a small group of conglomerates driven by the profit-driven demands of Wall Street.
- The environmental movement is weak and vulnerable, through a belief in civil authority and good faith. There is no articulated vision of the future that is commensurate with the magnitude of the crisis.
- The rise of the modern right in recent American politics is responsible for a market fundamentalism that grew in parallel with today's environmentalism. The Heritage Foundation, the American Enterprise Institute, and the Cato Institute all grew at the same time as the Sierra Club, the World Wildlife Fund, and so on.
- The environmental movement was successfully stigmatized as a group of unstable alarmists and bad-faith prophets by these same right-wing well-funded entities.
- The antienvironmental disinformation industry sprang up and neutralized the environmental movement through right-wing abuse.

- The capitalist world is serving up an ever-increasing volume of environmental assaults. Once-dead issues are resurfacing; for example, strip mining is being called mountaintop removal, nuclear power is now clean power, mineral development in pristine areas is viable, and coal is now clean even though many miners die each year because of lax enforcement of safety procedures. All are driven by an insatiable need for growth and profits.
- Environmental issues are increasingly complex and scientifically difficult, chronic, subtle, and slow to unfold.
- The regulatory and management apparatuses are huge and impenetrable.
- Regulatory slippage is occurring, because the sources of pollution are doubling in size. Problems in detecting warning signals and in overcoming vested interests lead to delay in regulation, often incurring damage that could have been prevented with higher sensitivity to environmental alarms.
- Limits that stem from a pragmatic, compromising, deal-with-the-effects approach lead to quick fixes that address symptoms but not underlying causes. The low-hanging fruit approach that improves looks is more tolerable, economically attractive, and politically easy but, like treatment for a cancer, is not a cure.

How can the Market be Transformed Into a Benign and Restorative Force?

The transformation of the market into a powerful instrument for environmental protection and restoration that limits imperialism of the market is a complex task. Public intervention has led to subsidies that are often perverse and do not take into account environmental costs. Scarce natural resources and environmental assets are often under priced and a wedge is driven between the private and social costs of production and consumption. Therefore, the true scarcity of resources production uses up the resource, or the damage caused is obfuscated, leading to overproduction and over consumption depleting resources.

The indirect costs of environmental damage include those to the downstream environment including people.[36] The Commons and the public good are enhanced through such amenities as biodiversity enjoyed by many. The tragedy of the Commons is evidenced when natural resources made available to all are exploited far beyond the optimal level. Thus, individually rational actions add up to a socially undesirable outcome.

The command and control regulations of the 1970s and 1980s tried to set a standard past which polluters could not go. However, market-based mechanism incentives would have led to earlier and better integrations of environmental objectives into business planning, forging an alliance between environmentalists and economists and business. Germany is now shifting the tax burden from work and wages to energy consumption and the resulting pollution.[37] Effluent charges and other environmental charges have further been developed in Europe. Cap and trade schemes in the US began in the 1990 amendments to the Clean Air Act with caps on sulfur emissions from power plants to reduce acid rain. A cost–benefit analysis requires valuation that is usually in dollars. "The basic problem with narrow economic analysis of health and environmental protection is that human life, health, and nature cannot be described meaningfully in monetary terms; they are priceless. When the question is whether to allow one person to hurt another, or to destroy a natural resource; when a life or landscape cannot be replaced; when harms stretch out over decades or even generations…then we are in the realm of the priceless, where market values tell us little about the social values at stake." (Priceless, by Frank Ackerman and Lisa Heinzerling).[38] Is neoclassical economics, a model based at its core on egoistic, anthropocentric, rationalistic, and linear thinking reductionist calculation, appropriate for making environmental choices?

We are running out of environment. Therefore, it should be very expensive to do environmental harm and inexpensive to do things that are environmentally harmless and restorative. Thus, governments should stop environmentally perverse subsidies. Governments should intervene to implement the principle of "the polluter pays."[39] Subsidies for agriculture (agribusiness), energy, transportation, water, fisheries, and forestry should be quantified. Right now these subsidies are globally equal to 850 billion USD annually. With the polluter-pays principle, any environmental consumer or despoiler is required to bear the full costs of all environmental damage caused to humans or nature, of all cleanup and remediation, and of expenses required to reduce impacts to sustainable levels. Such damage would include long-term and future health damage to humans through environmental degradation and pollution.

Moving to a Postgrowth Society

The struggle for subsidies is not humankind's permanent problem today. The problem of today is to use our freedom from pressing economic cares, at least in the industrial world, to live wisely and agreeably and well. The association between economic growth and poverty reduction is less close than we believe. Antipoverty strategies have much more in them than a commitment to economic growth. The GDP should be measured in terms of:

- Growth in production, meaning goods, services, and government expenditure;
- Growth in biophysical throughput, meaning capital stocks that become waste — a throughput is the origin of much of the economy's burden on the environment;
- Growth in human welfare, meaning numerous welfares, i.e. for everyone, including the Commons and all that the Commons entail.

Can we continue to grow at current rates by substituting green technologies? The US CO_2 levels can be reduced to safe levels if we reduce releases from fossil fuel use by 80% over the next 40 years. This equals about a 7% reduction each year for the next 40 years. One-half of the required rate of change is needed simply to compensate for the effects of economic growth. This would be like running down a very fast down escalator. The necessary reduction in atmospheric CO_2 levels today is not being accomplished by any world government or in any systematic way.

Governments are profoundly committed to promoting growth but not to reducing carbon emissions. In the next 20–30 years, the world economy will likely be twice its current size. No one is challenging growth as a *modus operandi* in the biosphere. Speed is required for technological change to stay ahead of growth. Just ask Apple. Development of international environmental law and regulation is painfully slow but the world economy and urbanization surge ahead. It took 20 years from agreeing on a phaseout to the actual phaseout of chlorofluorocarbons.

Growth is not delivering the social goods. Incomes are higher, but individual and social well-being is not improving — it is declining. Growth has equaled social unease, manipulation by marketers, obsessive materialism, environmental degradation, endemic alienation, and loneliness. "We seek fulfillment but settle for abundance" says Clive Hamilton in *Growth Fetish*.[40]

In ecological economics, the pollutants discharged and the environments into which they are discharged have an assimilative capacity and the harvesting of renewable resources is done at a sustainable rate.[41] Quantitative limits can be implemented by either a tax or a cap and trade mechanism. Thus, the natural capital is fully protected and regenerated. In ecological economies:

- There is more leisure and a shorter work week;
- There are greater labor protections;
- There is job security and benefits;
- There is retirement and health benefits;
- There are restrictions on advertising;
- There are new ground rules for corporations;
- There are strong social and environmental provisions in trade agreements;
- There is rigorous consumer protection;
- There is greater income and social equality;
- There is progressive taxation for the rich and higher income support for the poor;
- There is major spending on public sector services and environmental amenities;

- There is a huge investment in education, skills, and new technology to promote ecological modernization, and rising labor productivity to offset smaller workforces and shorter hours.

Now, there is freedom for the growth-at-all-costs paradigm and ruthless economy. Our current growth mania was not always. The acceptance of limits in the pursuit of growth means coming to terms with America's need to reconcile its love of liberty with its egalitarian pretentiousness. The rapid growth has been used to resolve this tension at the core of the American enterprise. This tension can be resolved in other ways. As Mahatma Gandhi said, "First they laugh at you, then they ignore you, then they fight you, then you win."

Well-Being

Thomas Jefferson was a man of the Enlightenment, when the "right" to happiness first came into being. The pursuit of happiness meant the pursuit of private pleasure *and* the public welfare.[42] Jefferson, most interpret, meant the coexistence of these two meanings. The double meaning, however, was soon lost in practice. It came to mean only the personal. Waves of immigrants came here to use America as the land of opportunity to pursue prosperity, pleasure, and wealth. Civic virtue was jettisoned and the pursuit of happiness and the rise of American capitalism became the justification for work and sacrifice, and a basis for meaning and hope that only loomed larger on the horizon of Western democracies. With this came a shift from production to consumption as the fulcrum of capitalism.[43]

Well-being, according to Diener and Seligman, includes pleasure, engagement, and meaning.[44,45] The positive relationship between national well-being and national per capita income disappears when one looks at only countries with a GDP per capita of over USD 10,000 per year. Therefore, once a country achieves a moderate level of income, further growth does not significantly improve perceived well-being. Peoples with the highest well-being are not those from the richest countries but those who live where political institutions are effective and human rights are protected, where corruption is low and mutual trust is high. Richer people in societies are happier, while societies that get richer do not get happier. Habituation leads us to think that more is better and more will make us happier. But this leads only to the hedonic treadmill. Advertisers recognize this and feed our addictions. But the true wellsprings of happiness are[46]:

- Belonging,
- Close and long-term social relationships,
- Family relationships,
- Stability in our financial situation,
- Work that nourishes us,
- Our community and friends,
- Our health,
- Our personal freedom,
- Our personal values.

What we are experiencing now is a famine of warm interpersonal relationships. And economic development that improved well-being over the millennia is no longer a source of well-being. The guiding principles that really matter must be continually reconsidered in terms of the ends they produce. Economics does not really have custody of how we think about well-being.

The hallowed search for happiness has been hijacked by a discomforting and frenzied activity. Joy becomes mania — a reckless pursuit, irritability, confusion, depression leading to anxiety, and competition, and social disruption. While economic output is up, satisfaction has decreased. Scrap the GDP, which is not a measure of anything, for the ISEW — the Index of Sustainable Economic Welfare.[47] Change the GDP to a measure of well-being. The HPI (the Happy Planet Index), if it were instituted, would put the US at the bottom of the list and Costa Rica near the top.[48]

Consumerism is paired with materialism. The material conditions of life have been elevated over the spiritual and social dimensions. Consumer sovereignty does not reign but is shaped by forces like advertising, cultural norms, social pressures, and psychological associations. Consumer spending has been a leading driver of environmental decline, including the decline of our own health. Our endless stream of needs drives the economy. In other words, consumers serve the economy and not the other way around.[49] Consumer debt in 1970 in the US was USD 525 billion. In 2004, it was USD 2225 billion. The biggest increase has been driven by the rising costs of the basics — housing, health care, food, and education. While real wages went up by zero between 2001 and 2004, the cost of the basics went up by 11%.[50] Since 1970:

- New house size became 50% larger;
- Electricity consumption per person rose by 70%;
- The municipal solid wastes generated per person increased by 33%;
- And since 1994 80% of all new homes have been exurban, with more than half on 10 acres or more.

We have been reluctant to face the consumption issue.[51] Green consumerism is beginning to drive corporations and what they produce. There has begun an effort to "dematerialize" the economy with more efficient use of resources, and to delink social welfare from output.[52]

(1) We need to increase consumer awareness and choice through school curricula, citizen engagement, and signal producers.
(2) We need to promote innovative policies that can provide incentives, assess more accurate prices, and eliminate subsidies for wasteful or unsustainable practices.
(3) We need to accelerate demand for green products in business, governments, institutions, and all major consumers.
(4) We need to demand corporate accountability for social accountability to investors and consumers through campaigns, boycotts, and shareholder advocacy in order to influence corporate behavior.
(5) We need to encourage sustainable business practices within NGOs, governments, and others to help companies "green" their products and services by:

- Mapping environmental footprints;
- Rethinking resource extraction, use, and recycling;
- Sustainable redesign of products;
- Analysis of supply chains and their environmental impacts.

However, even green consumption has environmental costs. And consumption linked to an environmental agenda has a problem — consumption would continue to expand as the privatization of the environmental crisis encourages upwardly spiraling consumption that translates into business as usual. Citizens must realize that consumption *is* the problem.[53] Only collective citizen action can reframe and shape the institutional and political forces where choices are constrained. There is tremendous potential for manipulating green consumers and perverting the process that equals a "greenwash".[54]

Market-based consumption is not tightly coupled with human welfare and life satisfaction. If hyperconsumption is damaging psychologically and environmentally, then we can improve our lives and environment by slimming down and doing with less. Consumption is an addiction that leads to alienation and passivity. When consumption is exalted, so is insecurity. Our denial of death is an attempt to transcend mortality through wealth. The institutional architecture of everyday choice, as in a mortgage, in health care, in education, or in energy consumption, needs to be challenged. Affluence is a shallowness that leads to a constantly shifting identity and to a split between heart and mind. It leads to a sense of misdirection of life's energy, and truly it is. We need to practice resurrection. And become whole again.

Corporations

Corporations are the principal actors on capitalism's stage. They have defining characteristics that drive their behavior:

- There is a separation of ownership from management — shareholders.
- There is limited liability, in which the shareholders are not personally liable to a firm's creditors.

- Corporations have a "personhood" that enables them to become individuals who enjoy the protection of constitutional provisions.
- Directors and managers have a duty to act in the best interest of the corporation and maximize the wealth of the shareholders. This has become a huge obstacle in the corporate evolution to a socially responsible institution.
- Nothing in its legal makeup limits what a corporation can do to others in pursuit of its selfish ends and, in fact, the corporation is compelled to cause harm when the benefits of doing so outweigh the costs. Only pragmatic concern for its own interests and the laws of the land constrain the corporation's predatory instincts and interests. All of these bad things that happen to people and the environment as a result of a corporation's relentless and legally compelled pursuit of self-interest are categorized as "externalities" — other people's problems.

There is an ongoing tug of war between corporate power and citizens' power.[55] However, it is not an equal match. Business can exert tremendous power directly in the political process through lobbying and campaign contributions. Today, about 35,000 lobbyists in Washington, DC represent corporate interests. PACs spent USD 15 million in 1974 and USD 222 million in 2005. The US Chamber of Commerce is the largest PAC. Corporate-owned media can shape public opinion and policy debate. Corporate tools of the trade include expensive issue advertising, business-oriented think tanks, well-funded studies, and policy entrepreneurs. Business leaders sit on nonprofit boards and contribute to fundraising. Business supports university and other research defining many things, including disease and treatment. This helps to explain why cancer prevention is at the bottom of the heap when it comes to expenditures for research into causation, especially environmental causation. The majority of environmental research into cancer causation is being done by privately funded nonprofit organizations, with the public acting as the main impetus.

Labor can strike but capital can leave an area or refuse to invest there if the "business climate" is not right. As long as regions and nations want to attract investment and growth, competing with one another, corporations will be served. Therefore, corporations are the dominant economic and political actors. Corporate leaders are regularly appointed to top positions in the executive branch, and corporate experts are listened to by Congress. Corporate owners and executives are a dominant class with the power to shape the economic and political framework within which other groups and classes must operate.[56]

Of the 100 largest economies in the world in 2000, 51 were corporations. In 1970, there were 7000 multinational corporations. In 2007, there were 63,000. Within these 63,000 corporations there were 90 million employees, and these corporations contributed 25% of the gross world product, driving the processes of economic globalization. In 1975, world trade accounted for less than USD 1 trillion in profits. In 2000, it accounted for USD 5 trillion. These multinationals have a huge impact on the global environment, generating one-half of the gases responsible for global warming. They control one-half of the world's oil, gas, and coal mining and refining.[58]

The globalization of market failure, and the control of vast resources and technical capabilities, both without the responsibilities of nationhood, enable these multinationals to move more quickly when a challenge or opportunity arises.[59] If they are unfettered by national or international laws, ecological understanding, or social responsibility, then enormously destructive acts take place. Their agility and their access to capital and resources allow them to innovate, produce goods and services, and influence the world on a scale and at a speed the world has never seen before.

Several hundred global corporations and banks have increasingly woven webs of production, consumption, and culture across borders. Aided by global bureaucracies that have emerged over the last half-century, the overall result has been a concentration of economic and political power that is increasingly unaccountable to governments, people, or the planet.[60] There has been a redesign of the planet's social, economic, and political arrangements since the Industrial Revolution. A power shift of stunning proportions is being engineered, moving real economic and political power away from national, state, and local governments and communities toward unprecedented centralization of power for global corporations, bankers, and global bureaucracies.[61]

The first tenet of globalization design is to give primary importance to the achievement of ever-more-rapid, never-ending corporate economic growth — a kind of hypergrowth like that of cancer — fueled by a constant search for access to new resources, new and cheaper labor sources, and new markets. The ideological heart of the model is free trade accompanied by deregulation of corporate activity. The goal is to remove as many impediments to expanded corporate activity as possible.[62]

Environmental deterioration is placed at the doorstep of these forces with ever-increasing consumption, exploitation of resources, and waste disposal as external problems. Export-oriented production is especially damaging, because it is responsible for an increasing global transport activity while requiring very costly and ecologically damaging new infrastructures like ports, airports, dams, and canals.

Steps must be taken to encourage voluntary corporate initiatives. Corporate accountability must be promoted through regulation and governmental controls at the national and international levels. The very nature of the corporation itself must be transformed. Corporations must be greened. New technologies must be solution-oriented. Pressure must be put on corporations to run a business based on environmental stewardship. Huge majorities in 20 countries now favor tougher regulations to protect the environment.[63] In the US, 66% of Americans say that they want to see corporations have less influence on the nation. And 38% of Americans see big business as the biggest threat to the future of the country.

New capitalists are seeking investments in responsible management and sustainable institutions.[64] They are seeking a triple bottom line — to support the economy, the environment, and society. They are seeking codes of conduct and product certification schemes at the national and international levels. There are now many voluntary codes of conduct:

- Global Reporting Initiative guidelines for corporate reporting on sustainability;
- LEED certification of new green buildings;

- The Forest Stewardship Council and the Marine Stewardship Council to certify and label eco fish and forest products;
- Environmental performance principles adopted by major banks;
- The U.N. Global Compact to list good behavior on labor, environment, and human rights issues;
- The ISO 14000 program.

These are a few among thousands of environmental groups, NGOs, and engaged academics, many of whom have global warming as a key driving issue.

Corporate greening is being driven by green consumerism, by lenders and insurers, and by blame- and-shame campaigns. Behind these actions are NGOs, existing governmental regulatory agencies and by the prospect of future regulation by those agencies, by sales, and by a general need to improve corporate standing as good citizens. The market for virtue has grown with the green revolution.[65]

To be reliably green, government action is needed:

- The corporate charter must be revoked if the corporation has grossly violated the public interest, and so there must be periodic public reviews.
- Unwanted corporations like Monsanto must be excluded or expelled.
- Corporate directors and top managers should be personally liable for gross negligence, and limited liability should be rolled back.
- The idea of a corporate personhood must be eliminated.
- Corporations should be excluded from politics; elections should be publicly financed; conflicts of interest should be stopped by ending the revolving door between government and corporations; and public oversight of political appointees should be performed.
- Corporate lobbying should be reformed; there should be no lobbying on public policy without board-of-directors oversight of the corporate policy decisions and lobbying expenditures.

The corporations of the future will be reconstituted to serve, promote, and be accountable to broader domains of society than just themselves and their shareholders. Shareholder primacy is the single greatest obstacle to corporate evolution. The gladiatorial culture of the corporation deifies competitive advantage, efficiency, and shareholder returns, and is not a culture that is compatible with a sustainable economy and a humane society. Wealth is a joint product of all resource providers — shareholders, employees, unions, future generations, the government, customers, communities, and suppliers. Each provide resources for wealth creation over time, and each has a right to expect returns on their contribution.

We need a whole new set of principles that serve the public interest, sustainability, equity, participation, and respect for the rights of human beings and all other forms of life. We need to reconnect meaning with science, and the heart with the mind.

Beyond Capitalism

Capitalism became the staging ground for a kind of "associationalist" socialism. Keynes said that the future would require "a somewhat comprehensive socialization of investment." Samuel Bowles has said that changes in science and technology are likely to bring fundamental changes in the institution of capitalism and/or lead to a qualitatively different economic system.[66] The information revolution and global warming are accelerating the impact of humans on the environment and raising challenges without precedent in human history. Many have done well and are reluctant to risk their privileged status. To experiment with institutional structures that might be more suitable for dealing with these challenges and closing the gap between rich and poor is fraught with emotional and political angst. But we are heading toward a world plagued by economic irrationality, buffeted by environmental crises, and divided into increasingly hostile camps of haves and have-nots.

Modern capitalism is driving the world to a point where there is a choice: either costly environmental measures that could serve as the *coup de grace* to the viability of the capitalist world economy or various ecological catastrophes brought on by the ceaseless accumulation of capital and growth inherent in capitalism. Capitalism is in crisis because it cannot find reasonable solutions to its current dilemmas, mainly the inability to contain ecological destruction.

The central political debate of the next 25–50 years is what will replace the capitalist system. Dryzek stated that the combination of capitalism, interest group politics, and bureaucratic states will prove "thoroughly inept when it comes to ecology."[67] The outcomes are overproduction and underconsumption leading to overaccumulation, global social polarization, crises of state legitimacy and political authority, and a crisis of sustainability.

America is slowly losing legitimacy, because the realities it produces contradict the values it proclaims. Capitalism's inability to sustain the environment is the biggest threat to its future. The alternatives have been socialism or communism, both of which are fading around the globe. But within capitalism there are a variety of national economic systems: the Scandinavian countries have a social-democratic capitalism with public control over capital investment with more comprehensive social programs, the market and the state; and Japan has a state capitalism with the state dominating the market. Probably, there is no future for socialism. So we need to identify a new nonsocialist operating system. How can we produce and distribute material wealth for the betterment of all?

Forms of policy should be to promote "the full realization of human potential through, in the first instance, proper appreciation of the sources of well-being. Reaffirmation is a necessary role of public ownership, without any expropriation of private property. This is anti-capitalist, though, in the sense that it argues that government and society would no longer cede special significance to the objectives or mutual claims of the owners of capital."[68]

Many Americans are already at work experimenting in local settings. This implies a movement at the grass-roots level for deep reforms. Washington, DC will not drive change. We are in the process of altering the "genome" of capitalism's and our own behavior.

Things that are helping to move our way of being in new directions include the ideas and realities that[69]:

- People own their own work;
- 48,000 co-ops are now operating in the US;
- 10,000 credit unions are now operating in the US;
- 1000 mutual insurance companies are owned by their policy-holders, with USD 80 billion in assets;
- The number of public trusts has increased exponentially;
- The top 1000 pension funds in the USD own USD 5 trillion in assets and are becoming very assertive on social and environmental issues;
- Cities and states are chartering municipal development corporations to provide health services and environmental management;
- Charities and nonprofits are getting into business to the tune of USD 60 billion annually earned by the 14,000 largest US nonprofits, making them corporate hybrids with ownership by workers, public ownership, and public and private enterprises that do not seek traditional profits, with greater local control, more sensitivity to employee, public, and consumer interests, and heightened environmental performance.

A new sector that is public or independent is evolving that focuses growth on high-priority human and environmental needs. The propositions that this new sector share are as follows[70]:

Proposition 1: Modern capitalism and the system of political economy is profoundly destructive and threatens the planet. The current system cannot accommodate solutions and, therefore, must change.

Proposition 2: Affluent societies have reached fruition regarding overcoming hardship and deprivation.

Proposition 3: Modern capitalism is no longer enhancing human well-being but is producing a stressed and ultimately unsatisfactory social reality; dissatisfaction with this social reality will force change.

Proposition 4: The international social movement for change, the irresistible rise of global anticapitalism, is stronger than many imagine; there is a coalescing of forces for peace, social justice, community, ecology, and feminism. It is a movement of movements.

Proposition 5: People are busy planting seeds of change through a host of alternative arrangements.

Proposition 6: The end of the Cold War has opened the door, creating political space for questioning capitalism.

A Profound Reorientation

We are now immersed in a "mode of consciousness that has established a radical discontinuity between the human and other modes of being and the bestowal of all rights on humans but not others. We have difficulty accepting the human (ourselves) as an integral part of the Earth community. We see ourselves as a transcendent mode of being. All other Earthly beings are instruments to be used or resources to be exploited for human benefit." (Thomas Berry)

Revolution by consciousness needs a process already underway in a population. And it needs the existing order, which is already dependent upon an earlier consciousness for its power, and, therefore, unable to survive a change in consciousness. These exist now in the US. This is responsible for the polarization we are now experiencing. At the same time, we need a rapid evolution to a new consciousness, because today's problems cannot be solved with today's mind, as disconnected as it is from the unchanging truth of the heart. Today's dominant worldview is simply too biased toward anthropocentrism, materialism, egocentrism, reductionism, rationalism, and nationalism to sustain changes needed.

Paul Raskin, in *The Great Transition Initiative*,[71] states that consumers, individualism, and domination of nature have given way to a new triad: quality of life, human solidarity, and ecological sensibility. Scarcity and survival has dominated existence. Now we have the historical possibility for a postscarcity planetary civilization. We need to move away from the orgy of consumption among the privileged and the desperation among the excluded. This is quality of life — living knowing that all are taken care of. Connectedness of the whole globe and the future (including future generations) is a manifestation of the capacity of reciprocity and empathy that lies deep in the human spirit and psyche when these are connected. This is human solidarity. The right to dominate nature is no longer sacrosanct. The deep sense of humanity's place in the web of life, and dependence upon it, is sacrosanct. This is ecological sensibility. All are connected to one another in what one could call the ceaseless creativity of the universe termed the Sacred — or the Great Chain of Being.

In redefining wealth, we can call the following true wealth: health, community, and the natural environment. To have these definitions become tangible, we must move from hoarding to sharing, from concentrated to distributed ownership, and from rights of ownership to responsibilities of stewardship.

Daniel Patrick Moynihan has stated: "The central conservative truth is that culture, not politics, determines the success of a society. The central liberal truth is that politics can change a culture and save it from itself." The religions of the world wield particular moral authority, and the environmental crisis calls on the religions to respond by finding or rediscovering their voice within the larger Earth community. Religions have played key roles in ending slavery, in the civil rights movement, in overcoming apartheid. Contemporary capitalism can be transformed as well. The market can be made to work for the environment rather than against it. Corporate behavior can be altered to meet real human and social needs. And government can be the principal means of doing this. Even though it is weak, shallow, dangerous, and corrupted, democracy in America is the best money can buy. And although our government is hobbled by its addiction to the GDP and its growth, our democracy holds the seeds of vision for a new democracy. Democracy at the local, community, and bioregional levels is needed, with members of particular geographic or political communities working together to build a future that is environmentally healthy and economically vibrant at the local and regional levels.

Close-by grass-roots local activists must still influence beliefs and behaviors of real human beings. The essence of democracy is deliberation rather than voting, interest aggregation, or rights. The essence of democracy is:

- Political equality for all participants;
- Interpersonal reasoning as the guiding political procedure;
- Public giving, weighing, acceptance, or rejection of reasons.

Deliberative democracy requires direct participation of citizens, and it requires types of dialogue mechanisms that can be used in the process. Deliberative democracy is self-government rather than representative government in the name of citizens. A national system of neighborhood assemblies with a national initiative and referendum process will provide empowerment of citizens to decide matters of common concern and to legislate the results themselves. Political accountability and democratic control must be given to a range of international issues, with individuals given multiple citizenships that are at once national, regional, and global. Democracy as a process must mirror the Great Chain of Being.

Adjudication of certain issues is necessarily retained at the global level of governance. The rights of regions to pursue diverse forms of development and democratic decision-making constrained only by their obligations to conform to global responsibilities and principles would be a driving mechanism. This would mean that there is direct citizen participation in governance, and that there is a decentralization of decision-making, and that people would feel a powerful sense of global citizenship, interdependence, and shared responsibility.

Now

Right now we need a far-reaching overhaul of American environmental politics:

- Environmental politics needs to be broadened, so that environmental concern and advocacy is extended to a full range of relevant issues with an agenda to expand and embrace a profound challenge to consumerism and commercialism and the lifestyles they offer, including a healthy skepticism of growth mania, focus on what society should be striving to grow, challenge to corporate dominance, and a redefinition of the corporation and its goals. This will require a commitment to deep change in the functioning and reach of the market and a democratization of wealth.

- There must be advocacy of human rights as a central concern where social justice and environmental concerns are focused as one cause. Many environmentalists have been persecuted, jailed, or murdered. Their rights should be vigorously defended. Environmental issues should be seen as human rights issues – that is, the right to clean water, air, sanitation, sustainable development, cultural survival, freedom from climate disruption and ruin, and freedom to live in a nontoxic environment free of toxic trespass, with all of these same rights preserved for future generations.

- We must address America's social problems directly and generously by providing and guaranteeing good jobs, income security, and social and medical insurance as alternatives to endlessly pumping up an environmentally destructive economy. Environmentalists must join up with others to address the crisis of inequality that is unraveling America. We are in crisis in the presence of unprecedented profits, soaring executive pay, huge incomes, increasingly concentrated wealth for a very small minority. With poverty rates near a 30-year high, stagnant wages despite rising productivity, declining social mobility and opportunity, record levels of people without health insurance, shrinking safety nets, and the longest work hours among the rich countries, Americans are suffering more and living in fear.

- Political reforms like campaign finance reform, election reform, and the regulation of lobbying are necessary for a revitalization of large-scale membership organizations that give citizens more leverage in the political process. Increased voter turnout, open primaries, nonpartisan redistricting, minimum free TV and radio time for all federal candidates meeting basic requirements, a reduction of perks for incumbents, and equal air time for competing political views are all necessary.

Environmental goals will not be reached unless the goals of many issues are reached. Unions, the working class, minorities, religious organizations, the women's movement, communities of shared fate, the environmental community, those working on domestic reform, those with a liberal social agenda, and those working for human rights, international peace, consumer issues, world health and population concerns, and world poverty and underdevelopment are all part of the environment. These causes must succeed in order for the environmental causes to succeed, because they are all connected.

Building a movement of joined forces will contribute to the emergence of a powerful citizen's movement for change. The best hope we have is a coalescing of civic, scientific, environmental, religious, student, and other organizations with enlightened business leaders, concerned families, and engaged communities networked together, protesting, demanding action and accountability from governments and corporations, and taking steps as consumers and communities to realize sustainability in everyday life. This is what the Occupy movement is really about. And although it looks disparate, the truth is that, consciously or unconsciously, the movement participants intuitively recognize that all of these issues are connected.

Today there are close to two million organizations in the world working toward ecological sustainability and social justice. This means that there are tens of millions of people dedicated to change. All of these organizations have these two basic tenets in common: the Golden Rule and the sacredness of all life.

The future can be remade. But we must know the full extent of our predicament in order to change. There are solid grounds for hope: global population growth is slowing; our scientific understanding has greatly improved; world poverty is decreasing; technologies can and are bringing improvement in manufacturing, energy, transportation, construction, and organic agriculture. There are new burgeoning capacities for leadership and effectiveness. Businesses are starting to see value in greening. A global civil society is emerging. And the seriousness of looming environmental threats is beginning to sink in. New forms of business and management are evolving. Consumers are beginning to downshift and go green. Student activism is reawakening. Faith communities of all kinds are taking up environmental causes. There is a growing worldwide endorsement of the Earth Charter, which speaks to:

- Being, not having;
- Giving, not getting;
- Needs, not wants;
- Better, not richer;
- Community, not individual;
- Other, not self;
- Connected, not separate, and ecology, not economy;
- Part of nature, not apart from nature;
- Dependent, not transcendent;
- Tomorrow, not today.

We must practice radical hope.

The Earth Charter Preamble[72]:

(1) We are Earth, the people, plants and animals, rains and oceans, breath to the forest and flow of the sea.
(2) We honor Earth as the home of all living things.
(3) We cherish Earth's beauty and diversity of life.
(4) We welcome Earth's ability to renew as being the basis of all life.
(5) We recognize the special place of Earth's Indigenous Peoples, their territories, their custom and their unique relationship to Earth.
(6) We are appalled at the human suffering, poverty and damage to Earth caused by inequality of power.
(7) We accept a shared responsibility to protect and restore Earth and to allow wise and equitable use of resources so as to achieve an ecological balance and new social, economic and spiritual values.
(8) In all our diversity we are one.
(9) Our common home is increasingly threatened.
(10) We thus commit ourselves to the following principles, noting at all times the particular needs of women, indigenous peoples, the South, the disabled and all those who are disadvantaged.

The Precautionary Principle Again

The Hippocratic oath, taken by doctors, first states: "Do no harm." In what is thought to be the oath for doctors of Chinese medicine, it is stated that first "the doctor takes care of people's lives." The combination of these two precepts holds the essence of the precautionary principle.

The precautionary principle as applied to environmental policy points out that it only makes sense to act with prudence to keep from harming ourselves and the Earth through our own technologies. Critics have pointed to all the "cherished things," such as free-ranging technological creativity, and resulting cherished things that would presumably be given up by such prudence. They say that this would lead to general paralysis. This is the religion-versus-science argument again. We must move beyond this linear way of thinking and broaden our *modus operandi* to one that is circular.

The precautionary principle originated in Germany more than 20 years ago, when private landowners noticed that their treasured forests were dying. They appealed to their government to do something and the German government began an all-out effort to cut back power plant emissions, which were producing acid rain. The effort was translated into German law, the *Vorsorgeprinzip*, which became enshrined in international law as the precautionary principle (Raffensperger and Tickner, 1999).

There are several versions of the precautionary principle but all are based on three core elements: potential harm, scientific uncertainty, and precautionary action. The 1992 Rio Declaration on Environment and Development states: "In order to protect the environment, the precautionary approach shall be widely applied by States according to their capabilities. Where there are threats of serious or irreversible damage, lack of full scientific certainty shall not be used as a reason for postponing cost-effective measures to prevent environmental degradation" (SEHN, 2002).

The US has officially supported most of the international accords that include the precautionary principle. However, in the past several years, strong opposition has been mounting in US industry and in government agencies supporting commerce. In January 1998, SEHN convened a small gathering of activists, scientists, and policy-makers to discuss using the principle as a basis for reforming environmental policy in the US. The statement produced by this gathering is called the Wingspread Statement, spoken of earlier in this text. The widely cited definition of the precautionary principle from this statement includes the following: "When an activity raises threats of harm to human health or the environment, precautionary measures should be taken even if some cause-and-effect relationships are not fully established scientifically." The Wingspread Statement went on to define three additional components of the application of the precautionary principle: "In this context the proponent of an activity, rather than the public, should bear the burden of proof. The process of applying the Precautionary Principle must be open, informed, and democratic and must also involve an examination of the full range of alternatives, including no action."

These components — shifting the burden of proof; assessing alternatives; and transparent, democratic action — have often appeared as a part of or alongside the precautionary principle in international treaties and various national statements. The Wingspread Statement brought them together and thus defined not only the principle itself but also something of the way in which it could be applied.

The precautionary principle has many practical uses and applications. And at bottom it brings values to the forefront of discussion. Invoking the precautionary principle is an acknowledgement that policy choices are value-laden, and it is an endorsement of certain values. The precautionary principle embodies certain values by exposing the contradictory values that currently govern decision-making processes. It can be effective only if certain values are allowed to enter into the decision-making process. The principle may be most effective if specific values, in the form of goals, are allowed to guide the entire process from beginning to end.

What we find ourselves involved in today is a contest of values. For example, the Chlorine Chemistry Council identified the precautionary principle as the greatest emerging threat to that industry as early as 1994 (Rampton and Stauber, 2001). And "Radical environmental groups brandishing the precautionary principle have prevailed upon governments in recent decades to assail and intimidate the chemical industry and, more recently, the food industry." (Miller and Conko, 2001). The economics-first paradigm is being countered in a way that is unprecedented. In the Wingspread Statement, the most explicit embodiment of values or ethics lies in "burden shifting." Who or what gets the benefit of the doubt: products or the people they might harm; perpetrators or possible victims; the advance of technology or the survival of ecosystems?

Democracy and transparency in the decision-making process also represent an ethical component: the right to know, the right to be included in decisions that affect one, and the duty to include all who are affected. These ethical considerations are a statement of values.

The term "*Vorsorge*" means, literally, "fore-caring." It implies preparing for a difficult future. It is proactive, whereas precaution seems more reactive in stance. The precautionary principle, or fore-caring, gives us a way to change our behavior, personally and collectively, by reminding us to acknowledge our mistakes, admit our ignorance, and act with foresight and caution to prevent damage. It singles out scientific uncertainty, because scientific uncertainty has often been the key argument against protective action. The precautionary principle calls for a humble recognition that the world is full of scientific uncertainties. It acknowledges that the Earth is made up of complex and interrelated systems vulnerable to harm from human activities in ways that we do not yet understand or even know how to ask about. Precaution, or fore-caring, is an expression of values that give priority to these vulnerable systems, including human bodies.

The European Union (EU) has implemented to some extent the precautionary principle within a narrow range. Where there is reason for concern, a go-slow approach has been instituted with some preventive action until you have better information and giving consumers a say. As a result, throughout the EU a social consensus has arisen around quality of life which includes many factors: culture, environment, health, esthetics, and so on, as well as economic prosperity. The interconnectedness of all of these expressions of life is the foundation of the web of life and is the Great Chain of Being. Cancers are a symptom of when these connections are broken. By healing these connections and making them whole again, we prevent most cancers and many other diseases.

References

1. National Cancer Institute. Surveillance Epidemiology and End Results (SEER). Incidence and mortality. www.seer.cancer.gov/statfacts/html/all.html
2. Cancer rates. *Heath and Environment*. Issue 17, Aug. 2009. www.healthandenvironmentonlinecom/issue-archive/cancer-rates
3. Cancer Prevention Coalition. US National Cancer Institute manipulates cancer statistics. App. II. www.preventcancer.org/losing/nci/manipulates.htm#stats
4. www.cancer.org/acs/groups/content/epidemiologysurveillance/documents/doc
5. Palkinghorne J. Reductionism. *Interdisciplinary Encyclopedia of Religion and Science*. www.dief.org/en/voci/104.asp
6. Darwin C. (2003) *On the Origin of Species by Natural Selection, or the Preservation of Favoured Races in the Struggle for Life*. Modern reprint. John Murry, London.
7. Cushing J. (1998) *Philosophical Concepts in Physics*. Cambridge University Press.
8. Clancy S, Brown W. (2008) Translation: DNA to mRNA to protein. *Nat Educ* 1(1).
9. Crick F. (1970) Central dogma of molecular biology. *Nature* **227** Aug. 8.
10. Adams J. (2008) The complexity of gene expression, protein interaction, and cell differentiation. *Nat Educ* **1**(1).
11. Kauffman S. Autonomous agents and adjacent possible theory (ADAPT). www.theoryofmind.org/pieces/AAAPT.html
12. Bandura A. Toward a psychology of human agency. Stanford University. www.Wexler.free.fr/library/files/bandura%20(2006)%20towards%20psychology
13. The Physics Classroom. Basic terminology and concepts. Work, energy, and power. www.physicsclassroom.com/class/energy/a511a.cfm

14. Lovejoy A. (1976) *The Great Chain of Being: A Study of the History of an Idea.* Harvard University Press.

15. Jergensen S. Muller F. (2000) *Handbook of Ecosystems Theories and Management.* CRC.

16. McCraw T. (1998) *Creating Modern Capitalism: How Entrepreneurs, Companies, and Countries Triumphed in Three Industrial Revolutions.* Harvard University Press.

17. Speth J. (2008) *The Bridge at the Edge of the World: Capitalism, the Environment, and Crossing from Crisis to Sustainability.* Yale University Press.

18. Myers N, Kent J. (2001) *Perverse Subsidies: How Tax Dollars Can Undercut the Environment and the Economy.* Island Press.

19. The International Society for Ecological Economics. www.isecoeco.org

20. Sustainable consumption. Simple living. The Sierra Club. www.sierra-club.org/sustainable_consumption/simpleliving

21. Living Economies Forum. People-Centered Development Forum. www.livingeconomiesforum.org/people-centered-development-forum

22. Lovins L, Lovins A, Hawken P. (2008) *Natural Capitalism: Creating the Next Industrial Revolution.* Back Bay.

23. Hawken P. (2010) *The Ecology of Commerce, Revised Edition: A Declaration of Sustainability.* Harper Collins.

24. Earth Community. Thomas Berry and the Earth Community. www.earth-community.org

25. Bruno S. (2006) *Wal-Mart World: The World's Biggest Corporation in the Global Economy.* CRC.

26. Ekins P. (1999) *Economic Growth and Environmental Sustainability: The Prospects for Green Growth.* Routledge.

27. EBM Tools Network. Ecosystem-Based Management Tools Network. Keeping water local — cost–benefit analysis of water resource planning, application of W.E.A.P. for holistic water resources management in Massachusetts. www.ebmtoolsdatabase.org

28. Cornell University News Service. July 13, 2005. Organic farming produces same corn and soybean yields as conventional farms, but consumes less energy, water and no pesticides, study finds. www.news.cornell.edu/stories/july05/organic.farm.vs.other.ssl.html

29. *The Corporation*. Film. 2004.
30. Robinson W. Globalization: Nine theses on our epoch. www.soc.ucsb. edu/faculty/robinson/assets/pdf/globalization.pdf
31. Schalte JE. (2000) *Globalization: A Critical Introduction*. Palgrave Macmillan.
32. Ausubel J *et al.* (1995) The environment since 1970. *Consequences* **1**(3).
33. US Environmental Protection Agency. Water: Water Quality Reporting (305b). National Water Quality Inventory Report to Congress. www. water.epa.gov/lawsregs/guidance/cwa/305b/index.cfm
34. US Environmental Protection Agency. Summary of the Toxic Substances Control Act. 15 U.S.C. 2601 *et seq.* (1976). www.epa.gov/lawsregs/laws/tsca.html
35. Toxics Release Inventory — US Environmental Protention Agency. www.epa.gov/TRI
36. Living Downstream, Walking Upstream. www.livingdownstream.com/about-movement
37. Organization for Economic Cooperation and Development. Germany. www.oecd.org/env/environmenta/countryreviews/2448059.pdf
38. Ackerman F. (2012) *Priceless: on knowing the prices of everything and the value of nothing*. Read How You Want.
39. OECD: The implementation of the polluter-pays principle. www.sedac.ciesin.columbia.edu/entri/texts/oecd/oecd-4.09.html
40. Hamilton C. (2004) Growth Fetish. Pluto.
41. Farber S, Bradley D. Ecological economics. www.fs.fed.us/eco/s21pre.htm
42. Hamilton C. The surprising origins and meanings of the "pursuit of happiness." www.hnn.us/articles/46460.html
43. Oslo Roundtable on Sustainable Production and Consumption. www.iisd.ca/consume/oslo004.htm
44. Kahneman D, Diener E *et al.* (2003) *Well-Being: The Foundations of the Hedonic Psychology*. Russell Sage Foundation.
45. Seligman M. (2011) *Fourish: A Visionary New Understanding of Happiness and Well-Being*. Free.
46. *Citizen Renaissance*. Chap. 7: The rise of well-being economics. www.citizenrenaissance.com/the-book-/part-three-where-we-are-heading

47. Friends of the Earth. ISEW explained. www.foe-co.uk/community/tools/isew

48. Happy Planet Index. www.happyplanetindex.org

49. Speth J. America the possible: breaking the chains of consumerism. Sep. 10, 2012 in *Common Dreams*. Comments on his book with a somewhat similar title. www.commondreams.org/view/2012/09/10–1

50. City-Data Forum. Has your wage increases kept up with inflation / cost of living increases? www.city-data.com/forum/economics/224751.

51. Earth 911. How to reduce your household waste. www.earth91.com/howto/how-to-reduce-your-household-waste

52. Understanding the green consumer. www.gdrc.org/uem/green-consumer.html

53. Dauvergne P. The problem of consumption. www.ideas.reprec.org/a/tpr/glewvp/v10y2010i2p1–10.html

54. Greenwashing Index. www.greenwashingindex.com

55. Ketola K. (2011) Corporate states or corporate citizens? Chess between corporations, states, and citizens with sustainable development at stake. *Int J Sustain Econ.* **1**: 107–122.

56. Palast G. (2003) *The Best Democracy Money Can Buy: An Investigative Reporter Exposes the Truth About Globalization, Corporate Cons, and High-Finance Fraudsters.* Constable, London.

57. www.corporations.org/system/top100.html

58. Global Issues. Corporations. www.globalissues.org/issue/50/corporations

59. Stiglitz J. (2008) The globe and mall. www.stwr.org/globalization/a-global-lesson-in-market-failure.html

60. Waugh R. Does one "super-corporation" run the global economy? Mail Online. www.dailymail.co.uk/sciencetech/article-2051008/does-super-corporation

61. Mander J. (2000) Economic globalization: The Era of corporate rule. E.F. Schumacher Society. Nineteenth Annual E.F. Schumacher Lectures.

62. Mander J. (2001) Economic globalization and the environment. *Tikkun Mag*, Sep./Oct.

63. Environmental Performance Index. Yale University. http://epi.yale.edu/

64. Davis S *et al.* (2006) *The New Capitalists: How Citizen Investors Are Reshaping the Corporate Agenda.* Harvard Business Review Press.

65. Vogel D. (2006) *The Market for Virtue: The Potential and Limits of Corporate Social Responsibility.* Brookings Institution Press.
66. US SIF. The Forum for Sustainable and Responsible Investment. www.ussif.org
67. Dryzek J. (2000) *Deliberative Democracy and Beyond Liberals, Critics, and Contestations.* Oxford University Press.
68. *Op. cit.* No. 40, p. 212.
69. Speth J. (2009) *The Bridge at the Edge of the World: Capitalism, the Environment, and Crossing from Crisis to Sustainability.* Yale University Press.
70. *Ibid.*
71. Great Transition Initiative. www.gtinitiative.org
72. Earth Charter Commission. The Earth Charter Preamble. www.earthcharterinaction.org/content/pages/read-the-charter.html

CHAPTER 9

Connections

> May all beings enjoy happiness and the root of happiness.
> May they be free of suffering and the root of suffering.
>
> May they not be separated from the great happiness devoid of suffering.
>
> May they dwell in the great equanimity free from passion, aggression and prejudice.
>
> — *metta* practice from the Vipassana
> tradition of Buddhism

What Is Health?

Although the linear scientific model has been posited to have improved the practice of medicine through the understanding of human biology, modern medicine has no definition for health. To a large extent the assumption is that health is the absence of disease and the symptoms of disease. Therefore, the maintenance of health has to a large extent become the management and treatment of disease. Prevention plays a small role in modern medicine. And prevention has come to be defined as a public health issue. In the case of cancers, there are no specific public health agendas for cancer prevention beyond early detection. There are water and air quality monitors in place but few known carcinogens are monitored in water or air although we are aware that carcinogens exist in each of these moving streams. There are no monitors for soil that are part of a public health mandate even though soil health is a major part of food safety and quality. And the manufacture and use of over 100,000 chemicals brought into the environment since the 1940s remain unlimited by any policies requiring knowledge of their potential dangers to health before they are manufactured, sold, or used.

Part of what drives public health actions, or inactions, is the medical and the medical insurance industry, and we know that these industries do not have a vested interest either scientifically, philosophically, or politically and economically in prevention of disease of any kind unless it is acute infectious disease backed by political capital. The profit motive drives all decisions, and prevention of disease is not very profitable. Nixon's "War on Cancer" mandated in 1971 that the National Cancer Institute (NCI) invest at least 10% of its research dollars each year in cancer prevention. But the NCI, according to its own statistics, has never invested more than 4% of its prevention research dollars in any given year. And then the research is on early detection and not causes, especially environmental and lifestyle causes.[1] The largest public health actions for chronic health issues that underlie cancer have come in the form of stopping the tobacco industry from advertising. And only recently has political action begun in regard to cardiovascular disease, obesity, and type II diabetes, all underlying chronic and functional diseases that are foundational for many cancers. These efforts have mostly to do with public service announcements initiated by the current administration but not with laws that would change the availability of the pseudofoods that contribute to addictions to these nonfoods and to these serious chronic diseases. We all know that to "just say no" does not work when it comes to addiction. And it is addiction to many of the foods in the center aisles of grocery stores that drives cardiovascular diseases and diabetes.

The definition of health in Chinese medicine is a more complex discussion. Chinese medicine is a perennial form, in that it has foundations in a holism that connects the concepts of Heaven and Earth. It understands the workings of life partly from a metaphysical and partly from a logical and perhaps instinctual (observable and logical) way. The metaphysical considerations of an introspective experience gained through organized meditation practices pit empiricism against rationalism. And the scientific research on behavior and symbolic logic pit environmental determinism against apriorism.

In Chinese medicine, the distinction between theories and models is obscure, whereas these define modern Western medicine. The theories of Chinese medicine can be seen as piles of interrelated models. Although often very logical, Chinese medicine is not deduced by logic but is discovered more by experiential philosophy — it is an expression of what is seen in nature and in the universe. It is ecological or environmental, if you will. Chinese medicine pays more attention to specific visual objects of both the outer and the inner vision, rather than to abstract objects like mathematical conclusions framed by statistics.

The models of Chinese medicine possess a layered or spherical four-dimensional structure that includes the transformations generated by time. Even so, the interrelationships amongst the models are very clear. These interrelationships intertwine intuition, emotions, and beliefs, and the grounding of spiritual experience in the philosophy and observational logic of the understanding of life. Although very sophisticated, Chinese medicine is very much common sense. This point of view has the capacity to reshape modern science. This is a much-needed change, because it is partlly the linearity coming out of the Age of Reason and so purely expressed in modern science and reductionism that is responsible for the environmental degradation in which we live and that treats the resulting diseases of that degradation but not the cause or the patient.

The association between the human and the universe is foundational to Chinese medicine. The disassociation of the human and the universe is foundational to Western medicine based in modern Western science. In Chinese medicine, the human body is a miniature of the universe. The internal mechanisms and relationships of the human body resemble those of the universe, with a similar cause-and-effect relationship. This is expressed elegantly in the *Neijing Tu* (the cover art for this book). It depicts the inner alchemical pathways of the human being and their relationship to the outer world and the universe.[2] The art of the practice of Chinese medicine is to understand how to handle all of these relationships in order to make an accurate assessment of a pathological situation, or an imbalance, of the human body not only in relationship to itself but also in relationship to the universe. It is a phenomenological analysis. It has to do with consciousness — of both the patient and the practitioner. It is a natural systems approach. Perhaps it could even be said that Chinese medicine is the antithesis of evidence-based medicine, although there is a great deal of evidence that it is successful in treating the diseases that Western medicine has defined. There is also evidence, which cannot currently be verified analytically, that Chinese medicine treats many imbalances that are not yet a definable disease in the Western medical sense. This inability to define a predisease or condition is because Western medicine relies heavily upon symptoms and only upon signs that are measurable through standard observation. It relies upon measurable signs and symptoms because it mainly treats disease; it does not prevent disease. And vice versa. Chinese medicine relies especially upon intensely minute palpation and observation. This minute palpation and observation evolves as a part of meditation and personal inner development, giving the best practitioners a deep relationship with the universe and the Sacred. These are deep listening skills that have traditionally been built into Chinese medicine. This reality makes Chinese medicine preventive medicine. Some Western medicine providers have these skills, as well. They were learned because those individual practitioners paid attention and gave themselves permission to develop the skills of deep listening.[3] In Buddhism, one of the foundations of Chinese medicine, this deep listening is translated as mindfulness.

Health, according to Chinese medicine, is a flexible and changing continuum of balance between all of the interrelationships within life. These relationships take into account the constitutional inheritance of a given human being. This inheritance is then enhanced or depleted by the ways in which that being lives. With the entry of Buddhism into China came another aspect of health in certain branches of classical Chinese medicine — karma playing a role in health. The soul brings with it certain injuries and strengths that set the stage for growth through living, a sort of energetic and spiritual inheritance based on reincarnation. It is the cause-and-effect parameter of Western science; for every action there is an equal and opposite reaction — balance. In other words, the advancement of the soul is important; and the life of the soul within the human body, which is the cathedral for that soul, sometimes coupled with human suffering, can be an impetus to the knowledge and wisdom for growth of the soul. The evolution of life is an important aspect of all Eastern religions and philosophies. The Roman Christian Church sought to exclude these perennial truths from every aspect of life, including science and religion. Placement of the knowledge of sacred truth in the hands of a few meant ultimate power. This historical reality may have contributed significantly to the separation of meaning and agency, which is the central dogma of modern Western science. It is perversely paradoxical that the medieval Christian church was partially responsible for taking the god or spirit out of how we scientifically understand the workings of life.

When the health of an individual is assessed according to Chinese medicine, many considerations are taken into account. These include the constitution or inheritance, the acquired constitution that reflects what that person did with their inheritance, the immediate environment the person lives in — (physical as well as familial and spiritual), the regional and larger environment they live in, and the times in which they live. How these ripples of influence affect an individual has to be taken into account when one is advising them how to maintain health and how they can become more healthy. From this perspective, health is a continuum and not an either-or process based solely on signs and symptoms. Personal actions, including food choices and family and work dynamics, and the influence of the surrounding environment on an individual are important. Health is seen as a continuum and, even as we age, we can become more healthy by making good choices, by balancing our karmic inheritance through knowing more and more who we are, and by growing emotionally and spiritually and acting on our regional environments to change things for the better for us all.

In this regard, Chinese medicine is part of the Sacred. Just as North American First Peoples and others retain within their memories spiritual sites as sacred, and just as rituals and talismans of power are sacred, and just as the Bible, the Torah, the Koran, and other books are sacred, so is Chinese medicine and many other forms of knowledge from perennial systems that have evolved over time. The Holy Land is everywhere and in everything, and is not only a specific concept of place. The kernels of all of these sacred realities of old remain as true today as they were even thousands of years ago. They are based on a connection to the Earth and sky that is deeply meaningful and truthful for today. This is what makes them sacred. And their loss is emblematic of the injury specific to our current dilemma. Sacredness in life is part of health.

Loss of family and connections, loss of clean air and water, loss of healthy soils and the clean and vibrant foods that healthy soils grow, loss of access for all creatures and all peoples of the Earth to life and natural resources and their particular interpretation of the meaning of life all contribute to loss of health. What happens to the least of these happens to all of us. In the First World, these losses have contributed to chronic illnesses and a lifestyle that in turn contributes to the modern cancer epidemic. It contributes to a moral trauma and universal grief from which we all now suffer. This book has tried to iterate from multiple points of view how we got here and how Chinese medicine paradigms can be used to shed a different light on a subject that is almost always spoken of from the point of view of conventional Western medicine, an expression of linear thinking. The issues brought up can be condensed into just a few categories.

The Carbon-Based Economy

The reliance of the developed world on nonrenewable energy sources like petroleum, natural gas, and coal drives not only the combustion engine but also industrial agriculture, the modern chemical industry, global trade and economics, the pharmaceutical industry, plastics, manufacturing, and by extension many other realms of living ending in impacts on health. These connections are the one main economic reason why there has not been a shift away from petroleum as the main driver of global business.[4] Without petroleum the chemical industry would be unable to provide to the pharmaceutical industry the elements of their drug manufacturing. Modern drugs to a large extent drive the definition of disease and vice versa, and therefore how diseases will be treated. Without petroleum agricultural practices and the food industry would not have been industrialized. The industrialization of vast tracts of land in the Midwest, the Amazon basin, and elsewhere has increased the need for petroleum-based inputs and for water. Without petroleum the endocrine-disrupting chemicals embedded in the chemical industry and the plastics industry would not be ubiquitously available and dumped. It is a vicious circle feeding on itself to the greater detriment of soil health, water resources, climate, food quality, and animal and human health. Not to mention the loss of species and human cultures through the loss of habitat and environmental degradation.

The industrialization of our food supply, made possible by a carbon-based economy, has produced foods not worthy of being called food. Many of our foods are manufactured as opposed to grown.[5] The manufacture of food requires petroleum for agricultural inputs, petroleum for plowing and reaping, petroleum for transportation of the food produce to the manufacturing plant, petroleum for producing the pseudofood and packaging, petroleum for transporting the packaged food product to the market, petroleum for carting away the waste and recycling that is generated, and petroleum for all of the advertising that attends this way of doing business. And, unfortunately, the food produced in this way is not worth eating and leads to type II diabetes and cardiovascular diseases, which underlie cancer.

Carbon trading is supposed to be a "green" solution to our problems.[6] But in effect, it privatizes the atmosphere, suggesting that the Earth's capacity to regulate its climate can be understood as a measurable commodity that can be bought, sold, and traded. It is predicated less on reducing emissions than on the desire to make carbon cuts as cheap as possible for large corporations. It maintains the essence of the current human-centered market model that has led us — and the planet — to the current crisis. Corporations and governments can buy their way out of needed structural changes to energy practice, production and consumption patterns allowing business as usual. The issues of power, social justice, inequality, and community control over local ecosystems are ignored.

Reliance on nonrenewable fuels is the main cause of global climate change. It is not just the burning of fossil fuels that is the problem. Extraction and ownership of the lands from which these nonrenewable fuels are removed has driven many wars and the rape of the Earth and of our seas. The loss of tree cover, the tilling of soils opening the land and releasing that vast carbon sink, the resulting increased need for water and depletion of waters — all of these contribute to global climate change through the point source of carbon-based enterprises.[7] The depletion that results alters and damages the ubiquitous San Jiao of the Earth and the *San Jiao* and *Source Qi* of the individual living on the Earth. We must move away from a life that requires carbon-based energies in order to sustain itself while simultaneously undermining and consuming itself. It is by definition insanity and the antithesis of health. To sicken one in two men and one in three women in the US with life-threatening cancers and then to focus on treatment for that disease without attending to prevention and the elimination of the causes is evil — the antithesis of the Sacred.

Corporate Culture and Globalization

Corporations are the largest and primary structures of a market economy. Because of an obscure law that evolved out of early 20th century legal proceedings, an individual corporation is treated legally as a person with all of the rights of a person, including the right to free speech. Although a corporation may, in fact, comprise many stockholders and many more people who carry out the workings of the corporation, all of those workings and goals are treated as though they represented one individual. As a result, the corporation is exempt from oversight and proceedings that would protect the public, the environment, and the political structures of a country because that corporation is free to exercise its free speech.[8]

Corporations in the market economy of capitalism are driven by the profit motive. The one job that corporations have is to make profit for the stakeholders. With profit as a driving force and the only goal in the multinational corporate-driven world — a world that is in the process of globalizing and owning and defining all intellectual property rights and ownership of all other resources — this means that what is sacred in all realms of life is up for sale. The defining and codification of knowledge drives research. And this research is the mechanism by which ownership is then extended through patenting law. Research within the modern linear scientific apparatus has the goal of providing information that can be owned and from which profit can be made. This applies not only to material resources but also to intellectual resources, including medical knowledge, farming knowledge, seed saving, seed sharing, water rights, and the right to a clean world in which to live. The corporation is seen as amoral even while being seen as an individual. But, in fact, many corporations are truly immoral. Only people are immoral.

Right now five corporations control global trade in grain.[9] Monsanto and Cargill are key players in GATT and the WTO.[10,10A] The WTO's major role is the legitimization of the patenting of life forms indigenous to the Earth and the Commons, and to ownership of these patents by multinational corporations.[11,12] It is a corporate myth that industrial agriculture is necessary for growing more food and reducing hunger. The WTO institutionalizes and attempts to legalize corporate growth based on harvests stolen from nature and of plants developed by people who live as a part of the natural world.[13] TRIP (the Trade-Related Intellectual Property Rights Agreement) criminalizes seed saving and seed sharing. But it is a myth that biotechnology and resulting patented seeds are cheaper than traditional farming techniques and seed saving. In truth, biotechnology and genetically engineered seeds and agribusiness increase the use of chemicals, increase the costs of seeds, hold invisible technology fees, and increase water use.[14] These impacts undermine the health of the global population. The seeds and plants engineered over the millennia by specific human populations for their specific soil and weather constraints are far superior to the genetically engineered seeds coming out of Monsanto for sale to the world and for use in industrial agriculture. Monsanto's main goal is to stifle the local heritage seeds and plants and ways of agriculture that have been feeding those peoples for thousands of years.[15] Monsanto's purpose is to profit. To add insult to injury, much of the research behind these seeds and industrial agriculture is funded through public educational institutions and is, therefore, paid for by the taxpayer. The patent laws in place to allow corporations to recoup research and development costs funded by the taxpayer are actually allowing them to post even greater profits. The land, air, water, and living communities of the Earth all pay for this. The corporations make profit.

One of the ways in which the corporate culture has been sold is through the language of progress. This is true in agriculture, in Western medicine and science, in manufacturing of new products, and in the extraction of resources from the Earth. It remains to be seen if true progress is occurring, particularly when industrial agriculture is responsible for the tremendous contamination of our waters and land while providing poor-quality foods and destroying diversity in foods and contributing to global climate change. These same industrial techniques cause disease by utilizing pesticides and other endocrine-disrupting chemicals that have been identified as carcinogenic. Modern science and medicine seeks to treat diseases caused by the way in which we live but fails to get rid of the underlying causes, because modern science and medicine has strong links to the purveyors of those very causes. The manufacture of many modern items is done at the expense of the water, environment, and air while producing items unnecessary for our lives and items that may never break down in nature, thus again and again contaminating the air, water, and Earth. Not to mention human and other animal bodies. The largest numbers of products now being made in the US are garbage and prisons — the true mark of unsustainability.[16] They are emblematic of the growth model, the true costs of which are hidden away. It is a model that truly needs to be challenged.

The interlocking economic structures that bind the direction of medicine and science to the interests of industry have been developing since the Age of Enlightenment. And the arrival of the atomic and chemical age that followed WWII has on a large scale produced carcinogens and other chemicals that contribute to the modern cancer epidemic. These carcinogens and endocrine disruptors are manufactured in such a diverse array and such large quantities that they are no longer confined to the workplace where they were conceived and manufactured. They have seeped via the ecology of the Great Chain of Being into the general environment, where we all come into intimate and daily contact with them. Making visible the links between cancer, environmental contamination, and the current economic structure of a globalizing world is a difficult task.

The striking rise in incidence of cancers in the 20th century is emblematic, in a negative sense, of the overall connectedness of all life and activity on the Earth. As the manufacture of chemicals from a petroleum-based economy has increased, so has the incidence of almost all solid tumors and hematopoietic cancers. In fact, the human environment has become an uncontrolled experiment when it comes to the introduction of suspected chemical carcinogens. There remains no unexposed control population to whom the cancer rates of exposed people could be compared. Each of us is exposed repeatedly to minute amounts of many different carcinogens and other chemicals through many different routes as the injured ecology of the Earth continues to function. Science loves order, simplicity, and the manipulation of a single variable against a background of constancy. When everything is changing all at once, the tools of science do not work well. The science of how these cumulative and combined chemical exposures affect the human and the animal body over time is almost nonexistent.

Redefining the Commons

As the world has gotten smaller, the Commons have gotten larger. What once in prehistory included the entire Earth as the Commons moved to tribal and geographic areas used in common by the local peoples, because the resources held within that ground were needed by everyone for sustenance. In modern times the concept of the Commons has become extinct, especially in the developed world; the European concept of private ownership and empire has pre-empted the concept of the Commons in most places. Concurrently, the arena of human life has become ubiquitous. What were once wild areas or areas held in common as natural areas for animal grazing, wood gathering, and medicinal plant and food gathering have become owned and peopled. And what is now common to everyone is once again everywhere. "Everywhere" includes air, water, soil, climate, the oceans and the fauna and flora that live in them, the mountains and the rain and snow that fall on them, the ozone layer, the aquifers, and everything and everyone that live on the Earth and the knowledge they hold. And so the Commons has shrunk to almost nonexistence and simultaneously swollen to include almost everything as the lowest common denominators of life are touched by globalization and by pollution.

Land and forests were the first resources to be enclosed via ownership and then converted from Commons to commodities.[17] It is part of a long history of empire and colonialism where enclosing a life support system is a primary step in privatizing the Commons for personal gain. This enclosure in the modern world has come to mean that ownership implies the right to use that enclosure, that land, that forest, that water, that air, that knowledge in any way necessary to gain profit. As the capitalist system of economy has become the *modus operandi* of nations across the globe, what it has meant is the rampant opening of the doors of greed.[18] The conversion of common resources into commercial resources has led to deforestation of the world, loss of biodiversity, erosion, water pollution, climate change, disease, and poverty.[19]

The Commons have always been a local commonly owned and utilized resource for land-based communities.[20] This shared resource involved a combination of rights and responsibilities among users, a combination of utilization and conservation, and a sense of coproduction and sharing with nature. The Commons have always been considered a part of the heritage of the individuals involved based not on property but on a bundle of relationships handed down from generation to generation. The loss of biodiversity resulting from the loss of the Commons has ended in the loss of potential medicines and the loss of a plant base for foods that can be grown in a sustainable manner. This leads to the loss of a way of living based on a system of sustainability.

The transformation of common property rights into private property rights implies the exclusion of the right to survival for large sections of Earth society, including fauna and flora. Under conditions of limited availability, uncontrolled exploitation of natural resources involves taking away resources from those who need them for survival. The prudent and restrained use of resources is part of all perennial cultures and is an expression of the Great Chain of Being. Natural resources include the culture of a people, the land and its bounty, and the knowledge evolved over time that makes up that group of people.[21] Capital investment has become the only form of investment for Eurocentric cultures. But non-Western indigenous communities recognize that investment can also be of labor and of care and of nurturance. Rights in these cultures protect investments beyond capital.[22] They protect the culture of conservation and the culture of caring and sharing, because built into the rights of use came also the responsibility to protect the resource. The hierarchical systems of Europe were vertically linear and those at the top had the most right to life, whereas in perennial cultures the structures were circular and horizontal and based on the sharing of the Commons without a linear hierarchy. The linear hierarchy of Eurocentric cultures versus the circular and horizontal relationships of perennial and indigenous cultures becomes the very map of this entire discussion. Whereas accumulation of wealth has been the main value in hierarchical cultures, sharing of wealth has been the main value in sustainable cultures. Sustainability and justice were built into the equity expressed by common ownership.[23]

This is why the indigenous peoples of North and South America were vulnerable to a holocaust in which they lost their lands and their right to life. In a 60-year period it is estimated that 50 million people died after the Europeans entered their lands.[24] Previous to that time, no extinctions except that of the megafauna occurred in the Americas. After the arrival of the Europeans, the number of fauna and flora that have been lost is uncountable.

The colonialism of the capitalist perspective of empire has not only been aimed at the Third World. Privatization of the modern Commons in the First World has resulted in the ability of corporations, the modern empires, to contaminate and degrade in various ways all of the elements necessary for life.[25] It has allowed a process by which manufacture exists for itself as long as a profit can be gained even when the product of manufacture is unhealthful and unnecessary. This is especially true of food products, cosmetics, medicine, clothing, and engineering. The first car ever built was an electric car. It has taken over 100 years to get back to the electric car, because oil drove the politics of transportation. Now even the developed world is paying the price for this colonialism of privatization by the modern corporation — a colonialism that is based on ownership of the Commons of all of the Earth.

Is it possible that the hierarchy of European cultures has driven the linear model of reductionism?[26] The model based on looking for the next-smallest item of truth is certainly vertical but lacks the outer or upward view and so must remain accurate but small in its observations. The ownership of these observations as expressed by IPRs (intellectual property rights) is diametrically opposed to indigenous knowledge systems. The cumulative innovation of millions of people over thousands of years can be "pirated" and claimed as "innovation" by Western-trained scientists or corporations. This is a modern form of colonialism unique to the West and inherently racist.[27] The lack of recognition of existing knowledge of other countries as prior art or science is a form of intellectual elitism and is thievery. It also limits all peoples' access to this knowledge for their own survival unless they can pay for it. This in turn drives poverty, diseases of poverty, and diseases of chronic illness and affluence caused by the global sickness of the profit motive.[28]

International conferences and efforts to enact laws to protect the rights of indigenous peoples and their knowledge have been taking place since the early 1990s. The issue of farmers' rights across the world has also been given attention and there is now legal recognition for farmers' innovations in contributing to the rich diversity of agricultural crops in the world.[29] One main objective has been to give farmers the right to control and access agricultural diversity so that they can continue to sustainably develop their farming systems and plant materials. The well-funded efforts of Monsanto and ADM and other large corporations that wish to control seed production and the means by which agriculture is done across the world are being confronted by well-organized nongovernmental organizations fighting to preserve sustainability in farming.[30]

The ownership of intellectual knowledge has been driven by reductionism. And biological reductionism has the inevitable consequence of biodiversity erosion and monocultures.[31] Second-order reductionism moves out of reductionist biology, expressing itself as genetic reductionism, amplifying the ecological risks of first-order reductionism, and introducing new issues such as the patenting of life forms and the definition of diseases only in terms of the currently understood lowest common denominator. Reductionist biology is a manifestation of cultural reductionism and devalues nonreductionist forms of knowledge and ethical systems related to living organisms.[32] This includes all non-Western agricultural and medical systems as well as disciplines that do not lend themselves to genetic and molecular reductionism. These disciplines have been developed over centuries and even millennia, and are essential for dealing sustainably with the living world.

Genetic engineering is taking us into second-order reductionism: not only is the organism perceived in isolation from its environment, but genes are perceived in isolation from the organism as a whole. And when modern medicine states that the injury in the disease of cancer is to the DNA, the precluding injuries that injured the DNA are not taken into account. As a result, no change in the way we do business occurs and the origin of these injuries remains invisible. This is not preventive medicine.

All of these reductionist concepts are emblematic of the removal of bits of knowledge from the Commons by making inaccessible the underlying truth of the whole. In fact, the Rockefeller Foundation served as a principal patron of this reductionist view of life through molecular biology from the 1930s to the 1950s. Warren Weaver, the director of the Foundation's natural science division, coined the term "molecular biology" in 1938.[33] The term was intended to capture the essence of the Foundation's program and its emphasis on biological entities' ultimate minuteness. The motivation of this agenda was to develop the human sciences as a comprehensive and explanatory framework of social control grounded in the natural, medical, and social sciences, aimed at restructuring human relations in congruity with the social framework of industrial capitalism. It was not only in Hitler's Germany that these ideas of natural selection and eugenics for the human race were in use. It was also here in the US.

The definition of truth as derived from the double-blind randomized placebo-controlled trial is only the beginning of the expressions of reductionism that remain alive and continue to evolve a new science that separates meaning and agency from scientific truths. As the primary functional tool in modern science and medicine, this current end place of reductionism disallows the evaluation of non-Western medical systems that are relational, circular, and horizontal and not reductionist. This effectively eliminates those systems of medicine from flourishing and from adding to the discussion of diseases and how they come about. This way of knowing truth is ultimately designed for the purpose of industrialization and ownership of the only "real" knowledge. It is immensely important that all knowledge be part of the Commons so that the truth of linear limited views of life can be observed, contrasted, analyzed, and made part of the ongoing and continuous process of *universal* understanding. The whole of knowledge must be available to everyone as a continually generated starting place for life and how we live it. The hiding or ownership of knowledge through IPRs for the purpose of gain is unethical, immoral, undermining, and destructive. It holds back the human race while pretending to be progressive. And the failure to evaluate in any meaningful way those truths from perennial systems, keeping them from being evaluated because of one way of thinking and knowing, is culturally elitist, and racist. These issues are problems of linear and hierarchical thinking. The explanations and conclusions derived from reductionism are problematic and limited as a result of hierarchical thinking. This way of knowing splits us from nature and makes us separate from nature, creating a vast cascade of injury that is at the root an expression of the split between heart and mind. It is a split where the mind rules the heart rather than the heart providing the foundation for the actions and conclusions of the mind.

Repairing the Split Between Humanity and the Natural World

"Ecstatic love is an ocean and the Milky Way is a fleck of foam on it." — Rumi

The meaning of this beautiful quote refers to the immensity of the Sacred. The Sacred is everything and everywhere. Consciousness is the evolving awareness of the Sacred and the result of living in it. The Sacred is all that surrounds us and is part of us. The spark of the Sacred that fuels this evolution of awareness comes through the *Source Qi* and emanates from the heart as defined in Chinese medicine. The mind, as an aspect of the heart, then becomes the window through which consciousness of the Sacred is perceived. The mind and the Sacred are both in every cell of the human body and in every cell of all of life. The more we can perceive this, the more evolved we become. Mindfulness. The more evolved we become, the more at one we are.

The quote also refers to the fact that if we humans annihilate the ability to live on this planet in its present form, the pervasive Sacred will somehow make arrangements for the human being and all other living beings to continue in some other place and/or in some other form or way. All meditation technologies have shared over the millennia images of other planes and other planets seen by training the mind and spirit to become one with the Sacred. One can be sure that the destruction of our world is not what is intended, because the Sacred intention is the evolution of consciousness and the experience of oneness. The destruction of our world would imply a lack of consciousness. But the laws of ceaseless activity will no doubt ensure the continuation of love; and humans and all other living creatures in this world are the outcome of the expression of love — ecstatic love.

The human body is the cathedral for this love, a ripple that extends outward and inward forever. It is home to the Spirit, the Sacred on the Earth. And as a physical manifestation it has certain requirements, including a surrounding atmosphere and material presence that supports life, the breathing in and out of *prana*, the taking in of sustenance, and the sustaining qualities of the community — not just the human community but the Earth community. In all of the travels related to our growth as human and spirit in this world, we move through the Great Chain of Being. Finding our original home is a metaphor for the wholeness that is emblematic of the Great Chain of Being. It refers to many things, including a physical space and a spiritual space. All of these spaces are sacred.

Going home is a profoundly charged concept for most humans. Going home also means finding home. And finding home means knowing the smells, the winds, the weather, the ceremonies that restore balance, the songs of gratitude, and the names of a place. Naming is very important in restoring our relationship with the Earth and finding one's place. The naming of our environment is a sacred activity. What makes it sacred is that the naming requires that we know our environment intimately, as one with it, and this intimacy generates truth and love.

Woman is the first human environment. Women, and the receptive, are our hope. Women must live according to natural law in order to remain healthy and give birth to healthy children. This goes for the feminine receptive principle in men as well. Men need to remember the vulnerability that has been beaten out of them both physically and emotionally. This vulnerability allows us all to listen. And listening is the first step in becoming one with the Sacred and restoring health on the Earth.

An industrial society does not listen, and it therefore is not sustainable because a society based on conquest and not on listening cannot survive when there is nothing left to conquer. Women know this, because they, along with the natural world, have been conquered for millennia and they know at the cellular level what this means. Much in nature is cyclical. Women are cyclical. Time itself is cyclical. The linear hierarchical thinking that comes out of a society based on conquest is not cyclical. It is linear and vertical, and when it reaches too high a height, it will fall. This in itself is a cycle. We must end this particular cycle. It is about restoration — something that women are very good at, restoration of balance and equality, of community, and restoration of a sustainable way of living for all.

In many indigenous traditions, it is considered a disgrace to take more than you need. Greed is a violation of natural law. It leaves you with no guarantee that you will be able to continue harvesting. And it means that you do not live your life in relationship with other individuals, with the land and everything on the land, and with the Sacred. It means one is living without listening. Developing a cultural practice that strives toward developing oneself as an individual and collectively as a society is part of natural law — the Yin and the Yang. Yin is listening and Yang is acting on what is heard.

Industrial thinking and law is based on the belief that humans are at the top of an evolutionary ladder and, as such, have full dominion over nature. It does not model itself on the cyclical and receptive structure of nature, although the humans within industrial societies are in truth part of nature. Industrial societies pattern themselves on linear thinking. Certain values permeate this way of thinking, especially the concept of progress defined by technological advance and economic growth. This inherently leads to a hierarchical perception that views the human as separate from nature.

There is an attitude that what is wild is opposed to what is cultivated and tame. There is a belief that "civilized" societies must tame the wilderness, saving small pieces of it here and there for recreational purposes. It is also believed that there is superiority of what is civilized over what is primitive (of the first order), and that indigenous peoples who live as a part of nature are therefore wild or primitive. In colonialism, this idea is taken to the extreme belief that "more civilized" people have the right to civilize "primitive" people and that civilizing them means separating them from the natural world and placing them in the constructed world. People who are viewed as primitive are almost always people of color and women, and people who are civilized are almost always those who are of European descent and male. This prejudice still permeates industrial society, which is also a product of European society. People of color who have embraced the industrial way of life are thought to have progressed. Those who are subsumed at the lowest level in this particular category are usually women and people of color — the modern-day slaves who do the worst work. This links this way of structuring society not only to linear hierarchical thinking but also to racism and sexism. Racism and sexism are linear and vertical ways of thinking. This makes some humans a part of the wild world — the inanimate world — when, in fact, they are living in an animate world of living connectedness, the real world.

Industrial society speaks a language of inanimate nouns.[34] Industrial language has changed things from being animate, alive, and having spirit, meaning and agency to being mere objects and commodities of society. The inanimateness of the natural world allows an industrial society to view the natural world as ownable and as a commodity to be manipulated. This is linear thinking and separates us from nature and from the Sacred.

Capitalism itself is a system that combines labor, capital, and resources for the purpose of accumulation. Since the goal of capitalism is accumulation, the capitalist's method is to take more than is needed in order to perpetuate growth of the economy, which in turn requires persistent consumerism. This very idea makes capitalism inherently out of harmony with natural law.[35] Whereas industrial societies practice conspicuous consumption, land-based societies practice conspicuous distribution.

The extinction of more species in the past 150 years than the total number of species from the last Ice Age to the mid–19th century, and the extinction of about 2000 different indigenous peoples of the Western Hemisphere alone,[36] is emblematic of linear thinking as manifested by a linear and industrial worldview. The rate of extinction in the Amazon rainforest, for example, has been one indigenous people per year since 1900. If one looks at world maps showing cultural and biological distribution, one will find that where there is the most cultural diversity, there too is the most biological diversity. It is a direct relationship. Therefore, cultural diversity is as important to sustainability as is biological diversity.[37] They are linked. And what links them is the fact that the peoples living within diverse cultures are still connected to nature and, as an extension, to their definition of the Sacred.

Industrial cultures from the European heritage are based on the denial of viable native cultures. As a result, if you have no victim, you have no crime.[38,39] Land-based peoples have not existed as full human beings with human rights, with the same rights to self-determination, to dignity, and to land — to territorial integrity — that other people have. The same can be said of women, including women in the First World. This loss of human rights has allowed usually white settlers to deny that a human holocaust ever took place. The holocaust has been first in human terms, and over time in terms of the fauna and flora with which those people lived. The estimation by contemporaries of Columbus is that in the Western Hemisphere alone 50 million people perished in a 60-year period. It is probably the largest holocaust in world history. The natural world has remained silent while all of this has happened. The indigenous human world is only now beginning to find its voice. We have much to learn from these people. They know how to survive within nature and within the Sacred. We do not.

The interlocking interests between all peoples' ability to survive and indigenous peoples' continuing cultural sustainability are key. Land-based peoples have lived sustainably on this Earth for thousands of years. For them this world is owned collectively. It is a community land trust. We do not own this land but we do belong to it because we humans evolved here on the Earth and in relation to it and its environments. We are all indigenous. We would not be who we are without this land. This implies responsibility for each other and to each other. In many cultures, people who transgress against the natural laws are collectively punished. They are not jailed away from the society of others but remain in relationship to each and every member of that society being reminded daily what is expected of them. If they still do not get the message, they are banished. The constant reminder to all, including the transgressor, is part of the healing. Relationship is the keyword of sustainability — relationship to each other and relationship to the land as a collective resource. This relationship requires that we become one with nature again.

The traditional ecological knowledge of land-based and indigenous peoples is essential for the future. They have lived by this knowledge for thousands of years. For example, the Northwest coast Haida say that they can take a plank off a cedar tree and leave the tree standing and alive. Weyerhaeuser cannot do this. In all of this land there are still native peoples struggling to make a living from the land; they are struggling only because we have relegated them to the poorest lands available. Only when their land holds some mineral or oil or uranium do we pay attention and work to steal from them once again. We do not approach them and listen to them for knowledge about sustainable living in our particular lands and communities. The truth is that there is no such thing as sustainable development. The only sustainable way of life is through community.

Community requires the knowledge of other people's lives. This knowledge allows us to know that consumption at the current levels means constant intervention in other peoples' land, countries, and resources. It is meaningless to talk about human rights unless you talk about consumption. The colonial activities necessary for satisfying our current lifestyle habits mean that these relationships are impossible and peace will never come to this world. These relationships are necessary in a world where we are at one with nature and with the Sacred.

All of the Earth's ecosystems are being systematically transformed into a market model where there is a "holder" and the "consumer." Environmental property rights exist where the consumer pays the holder or owner for protecting the biological diversity of an ecosystem property in accordance with an agreed price. Nature is being privatized, be it a wetland, lake, forest or mountain. There is also a strong trend to turn the world's freshwater supplies into a private commodity in the name of conservation. Water permits are being converted into water property rights. Chile has now sold most of its water rights in the South to a private Spanish company.

The Earth-Centered Model

The Universal Declaration of the Rights of Mother Earth[40] promotes an Earth-centered model that would protect biological diversity as a global Commons and a strictly managed and more equitably shared public trust. The model goes beyond Commons law, in that it recognizes the inherent rights of the environment itself, other species, and water itself outside of their usefulness to humans. This is being called Earth democracy. The Rights of Nature declaration has been used in Pennsylvania, where natural ecosystems and natural communities within a specific borough are being viewed as "legal persons" for the purpose of stopping the dumping of sewage sludge on wild land. Earth rights have been used throughout New England to prevent bottled water companies from setting up shop in local areas. In 2006, the Indian Supreme Court ruled that protection of natural lakes and ponds is akin to honoring the right to life — the most fundamental right of all, according to the Court. And, in 2008, Ecuador's citizens voted two-thirds in support of a new constitution that says; "Natural communities and ecosystems possess the unalienable right to exist, flourish and evolve within Ecuador. Those rights shall be self-executing, and it shall be the duty and right of all Ecuadorian governments, communities, and individuals to enforce those rights."

The preamble to the Rights of Mother Earth declaration acknowledges our profound dependence on and relationship with the Earth, and that the Earth is an "indivisible community of diverse and interdependent beings with whom we share a common destiny and to whom we must relate in ways to benefit Mother Earth." This book concludes with two extracts from the declaration. We are many tribes of being. And many species/tribes have been lost in the last 500 years because of the way in which our one tribe lives. Now, we are losing many members of our own tribe, men and women and children, to cancers and other diseases that are preventable. The numbers lost and their suffering are unbearable. If we do not recognize our failures, then we cannot change and rescue our Earth and, therefore, ourselves.

Article 2. Fundamental rights of mother Earth

Mother Earth has the right to exist, to persist and to continue the vital cycles, structures, functions, and processes that sustain all beings.

Article 3. Fundamental rights and freedoms for all beings

Every being has:

(a) The right to exist;
(b) The right to habitat or a place to be;
(c) The right to participate in accordance with its nature in the ever-renewing processes of Mother Earth;
(d) The right to maintain its identity and integrity as a distinct, self-regulating being;
(e) The right to be free from pollution, genetic contamination and human modifications of its structure or functioning that threaten its integrity or healthy functioning;
(f) The freedom to relate to other beings and to participate in communities of beings in accordance with its nature.

May all beings be happy.
May all beings be free from suffering.

References

1. Davis D. (2007) *The Secret History of the War on Cancer.* Basic.
2. Despeux C. (2008) *Neijing Tu and Xiuzhen Tu.* In *The Routledge Encyclopedia of Taoism.* Routledge.
3. The Mindful Society. Deep listening. www.mindful.org/deep-listening
4. Youngquist W. The post-petroleum paradigm — and population. www.jayhanson.us/page171.htm
5. Kenner R. *Food, Inc.* Film. Shown on *PBS.* www.pbs.org/foodinc/#. ulpywobirtm
6. Carbon Trade Watch. www.carbontradewatch.or
7. *Water Encyclopedia: Science and Issues.* Pollution sources: point and nonpoint.
8. NPR. What is the basis for corporate personhood? www.npr. org/2011/10/24/141663195/what-is-the-basis-for-corporate-person-hood.html
9. Greenpeace International. Corporate control of agriculture: background. www.greenpeace.org/international/en/campaigns/agriculture/problem/corporate
10. World Trade Organization. www.gatt.org
10A. WTO announces formalized slavery model for Africa. www.gatt.org
11. The International Property Rights Agreement and Plant Varieties. Factsheet 6 — The Agreement on Intellectual Property Rights. catalogue. gret.org/publications/ouvarages/en/F06en.html
12. Third World Network Briefing. Ten questions on TRIPS, technology, transfer and biodiversity. www.twnside.org/sg/title/trips10-cn.htm
13. Shiva V. (2000) *Stolen Harvest: The Hijacking of the Global Food Supply.* South End Press.
14. Food and Water Watch. The bad seeds: The broken promises of agricultural biotechnology. www.documents.foodandwaterwatch.org/doc. GM101.pdf
15. Mountainxpress.com Local organic seed growers take on Monsanto in federal court. www.mountainx.com/article.40000/local-organic-seed-growers-take-on-monsanto
16. Ranking America. How does the United States rank ... www.rank-ingamerica.wordpress.com/how-does-the-united-states-rank-in

17. Hardin G. (1968) The tragedy of the commons. *J Sci.*

18. Alighieri, Dante. *Divine Comedy.* The Nine Circles of Hell (Dante's Inferno). Circle Four (Greed). Princeton Dante Project. www.etcweb. princeton.edu/dante/index.html

19. Holzman D. Accounting for nature's benefits: The dollar value of ecosystem services. *Environ Health Perspect* **120:** a152–a157.

20. LaDuke W. Our Home on Earth. Environment International. On the commons. www.onthecommons.org/magazine/our-home-Earth

21. United Nations Environment Programme (UNEP). Recognizing and strengthening the role of indigenous people and their communities. Basis for action. www.unep.org/documentsmultilingual/default_ asp?documentID=52&articleID

22. USDA and the Natural Resources Conservation Services. Indigenous stewardship methods and NRCS conservation practices. www.fws.gov/ nativeamerican/graphics/nrcs_indigenous_stewardship_methods

23. Diversity, critical multiculturalism, and oppression. Durie. www.cswe. org/file.aspx?id=44654

24. Mann C. (2005) *1491: New Revelations of the Americas Before Columbus.* Knopf.

25. Alavi H. Colonialism and the rise of capitalism. www.scribd.com/ doc/19084211/colonialism-and-the-rise-of-capitalism

26. McKelvey W. (2003) Transcendental foresight: using complexity science to foster distributed seeing. In Tsoukas H, Shepherd, J (eds.), *Probing the Future: Developing Organizational Foresight in the Knowledge Economy.* UK.

27. Shiva V. (ed.). (1995) *Biopolitics: A Feminist and Ecological Reader on Biotechnology.* Zed, London, New Jersey.

28. Jose Manuel Durao Barroso, President of the European Commission. Eiropean Partnership for Action Against Cancer. Addressing the E.C. Brussels; Sep. 29, 2009. www.europa.eu/rapid/pressreleasesaction.do? reference=SPEECH/09/423&format=html&aged=0&language=en

29. *La Via Campesina.* International Peasants' Movement. Human Rights Council: Towards a better protection of the rights of farmers and peasants. www.viacampesina.org/en/index.php/main-issues-mainmenu-27/ human-rights

30. Food democracy now! America's family farmers fight Monsanto's scorched Earth legal campaign of threats and intimidation. July 5, 2012. www.fooddemocracynow.org/blog/2012/jul/5/scorched-Earth-legal-campaign

31. Giulio A, Levin S. The multifaceted aspects of ecosystem integrity. *Conservation Ecology* (online) **1(1):** 3.

32. Dockendorff C. The long way from non-reductionism to transdisciplinarity: critical questions about levels of reality and the constitution of human beings. MetaNexus.net

33. Kay L. (1993) *The Molecular Vision of Life: Caltech, The Rockefeller Foundation, and the Rise of the New Biology.* Oxford University Press.

34. Hannum H. (ed.). (1997) *People Land, and Community.* Yale University Press.

35. Magnuson J. (2007) *Mindful Economics.* Seven Stories.

36. LaDuke W. We are still here: the 500 years celebration. www.ratical.org/ratville/aos/500yrsnukes.html

37. Unesco and UNEF. Cultural diversity and biodiversity for sustainable development. World Summit on Sustainable Development, 2002. www.unesdoc.org/images/0013/001322/132252e.pdf

38. Rohrbach P. (2009) *German World Policies* (1915). Cambridge Scholars.

39. Lindqvist S. (2002) *"Exterminate All the Brutes": One Man's Odyssey into the Heart of Darkness and Origins of the European Genocide.* The New Press.

40. Universal Declaration of the Rights of Mother Earth. www.climateandcapitalism.com/2010/04/27/universal-declaration-of-the-rights-of-mother-earth.html

Addendum

Books Worth Reading

1. *Living Downstream: An Ecologist Looks at Cancer and the Environment* By Sandra Steingrabber. Addison-Wesley, 1997.
2. *A Small Dose of Toxicology: The Health Effects of Common Chemicals* By Steven Gilbert. CRC, 2004.
3. *Having Faith: An Ecologist's Journey to Motherhood* By Sandra Steingrabber. Berkley Books, 2001.
4. *Silent Spring* By Rachel Carson. Houghton-Mifflin, 1962; Mariner, reprint edition, 1994.
5. *Better Basics for the Home: Simple Solutions for Less Toxic Living* Anne Berthold-Bond. Crown, 1999.
6. *The Shock Doctrine: The Rise of Disaster Capitalism* Naomi Klein. Picador Publishing, 2008.
7. *Human Frontiers, Environments and Disease: Past Patterns, Uncertain Futures* Tony McMichael. Cambridge University Press, 2001.
8. *Inescapable Ecologies: A History of Environment, Disease, and Knowledge* Linda Nash. University of California Press, 2007.
9. *Environmental Toxicology: The Legacy of* D.A. Christie and E.M. Tansey, editors. Wellcome Trust Centre for the History of Medicine at UCL, 2004.
10. *Noah's Choice: The Future of Endangered Species* Charles Mann and Mark Plummer. Knopf, 1995.
11. *Free Market Environmentalism* Terry Anderson and Donald Leal. Palgrave Macmillan, 2001.
12. *Discordant Harmonies: A New Ecology for the Twenty-First Century* Donald Botkin. Oxford University Press, 1990.
13. *The Real Environmental Crisis: Why Poverty, Not Affluence, Is the Environment's Number One Enemy* Jack Hollander. University of California Press, 2003.
14. *Break Through: From the Death of Environmentalism to the Politics of Possibility* Ted Nordhaus and Michael Shellenberger. Houghton Mifflin, 2007.
15. *The End of Nature* Bill Mckibben. Random House, 2006.
16. *Walden: A Fully Annotated Edition* Henry D. Thoreau. J. Cramer, editor. Yale University Press, Paperbacks 2004.
17. *Biomimicry: Innovation Inspired by Nature* Janine Benyus, William Morroy 2003.
18. *Capitalism As If the World Matters* Jonathan Porritt. Earthscan, Routledge Publishing, 2007.

19. *Development as Freedom* Armartya Sen. Anchor Press, 2000.
20. *The Hungry Spirit: Beyond Capitalism — The Quest for Purpose in the Modern World* Charles Handy. Broadway Books, 1999.
21. *No Logo: No Space, No Choices, No Jobs* Naomi Klein. Picador Press, 2002.
22. *Sand County Almanac: And Sketches Here and There* Aldo Leopold. Oxford University Press, New York, 1949.
23. *Tree: A Life Story* David Suzuki. Greystone Books, 2007.
24. *Naturalist* Edward O. Wilson. Island Press, 2006.
25. *Bury My Heart at Wounded Knee: An Indian History of the American West* Dee Brown. Holt Paperbacks, 2007.
26. *A Short History of Progress* Ronald Wright. Dacapopress, 2005.
27. *The Weather Makers: How Man Is Changing the Climate and What It Means for Life on Earth* Tim Flannery. Grove, 2006.
28. *Staying Alive: Women, Ecology and Development* Vandana Shiva. Zed, 1989.
29. *The Nazi Doctors: Medical Killing and the Psychology of Genocide* Robert Jay Lifton. Basic, 1986.
30. *Soul Murder: The Effects of Childhood Abuse and Deprivation* Leonard Shengold. Ballantine Books, 1991.
31. *Dharma Rain: Sources of Buddhist Environmentalism* Stephanie Kaza and Kenneth Kraft, editors. Shambhala, 2000.
32. *The Food Revolution. How Your Diet Can Help Save Your Life and the World* John Robbins. Conari Press, 2010.
33. *From Rage to Courage* Alice Miller. W. W. Norton, 2009.
34. *The Return of the Mother* Andrew Harvey. North Atlantic, 1995.
35. *Betrayal of Trust: The Collapse of Global Public Health* Laurie Garrett. Hyperion Publishing, New York, 2000.
36. *The Little Black Book of Violence: What Every Young Man Needs to Know About Fighting* Laurence Kane and Kris Wilder. National Book Network, 2009.
37. *Mothers, Monsters, Whores: Women's Violence in Global Politics* Laura Sjoberg and Caron E. Gentry. Zed, 2007.
38. *Revolutionizing Motherhood: The Mothers of the Plaza de Mayo* Marguerite Guzman Bouvard. Rowman and Littlefield Publishing, 2002.

Websites Worth Visiting

1. Breast Cancer Fund. www.breastcancerfund.org
2. Campaign for Safe Cosmetics. www.safecosmetics.org
3. Collaborative on Health and the Environment. www.cheforhealth.org
4. Environmental Health News. www.environmentalhealthnews.org
5. Environmental Working Group. www.ewg.org
6. Household Toxins. www.householdtoxins.org

7. Skin Deep Report. www.ewg.org/reports/skindeep
8. Washington Toxics Coalition. www.watoxics.org
9. Physicians for Social Responsibility. www.psr.org
10. Greenwire. www.eenews.net/gn
11. Nature Conservancy. www.nature.org
12. Climatewire. www.eenews.net/cw
13. Live Science. www.livescience.com
14. Propublica. www.propublica.org
15. Daily Climate. www.dailyclimate.org
16. Center for Food Safety. www.centerforfoodcsafety.org
17. Navdanya. www.navdanya.org
18. Earth Democracy. www.navdanya.org/earth-democracy
19. Mother Jones. www.motherjones.com
20. Science News. www.sciencenews.org
21. Politico. www.politico.com
22. The Guardian. www.guardian.co.uk
23. National Fish and Wildlife Foundation. www.nfwf.org
24. Science. www.sciencemag.org
25. National Geographic News. www.news.nationalgeographic.com
26. Climate Desk. www.climatedesk.org
27. Living on Earth. www.pri.org/living-on-earth.html
28. National Public Radio. Morning Edition. All Things Considered. www.npr.org
29. Fast Company. www.fastcompany.com
30. Yale Environment 360. www.e360yale.edu
31. Chemical and Engineering News. www.cen.acs.org
32. California Watch. www.californiawatch.org
33. Center for Public Integrity. www.publicintegrity.org
34. Energy Wire. www.eenews.net/ew
35. NIEHS. National Institute for Environmental Health Safety. www.niehs.nih.gov
36. NTP. National Toxics Program. www.ntp-server.niehs.nih.gov
37. GDRC. Global Development Research Center. www.gdrc.org
38. Center for Environmental Health. www.ceh.org
39. Change.org. www.change.org
40. Science and Environmental Health Network. www.sehn.org
41. Collaborative on Health and the Environment. www.healthandtheenvironment.org
42. National Tribal Environmental Council. www.ntec.org
43. Inter-Tribal Environmental Council (ITEC). www.itecmembers.org
44. Honor the Earth. www.honorearth.com
45. Native Waters. www.nativewaters.org

Index

2,4-D   33, 256
15 years   87

abnormal nutrition   412
Abrahamic   201
Abuse   307
acceptable risks   433
ACE inhibitor   332
acetonitrile   83
ach (air changes per hour)   82
acquired constitution   493
ACTH   61
acupuncture   47
addiction   76, 490
additives   140
adenomatous polyps   147
adhesive removers   79
adjacent possible   443
ADM   31
adrenal hormone   318
adrenal HTN   323
aerosols   79
affirmation   212
Africa   22
Agency   442, 449
Age of Reason   405
agrarian   405
agribusiness   132
air pollution   78, 459
Alcohol   335
aldehydes   83
aldrin   252
Alice Miller   307

alkalinize   186
alkylphenols   253
allergenic   90
allergic asthma   96
Allium   332
alveolae   113
amino acid sequences   443
anaerobic bacteria   142, 149
Androgens   318
anger management   317
Angina pectoris   336
angiogenesis   121
angiomas   187
animal fat   147
animal husbandry   405
anorexia   52
Anorexia nervosa   209
anthropology   402
Antiacids   151
antidepressants   225
antienvironmental   459
Antihistamines   238
antioxidants   86
Antipoverty strategies   462
Antispasmodics   105
anxiety   220
Anxiety states   229
Aquarian Age   404
aquifers   32
archeology   401
Asbestos   82
asbestosis   82
aspartame   149

asthma   78
Astragalus   122
astronomy   402
Aswan Dam   36
Atelectasis   113
atherosclerosis   325
Atherosclerotic plaques   342
Atrazides   141
atrazine   32, 141, 246, 412
atrazine herbicides   262
attack arrays   424
Attack of EPIs   346
autocatalytic   443
autohypnosis   307

Bacillus thuringensis   138
ba zheng   424
because   203
before   246, 395
Benzene   79, 257
benzodiazepines   237
benzpyrene   412
beta blocker   332
betacarotenoids   147
bile acids   142, 149
binding of phlegm   91
binding phlegm   110
bioaccumulative   22
biodiesel   31
biodiversity   33, 133
biological contamination   138
biological diversity   508
biological reductionism   503
biomass   42
biopiracy   135
biotechnology   137, 497
bisphenol-A   253, 275
black men   318
Blazing heat in the yangming   176

blood-cracking   106
blood dryness, blood stasis   49
blood gases   89
blood glucose levels   174
bloodline   215
blood oxygenation   50
blood stasis   89, 340
blood sugar level   173
BMI   278, 318
body armor   210
body temperature   185
bonding   320
boundary conditions   445
boundary issues   211
BPA   253
brain chemistry   146
Breastfed babies   275
bright gate   416
Bronchial asthma   89, 96
bronchial reflex   96
bronchiectasis   112
bronchitis   78
Bronchodilators   95, 113
bronchospasm   92
BT   138
Building foods   186
bulimia   53
bulimia nervosa   209
bundle of relationships   500
burden shifting   483
Burkitt's lymphoma   64
burms   42

CAD   336
Calcified deposits   187
calcium   173
calcium channel blockers
     147, 332
calling   217

cancerization 42, 87
cancer prevention 489
Candice Pert 61
candidiasis 162
Cap and trade 461
capitalism 450, 496
capitalistic society 422
capitalist perspective
of empire 501
Capsella 332
carbon-based economy 495
carbon-based fuels 32
carbon disulfide 83
carbon emissions 463
carbon sinks 22
Carbon trading 495
carcinogen 249
carcinogenic 21, 428
cardiopulmonary diseases 89
cardiovascular disease 76, 490
caregivers 204
Cargill 497
Cartagena Biosafety Protocol 431
ceaselessly creative 446
ceaselessly creative
phenomenon 443
central dogma 443
centralization of power 470
Cervical cancer 75
CFCs 429
chang feng 150
channel 85
charbroiled 153
chemical additives 140
chemical carcinogens 64
chemical exposure 412
Chest X-ray imaging 87
CHF 345
child-rearing 204

child sexual abuse 277
Chinese medicine 46
chlordane 256
chlorinated compounds 261
Chlorinated pesticides 274
chlorination 38
Chlorine 38
Cholesterol 339
Chong 95
chong and ren 248
Chronic bronchitis 112
chronic malarial infection 64
chronic pain 225
chyme 158
CINs 75
circular and horizontal 501
circular thinking 441
city states 405
civilized 309
cleansing foods 186
climate change 22, 78
clumping 218
coastal wetlands 26
cocaine 86
cock's crow diarrhea 168
coconstruct 447
coconstructing 448
coconstruction 449
cocreate 448
coevolution 449
cold wheezing 106
coliforms 39
Colitis 167
collective knowledge 135
colonialism 24, 309, 500
Colonic polyps 149
colorectal cancer (CRC) 141
common property rights 500
Commons 23, 133, 499

community land trust   509
competitive   314
complex carbohydrates   147, 173
concept of progress   507
conditioning   311
congealed blood   49
conglomerates   459
connection   494
Consciousness   442, 444,
   448, 505
Conservation   423
constitutional inheritance   492
constraint   209
consumer society   450
Consumptive insomnia   243
contaminants   21
contest of values   482
continuum   492
contraception   203
contraceptive therapies   251
control population   421
cooperation   316
co-ops   474
COPD   78
coping mechanisms   86
coral reefs   26
Coronary artery disease   335
corporate accountability   466
Corticosteroids   95
Cortisol   52, 228, 278
cosmic activities   402
cosmic organism   402
counterflows   85
coupled organ relationship   85
cranial rhythm   63
cranio-sacral   59
creativity   449
credit unions   474
crisis of femininity   215

Crohn's disease   153, 170
Cryptosporidiosis   39, 170
CT scans   87, 249
cultivating the breath   417
cultural diversity   422, 508
cultural habituation   212
cultural sustainability   509
cultural task   448
Cultural transformation theory   302
culture war   429
cyclical   506
cysterna chyli   59
cystic fibrosis   113
Cysts   187

daidzen   256
Damp accumulations   53
damp–heat   85, 149
dampness   53, 220
damp phlegm   319
damp/phlegm stasis   152
DDE   35, 246
DDT   35, 246, 412
dead zone   30
decanol   83
Decentralization   136, 454
deep listening skills   492
defensive mode   316
Deficient heart Qi, heart blood,
   and heart Yin   232
definition of work   445
deforestation   22
Deliberative democracy   477
Department of the Interior   458
Depression   209, 220
depurate   35
deregulation   454, 470
desertification   22
destructiveness   315

detoxification 186
developed world 494
developmental 428
developmental defects 411
diabetes 78, 324
Diagnosis 161
dieldrin 255
dietary and lifestyle habits 342
differentiation 212
diffusing and descending
   functions 85
Digestive fire 172
dioxin 261, 280, 412
Directive 2003/74 428
discovering 321
discrimination 315
disease resistance 134
disenfranchised 132
disinfectants 79
disowned 315
ditestosterone 318
Diuretics 333
diversity 133, 443, 449
DNA 442
DNA methylation 407
DNA mutation 207
DNA repair genes 407
doing 440, 449
Domestic abuse 213
dominance 314
dominator culture 315
dominator model 302
dominator societies 303
Do no harm 481
downstream 461
Drive–Shame Binds 209
drought tolerance 134
Drug-resistant strains 38
dynamic heat exchanger 50

Dyspareunia 160
Dysphagia 159
dyspnea 113

early detection 489
early menarche 267
Early-onset asthma 93
Early puberty 267
Earth community 422, 440
Earth democracy 423, 511
EBV 55
ecological disorder 281
ecological economics 452
ecological footprint 453
ecological sensibility 475
economic democracy 423
ecosystems 57, 445
EC Treaty 426
EDCs 410
Effluent charges 461
EGME 257
egocentricity 314
emergence 441
emergent 448
emergent properties 443
emergent universe 446
EMFs 265
empathy 313, 476
emphysema 78
empire 500
encoded proteins 442
endless creativity 447
endocrine 428
endocrine-disrupting 141
endocrine-disrupting
   chemicals 263, 495
endocrine disruptors 39,
   219, 412
endocrine system 57

endogenous   149
endogenous estrogens   247
endorphins   61, 146
energetic center   416
energetic injuries   207
energetic medicine   47
energetics   417
enterocytes   141
environmental agents   408
environmental charges   461
environmentalism   458
environmentally perverse
   subsidies   461
Environmental obesogens   274
environmental restoration   453
environmental stewardship   470
environmental toxins   409
Environmental Working
   Group   32, 140
EPA   79, 458
EPI   97
epidemics   132
epigenetics   407
epigenetic tags   409
epigenetic transgenerational
   phenotype   411
epigenome   408
Epimutations   407
epochs   401
Epstein–Barr virus   64
ER-alpha   413
ER-beta receptors   413
Erectile dysfunction   340
erotic marketing messages   278
ERT   250
Essential HTN   323
esters   83
estradiol   250
Estradiol 17 beta   428

estriol   250
Estrogen   210
estrogen receptors   410
estrone   250
estuaries   26
Ethanol   31, 143
ethereal body   47
etheric body   206
ethnicity   206
eugenics   504
European Union   83
ever-changing cycle   442
evidence-based medicine   492
Evolution   401, 441, 442
evolution of consciousness   505
evolution of the universe   440
evolving consciousness   444
Exercise   276
existence of meaning   446
exogenous   149
external costs   136
external exposures   245
externalities   468
extinction   508
extinction event   402
extracellular fluids   60
ex utero   410

F1 generation   410
F3 generation   412
familial polyposis syndrome   141
farmers' rights   502
fascia   57
fasting insulin   185
Father absence   277
fat-soluble   35
fatty reservoirs   64
fecal transit time   142
fei wei   113

feminine receptive   506
Feminism   211
Fenugreek   162
Fetal toxicology   249
fetus   409
FEV   94
Fiber   142
fibrinogen   49
Fibromyalgia   160
fight or flight   324
fire   85
Fire and phlegm fire   232
fire poisons   54
fire retardant   82
five-phase ko cycle   51
five phases   445
five-phase theory   84
flame retardants   253
fluoroscopy   249
foliar techniques   35
follicular   221
food additives   64
food chain   139
food dyes   140
Food stagnation   170
Forest Stewardship Council   471
Formaldehyde   79
Formula-fed infants   275
fortress mentality   317
fortress world   453
four levels   248
four toos   238
free trade   470
fumigant   261
fumigate   34
fungicides   79, 412

GABA   270
Galileo   446

gallbladder cough   112
gao   59, 96
Garlic   122
gastroesophageal reflux   112
gastrointestinal tube   140
gate of breathing   57, 416
gate of light   58
GATT   497
GDP   465
GE   136
genes   407
genetically engineered   134
genetically engineered seeds   497
genetically modified foods   33
genetic predisposition   246
genistein   256
genotoxic   428
geology   401
germ line   411
giardiasis   170
gladiator sports   312
global agribusiness   137
global bureaucracies   469
global civilization   447
global climate change   496
global corporations   469
global crisis   45
global ethic   450
global grief   450
globalization   132
Global Reporting Initiative   470
global shen disturbance   231
global social polarization   473
Global warming   90
global wound   47
glucocorticoid receptors   409
Glutathione   147
glycogen   175
GMOs   428

GnRH   269
God   449
Golden Age   404
Great Chain of Being   27, 230,
   424, 433, 442, 445, 501, 506
Great Lakes   458
Great Months   402
great void   320
Great Year   402
Greed   507
Green consumerism   466
greenhouse gas   22
green space   41
Green tea   121
green technologies   462
greenwash   467
grief   314
gross world product   469
Ground level ozone pollution   78
groundwater   133
Groundwater depletion   37
growth   450
growth through living   492
gut motility disorders   158

habituated   209
Hammurabi   405
Happy Planet Index   465
hara   161
Hawthorn berries   332
HBV   55, 383
HCV   55, 383
HDL   318
healing arts   405
health   489
Heart and kidney disconnect   179
heart and mind   321
heart cough   112
heart disease   340

heart–kidney axis   64, 230, 322
heart–liver–kidney axis   317
heart–lung connection   89
heart Qi deficiency   222
heart Qi stasis   218
heart wrapping channel   57
Heaven   416
heaven Qi   58, 417
heavy metals   412
HEG   269
hematopoietic cancers   418
hepatitis   157
Heptachlor   261
herbicide resistance   136
herbicides   412
herbiciding weeds   32
heritage foods   138
heroic dream   217
hexachlorobenzene   275
hierarchy   309
high-fructose corn syrup   143
high trophic levels   27
Hippocratic oath   481
Histamine   94
history   440
Hitler   309
holocausts   311
Homo sapiens   403
honeybee   33
honey pill   116
hormonally sensitive tumors
   implies   246
hot wheezing   106
HPA   409
HPV   55
HRT   250
HSV   55
huang   59, 96
Huang Di Neijing Su Wen   149

hua tou jia ji   97
Human agency   443
human genome   406
human holocaust   509
human solidarity   475
humility   449
Hun disturbance   240
hybrid seed   29, 134
hydraulic civilization   29
hydrology cycle   25
Hygiene   405
hypercholesterolemia   247
hypercholesterolenemia   324
hyperinsulinemia   143, 174, 247
Hyperinsulinism   271
Hyperlipemia   340
Hypertension   147, 322

IARC   251
IGF-1   264
IGg   150
IGm   150
imagination   444
imaginative play   217
imbalance   491
immoral   497
immune function   318
immunotoxic   428
imperialism   135
inclusion   423
increase   341
Index of Sustainable Economic
   Welfare   465
indigenous   133, 309
indigenous communities   501
indirect costs   461
indoor pollution   79, 80
industrial agricultural   417
industrial agriculture   136

industrial farming   134
Industrialization   29
industrialized fleets   28
Industrial Revolution   447
Industrial societies   507
Inflammation   218
inflammatory bowel disease   153
inflammatory reactions   61
informational substances   60
inner conflict   207
inner development   492
insecticides   79, 412
insomnia   220
insulin   182, 334
insulin growth factor (IGF)   143
insulin resistance   143, 274
integrated pest management
   (IPM)   80
intellectual property   423
intellectual property rights   496
Intercostal chondritis   86
internal/external exercise   58
internal wind   86
international environmental
   law   463
interpenetrating environmental
   stressors   281
interpersonal bonds   213
interpersonal need   211
Interpersonal Need Shame
   Binds   211
interpretation of DNA   407
In the working too much   240
intimacy   316
intrinsic worth   422
in utero   410
inverted fire   150
Invisible phlegm   98
Ionizing radiation   64, 249

IPRs   135
Iroquois Confederacy   199
Irradiation   412
ISO 14000   471

Jade Screen   102
Jews   311
Jing   321, 416
juvenile onset diabetes   174

ketones   83
kidney and Source Qi
   deficiency   319
Kidney and spleen Yang
   deficiency   346
kidney Qi deficiency   221
kidneys root the Qi   88
kidney Yang deficiency   158
Kiiko Matsumoto   96
Kisspeptin   270
knotted Qi   208
knowledge systems   423
ko cycle   84
kyphosis   96

labor unions   454
language of progress   498
latent pathogenic factors   53,
   150, 218
latent pathogens   219
Late-onset asthma   94
law of ceaseless cycles   41
learn   321
LEED   470
legionella   39
Leptin   270
lightning rod   311
limitation   314
lindane   252

lineage-specific   411
linearity   46
linear scientific model   489
linear thinking   440, 442, 507
Ling Shu   57, 416
lipophilic   64, 210
listening   506
liver and heart constraint   319
liver blood deficiency   86
liver channel   320
liver constraint   51, 85, 340
liver/heart Qi stasis   227
liver–lung relationship   85
liver Qi   208
liver Qi stasis   101, 218
liver Yang deficiency   86
Liver Yin deficiency   86
living   148
Living knowledge   423
Low blood sugar   181
lower Jiao   88
lower trophic levels   27
lowest common denominators   500
Lung   50
lung cancer   77
lung cold   86
Lung dryness   113
lung heat   179
lung Qi depression   91
Lung Qi stasis   218
lungs govern the Qi   88
lung wilt   113
lymph   57
lymphocytes   61
Lynch syndrome   141

macrocosm   47
Maitake   122
malathion   256

mammogram 250
mangroves 26
marijuana 86
Marine Stewardship Council 471
market fundamentalism 459
market world 453
masculinization 137
master of the heart 57, 416
material and spiritual
  wisdom 419
matter-versus-spirit 441
MCF-7 breast cancer cells 263
meaning 440, 442, 444, 449
mechanistic action 445
mechanization 134
meditation 417, 492
meditation technologies 505
megadrought 402
Melatonin 238, 270
mesenterium 59
mesothelioma 82
messenger molecules 60
Metal (lung) 84
metastatic 121
metastatic breast cancer 228
methoxychlor 412
Methylene chloride 79
MHC 414
microclimate 42
microflora 149
microinvesting 216
microns 77
micronutrients 148
middle Jiao 88
Mind and heart 326
mind–body connection 410
mindfulness 492
mingmen 58, 416
ming men fire 158

Minoan culture 404
minute palpation 492
misogyny 210, 214
Mississippi Delta 30
modern cancer epidemic 498
modern corporation 450
modern-day slaves 507
modernism 457
modern medicine 489
Modern science 440
molecular biology 443, 503
monocrops 29
monocultural 133
monoculture 134
monopolize 423
Monsanto 31, 497
mood disorders 409
moral imperative 433
Moral law 449
moral trauma 316, 450
Mother Earth 511
Mother principle 302
mother–son relationship 227
moving Qi between the
  kidneys 415
moxa 95
Mucus 187
multifactorial disease 22, 219
multinational corporations 456,
  497
multinationals 469
municipal development corporations 474
mutagen 249
mutagenesis 412
mutation 54
mutual insurance companies 474
MWS 251
Myocardial infarction 336

naming   506
Nan Jing   57, 416
Nan Jing Source theory   416
naphthalene   83
naso technique   331
National Cancer Institute   490
National Pesticide Information
   Center (NPIC)   81
National Water Quality Assessment
   (NWQA)   35
natural capital   463
Natural capitalism   453
natural selection   441
natural systems   492
natural world   507
NCI   490
Neanderthals   403
Nei Jing   84, 221
Neijing Tu   491
neoplasms   75
neuronal communication   60
Neuropeptides   146
neuropharmacology   60
neuroscience   61
neurotransmitter science   410
New capitalists   470
new sustainability world   453
NFTC   428
niches   448
nicotine receptor sites   86
NIEHS   257
nitrates   140
nitrites   140
nitrogen oxides   78
NK cell   122
non-Hodgkin's lymphoma   33
nonjudgmental   317
nonrenewable energy   494
Nonresponse   368

nonviolence   317
nonviolent conflict resolution   314
Nonviolent empowerment   316
Norepinephrine   237
NREM   236
Nurse's Health Study   260

obesity   210, 272, 318, 490
objects of sex   209
observation   492
obsessive–compulsive
   disorder   229
off-breathe   79
Ogallala Aquifer   32, 143
Old European Neolithic   302
Old Testament prophets   405
Omega-3 fatty acids   334
omega-3s   142
open-pollinated   138
oral contraceptives   252
Organ agitation   220
organic pollutants   79
organochlorine compounds   255
organochlorine pesticides   259, 319
organochlorines   252
Organotins   275
organ toxin   150
Origin of Species   442
orthoaminoasotoluol   412
orthopnea   109
osteopathy   59
overdrafts groundwater   37
oxidative stress   186
Oxygenation   39

PAC   468
pack years   113
PAHs   247, 253, 260
paint strippers   79

Panax ginseng   122
panic disorder   229
PAP smear   75
Parabens   253, 256
parenting   218, 409
particulate matter   77
partnership model   302
partnership societies   303
patent   423
patent laws   498
Pathogenic Qi   91
pathological constitution   98
Paul Ekins   454
Paul Rohrbach   24
PBDEs   82, 83
PEFR   94
people-centered growth2   452
Perchlorethylene   79
perennial   24
perennial philosophies   402, 439
perennial sciences   415
perennial truths   493
pericardium channel   57
persistent stress   323
personal culture   211
perverse subsidies   456
Pesticides   33, 80, 410
petrochemical inputs   29
petroleum   495
petroleum-based   134
petroleum-based economies   447
phenomenological analysis   492
phenotype   408
phlegm   53, 85, 220
phlegm–dampness   339
Phlegm stasis   90
phthalates   83, 253, 274, 412
Physical punishment   314
Phytoestrogens   256, 276

pineal gland   270
Placental extracts   256
placental tissue   254
plastics   412
plum-blossom   105
Plum pit Qi   220
pluralistic systems   423
p-nonyl-phenol   252
poisonous pedagogy   307, 313
policy reform world   453
pollen   90
polluter-pays principle   462
polysaccharides   122
postgrowth society   452
postscarcity   475
posttraumatic stress disorder   229
potassium-to-sodium ratio   334
poverty   132, 206
powerlessness   214
PP   429
precancerous environment   187
precautionary principle   81,
   424, 481
precocious puberty   269
Prednisone   95
prematurity   271
Prempro   251
prenatal Qi   418
Prescriptions from the Golden
   Chamber   221
Prevention   489
priceless   461
Prilosec   173
Primary sudden cardiac
   arrest   336
primitive   507
private ownership   499
private property rights   500
processed meats   147

processional epochs   402
profit motive   456, 490, 496
progesterone   250
programming   208
proliferative   210
promote   61
promoting factors   247
prosocial values   314
prostate cancer   317, 410
PSA level   318
pseudofoods   133, 490
psychiatric disorders   230
psychic injuries   215
psychic murder   307
psychic split   133
psychoemotional imbalances
  322
psychological abuse   409
psychological predisposition   225
psychological stress   409
psychoneuroimmunology   62, 410
psychopath   309
Psyllium   162
pubarche   268
public health   489
public trusts   474
pulmonary heart disease   117
pulmonary tuberculosis   116
purging and draining   424
purification   185
purpose shame binds   217
PVC   254, 261

Qi   230
Qi and blood stasis   84
Qi deficiency of the heart
  and spleen   346
Qi dynamic   91
qigong   47

Qi-level heat lingering in the
  superficial yangming   243
Qing hao bie jia tang   381
Qing wen bai du yin   382
Qi transformation mechanism   209
quality of life   475
quantum uncertainty   440
Quercitin   162

RA   78
race   318
racism   25, 508
racist   502
rad   250
radiation-induced cough   105
radically unpredictable   446
radionuclide   249
Rage   132
Rage and violence   314
rainforests   22
rales   109
RAST   94
rationality   315
rBGH   264, 280
rBST   264
receptive   43, 137, 200, 506
recharge   23
reciprocity   476
recombinant bovine growth
  hormone   264
recombinant bovine somatotrophin
  264
recycling   40
reductionism   29, 440, 447
reductionist thinking   441
Regulatory slippage   460
rehabilitation   424
reishi   122
Relapse   368

release of energy   445
REM   236
Renal HTN   323
renewable resources   463
reparent   317
replicates   443
repression   311
reproductive cycle   203
Reproductive decisions   218
reprogram   411
resource   451
respiratory allergies   78
revelation   446
Riane Eisler   302
Rice bran   162
Rights of Nature   511
right to know   430
Rio Declaration on
    Environment and Development
    481
Risk assessment   431
risk of harm   430
RNA   442
Robert's formula   162
rodenticides   79
Root vegetables   173
rotting and ripening   171
Round-Up Ready   33, 134

saccharin   149
sacred   447, 449, 494
sacred consciousness   448
sacred creativity   449
sacred feminine   211
sacred truth   493
Sadism   313
salination   22
Sanitary and Phytosanitary
    Agreement   426

San Jiao   26, 149, 248, 415, 496
scapegoat   311
scarcity   451
Science and Environmental Health
    Network   426
scientific materialism   406
Scientific uncertainty   432
sea grass   27
Seaweeds   183
Secondary HTN   323
secretory organs   57
sedimentation   23
SEER data   250
SEHN   482
selective advantage   444
Selenium   147
Self-affirmation   215
self-consistent   448
self-consistent community   448
self-empowerment   317
self-hatred   206
Serotoninergic   237
serum cholesterol   318
serum testosterone   318
set point   184
Seven-star   105
seventh generation   420,
    424, 433
sex determination   412
sexism   508
sex trade   216
sexual intimacy   320
sexual orientation   206
shamebinds   207
Shang Han Lun   54
shen   58, 230, 321, 416
shiitake   122
sigmoidoscopy   161
single-motherhood   206

sinking spleen Qi   151
Skin tags   187
slavery   216, 315
small heart   58, 419
Smoking   51, 84
social accountability   466
social consensus   483
social costs   460
social-democratic   473
social greens world   454
social well-being   463
sociocultural factors   318
soil diversity   35
Soil erosion   31, 136
Soil microbes   36
Soil solarization   34
solution-oriented industries   452
soul   492
soul murder   306
Source   414, 415, 424
Source Qi   55, 57, 117,
    418, 496
Source theory   59, 415
sperm count   412
spiritual inheritance   492
spiritual laws   405
spleen–kidney–heart axis   55
spleen/pancreas   171
spleen Qi deficiency   221
Spleen-Yin deficiency   107, 153
split   214, 307, 449
splitting off   311
Stagnation   232
Starlink   138
stasis of Qi   50
state capitalism   473
Steaming bone disorder   178
Stevia   143
still falls   218

stomach fire   180
Stomach Yang deficiency   155
stress   318
subsidies   451, 462
Sucrose   143
Sugar   334
sunscreens   263
suppressor genes   407
supremacy   314
susceptibility   408
sustainability   451
sustainable development   456
sustainable farming   34
Sustained   368
Su Wen   56
Swallowing phlegm disease   156
Sweeteners   183
switched on or off   407
synthetic fertilizers   34
synthetic hormones   264

Tagamet   173
taijiquan   47
taiyin   107
tamoxifen   256
tan Yin   102
Tao   229, 416
TAP   414
TCDD   261
technology of progress   304
Teleological language   444
Television   278
Ten Commandments   450
termiticides   79
terrain   55
testicular cancer   412
testosterone   314
TEXB-alpha   252
Thallus eckloniae   332

The Commons   422, 461
The Great Transition Initiative   475
the hydraulic pumping mechanism
   of the diaphragm   51
Thelarche   268
The liver   51
The National Health and
   Nutrition Examination Survey
   (NHANES)   267
thermographically   42
the Sacred   444, 505
The Source   433
The spleen   52
Thick phlegm   112
Thick yellow phlegm   111
thinking too much   239
Thin phlegm   112
Thin white phlegm   111
Third Reich   309
Third World   134, 501
throughput   462
thymus gland   59
tissue organization field
   theory   248
Tobacco   75
tolerance   449
toluene   257
too much anger   242
too much food   241
topsoil   133
totalitarian regime   309
tou tong   326
Toxics Release Inventory   459
Toxic Substances Control Act   459
toxin exposure   319
toxins   54
tracks of injury   53
traditional ecological
   knowledge   509

transformation and transportation
   227
transforming phlegm   91
transgenerational   408
Transparent/clear phlegm   111
transverse rebellion   151
Treatment   179
trends of destruction   458
trichloroethylene   257
triglycerides   318
TRIP   497
triple bottom line   470
tumor   407
tumor suppressor genes   141
Tums   173
turbid blockage   342
type II diabetes   53, 325, 490

ulcerative colitis   153
umbilical cord blood   254
unconscious   315
unconscious programming   207
unemotional   314
U.N. Global Compact   471
universal   504
Universal Declaration of the Rights
   of Mother Earth   510
unsustainability   498
Upanishads   405
upper Jiao   88
upward steaming of fire   112
US Chamber of Commerce   468
USDA   31, 135, 140

values   440, 442, 449
Vedas   405
vengeance   314
ventilation rate   82
vertically linear   501

vinclozolin   410
violence   313
viscosity of blood   49
vitamin D   147
Vitamin E   148
VOCs   78
void of the heart   229
vulnerability   213

Wang Shu He's   419
war   315
warming needle   112
war on cancer   200, 400
Wasting and thirsting disorder
   177
water–fire duality   419
water stagnation   156
water within fire   65
Wei (protective) Qi   149
Wei Qi   52, 90, 236
Well-being   464
wellsprings of happiness   465
Wen Bing Xue   54
Western diseases   54
Western medicine   46
Whipple procedure   156
white men   318
WHO   78
whooping cough   105
wild   507
wind   149
wind–cold   104, 168
wind–heat   104, 150

wind–heat toxins   153
Wingspread Conference   426
Wingspread Statement   482
wisdom traditions   205
Wisdom truths   24
wood (liver)   84
World Bank   23
world economy   450
WTC   80
WTO   497

xenobiotics   408
xenoestrogenic   35, 218
Xenoestrogenic   210
xenoestrogenic endocrine
   disruptors   229
xenoestrogens   247, 412
Xenoestrogens   252
X-rays   249
xuan yun   326

Yang   85
Yang deficiency   90, 91
yangming   107
yangming channel   154
Yin   26, 85, 200
Yin fire   106
Ying   52
Ying (nutritive) Qi   149
Yuan Qi   64

zang organ   85
Zeranol   265